AGING AND GENERATIONAL RELATIONS

AGING AND GENERATIONAL RELATIONS

Life-Course and Cross-Cultural Perspectives

TAMARA K. HAREVEN
Editor

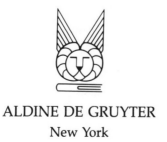

ALDINE DE GRUYTER
New York

About the Editor

Tamara K. Hareven is Unidel Professor of Family Studies and History at the University of Delaware. She is co-editor with Andrejs Plakans of the *History of the Family: An International Quarterly,* which they founded in 1996. Dr. Hareven is the author of several books and has edited collections on the history of the family, work and family, the life course, and aging. Among her best known books are *Amoskeag: Life and Work in the American Factory City* (1978); *Family Time and Industrial Time* (1982); and *Transitions: The Family and the Life Course in Historical Perspective* (editor, 1978).

Dr. Hareven has been the recipient of grants from the Ford Foundation, the National Endowment for the Humanities, the Social Science Research Council, and the National Institute on Aging. She has been a Fulbright scholar to India and Japan.

ALDINE DE GRUYTER
A division of Walter de Gruyter, Inc.
200 Saw Mill River Road
Hawthorne, New York 10532

This publication is printed on acid free paper ∞

Library of Congress Cataloging-in-Publication Data
Aging and generational relations over the life course. Selections
    Aging and generational relations : life-course and cross-cultural
perspectives / Tamara K. Hareven, editor.
        p.   cm.
    Contemporary essays excerpted from a larger volume entitled: Aging and generational relations over the life course.
    Volume resulted from the International Conference on Aging and Generational Relations over the Life Course . . . Univ. of Delaware, October, 1992.
    Includes bibliographical references and index.
    ISBN 0-202-30560-0 (pbk. : alk. paper)
    1. Aged—Family relationships—Congresses.   2. Aged—Care —Congresses.   3. Aging—Social aspects—Congresses.
    4. Intergenerational relations—Congresses.   I. Hareven, Tamara K.
    II. International Conference on Aging and Generational Relations over the Life Course (1992 : University of Delaware)   III. Title.
    HQ1061.A4557   1996
    305.26—dc20   96-9281
                                                                      CIP

Manufactured in the United States of America

10   9   8   7   6   5   4   3   2   1

Contents

List of Contributors

Kathleen Adams

Department of Liberal Arts
Wheelock College

Toni C. Antonucci

Institute for Social Research
University of Michigan

Marzio Barbagli

Department of Sociology
University of Bologna, Italy

Ming-Cheng Chang

Taiwan Provincial Institute
of Family Planning
Taichung, Taiwan

Napaporn Chayovan

Institute of Population Studies
Chulalongkorn University
Bangkok, Thailand

Rand D. Conger

Center for Family Research
in Rural Mental Health
Iowa State University

Glen H. Elder, Jr.

Department of Sociology
University of North Carolina
Chapel Hill

David J. Eggebeen

Population Issues Research Center
Pennsylvania State University

Vicki Freedman

Population Epidemiologist
RAND Corporation
Washington, D.C.

Anne-Marie Guillemard

University of Paris (Panthéon-
Sorbonne), and
École des Hautes Etudes en Sciences
Sociales, Paris, France

Tamara K. Hareven

Department of Individual
and Family Studies and History
University of Delaware

Albert I. Hermalin   Population Studies Center
                                   University of Michigan

Dennis P. Hogan   Population Studies
                                      and Training Center
                                   Brown University

James S. Jackson   Institute for Social Research
                                   University of Michigan

Rukmalie Jayakody   Institute for Social Research
                                   University of Michigan

John Knodel   Population Studies Center
                                   University of Michigan

Kiyomi Morioka   Department of Sociology
                                   Chiba University
                                   Chiba, Japan

Mary Beth Ofstedal   National Center for Health Statistics
                                   Washington, D.C.

Elizabeth B. Robertson   Prevention Research Branch
                                   National Institute on Drug Abuse

John W. Riley, Jr.   Consulting Sociologist
                                   Bethesda, Maryland

Matilda White Riley   Senior Social Scientist
                                   National Institute on Aging

Siriwan Siriboon   Institute of Population Studies
                                   Chulalongkorn University
                                   Bangkok, Thailand

Sean R. Snaith   Population Issues Research Center
                                   Pennsylvania State University

Beth J. Soldo   Department of Demography
                                   Georgetown University

Peter Uhlenberg   Department of Sociology
                                   University of North Carolina
                                   Chapel Hill

Introduction
Aging and Generational Relations Over the Life Course

This volume addresses one of the crucial social issues of our times—
the support that older people receive from their adult children and from
other kin. As the concentration of elderly people in the population increases and as life continues to be extended, the problems of generational assistance in the later years of life will become an even more central
issue in the aging society. It is not surprising, therefore, that the relations between the generations have recently become an important topic
in social science investigations. This interest has been further height-
ened over the past two decades by an intense concern among social
scientists and the public, with the family and the problems experienced
in the relations between generations. Since the family is a major arena in
which generational relations are acted out, one needs to focus on familial, as well as on social-structural and institutional contexts. The study of
generational relations thus requires a multidimensional approach: exter-
nally, it involves an examination of the interaction of individuals and
families with social institutions and with the historical processes affecting them; and internally, it requires an examination of the relations
within the family and the wider kin group (Hareven, 1991).

The chapters in this volume revolve around the following interrelated
themes: interaction of early life transitions of individuals and families
with later ones, and their impact in old age; coresidence among generations; life course antecedents in shaping intergenerational supports in
the later years of life; assistance to aging parents from children and other
kin who do not coreside; the institutional contexts affecting generational
assistance and reciprocities in old age; and the impact of social change
on generational relations. Following a life-course and comparative perspective, the essays help redress some of the misconceptions and myths
that have clouded our understanding of generational supports and provide a picture that does justice to the complexity in specific societies and
cross-culturally.

MISCONCEPTIONS AND MYTHS
ABOUT GENERATIONAL RELATIONS

A main misconception about generational relations in later life involves the question of who actually provides support for the elderly, and what form does this support take? On the one hand, family members assume that the public sector carries major responsibilities of care for the aged; on the other hand, the state assumes that the family is responsible for major areas. This confusion in the assignment of responsibilities often means that elderly people land between the family and the welfare state without receiving proper supports from either. In part, this confusion is exacerbated by a myth about the extent of family caregiving in the past.

According to the myth, a golden age once existed during which members of the older generation coresided with their children and other kin, and elderly people were secure in receiving support from their family members. The myth further assumes that industrialization and urbanization eroded kinship ties and diminished generational supports. Historical research over the past three decades, including the findings presented in the essays in this volume, has helped challenge these myths. In reality, the dominant form of household structure in Western Europe and in the United States in the preindustrial period was nuclear. Coresidence of three generations was *not* the dominant pattern in these societies; hence, industrialization did *not* bring about a nuclear household pattern. Three generations rarely lived together in the same household, although elderly parents often resided in a separate household nearby and were engaged in a variety of mutual supports with their adult children. Coresidence was more prevalent, however, in later life, primarily when elderly parents were too frail to maintain a separate residence (Laslett, 1977; Hareven, 1994; Kertzer & Laslett, 1995; Chudacoff & Hareven, 1978; Smith, 1981.)

Contrary to prevailing myths, elderly people in western society have never experienced a golden age. Both in preindustrial Europe and in colonial America, aging parents entered into contracts with inheriting sons in order to secure basic supports in old age. (Demos, 1978). Generational supports and relations with wider kin were based on voluntary reciprocity, not on rigidly enforced customs or laws. In order to understand how these patterns changed over time, it is necessary to take into account the cultural values governing reciprocal relations among kin in different time periods and among various groups within the same culture.

A full understanding of generational relations in the later years of life has also been handicapped by earlier researchers' reliance on surveys and census schedules that are limited to one point in time. By contrast, the life-course perspective that informs the chapters in this volume provides a dynamic approach to understanding earlier life antecedents of generational supports. As will be shown below, the life-course approach has contributed a historical and developmental perspective on the phenomenological, social-structural, and behavioral aspects of intergenerational relations. As some of these chapters show, relationships of mutual support among the generations were formed early in life and carried into old age after being modified by various events over the life course.

A LIFE-COURSE PERSPECTIVE

A life-course perspective provides both a developmental and historical framework for the study of intergenerational relations. It enables us to understand how patterns of assistance and support networks were formed over the life course and were carried over into the later years; how they were shaped by historical circumstances and by the actors' cultural traditions; and what strategies individuals and families followed in order to secure future supports for later life.

In its emphasis on interaction with historical time, the life-course approach provides an understanding of the location of various cohorts in their respective historical contexts. Specifically, it enables scholars and policymakers to examine the historical circumstances that have affected the lives of the members of different cohorts, and that help explain the differences in the experiences shaping their respective life histories. Relations of mutual support are formed over time and reshaped by historical circumstances, such as migration, wars, and the decline or collapse of local economies. Patterns of providing support and expectations for receiving support in old age are part of a continuing interaction among parents, children, and other kin over their lives as they move through historical time. Rather than viewing old people as a homogeneous group, a life-course perspective illuminates the ways in which their problems, needs, and patterns of adaptation were shaped by their earlier life experiences and by the historical conditions affecting them. The earlier life-course experiences of each cohort, as shaped by historical events, also affect the availability of resources for their members and their modes of assistance and coping abilities in later life.

A life-course perspective provides a framework for understanding variability in the patterns of support in later life, as well as differences in the expectations of the recipients and the caregivers, who are influenced by their respective social and cultural milieux. Generational assistance is shaped by values and experiences that evolve or are modified over the entire life course. For example, in the United States, ethnic values of premigration culture call for a more exclusive dependence on filial and kin assistance than do more contemporary attitudes, which advocate reliance on supports available from government programs and community agencies. Such differences in values are expressed in the caregiving practices and attitudes of successive cohorts. As Tamara Hareven and Kathleen Adams point out in their chapter, earlier life-course experience affected by historical circumstances guided the preferences expressed by members of different cohorts for different types of sources of support for elderly parents and for their involvement in parental care.

Underlying the life-course approach are three major dimensions, all of which revolve around timing: individual timing of life transitions in relation to external historical events; the synchronization of individual life transitions with collective familial ones; and the impact of earlier life events, as shaped by historical circumstances on subsequent ones. The timing of transitions involves the balancing and timing of an individual's entry into and exit from different family, work, and community roles over the life course. It addresses the question: How did people time and sequence their family, work life, and educational transitions in the context of changing historical conditions? In all these areas, the pace and definition of "timing" hinge upon the social and cultural contexts in which transitions occurred. For example: the timing of the transition to adulthood—leaving school, starting work, leaving home, getting married, setting up a separate household and becoming parents—has varied considerably over time and in different societal settings. While age is an important determinant of the timing of transitions, it is not the only significant variable. Changes in family status and in accompanying roles are often as important as age (Hareven, 1978; Hareven & Masaoka, 1988).

Central to the life course approach is the concept of linked lives. Generational relations in later life are interconnected with experiences and transitions from earlier life. From a life course perspective one views "old age" as part of an overall process of generational interaction in the context of changing historical events, rather than as an isolated stage or experience. Various stages and transitions in the life course are interlocked across generations. The synchronization of individual life transitions with collective family transitions involves most notably the juggling of multiple family and work-related roles over the life course. Individuals engage in a variety of familial configurations that change over life and vary under different historical conditions. Within a familial setting, the life transitions of the younger generation are intertwined with those of the older generation. For example, the timing of leaving home and marriage in early adulthood is interrelated with the timing of the older generation's transitions into retirement or with inheritance. This is precisely where the interdependence among generations is crucial.

The strategies that parents and children followed in determining exchanges and transfers in their reciprocal interactions over the life course represent, therefore, an important theoretical and empirical theme. For example, how did parents control their children's timing of leaving home and marriage? As Antoinette Fauve-Chamoux (1996) points out, for residents of nineteenth-century villages in the French Pyrenees, inheritance determined the timing of the heir's succession. But, parental strategies took different forms for the mate selection and the timing of each child's marriage, depending on whether it was the inheriting son or a noninheriting son or daughter who was marrying. Similarly, David Kertzer and Dennis Hogan (1996) emphasize the significance of inheritance in regulating coresidence and generational supports in a nineteenth-century Italian sharecropping village. They found important differences between wage earners and sharecroppers in the use of inheritance in exchange for supports in old age and their impact on the familial and economic status of women.

The task of synchronizing individual transitions with familial ones can generate tensions and conflicts, especially when individual goals are at odds with the needs and dictates of the family as a collective unit. As evidenced in several of the chapters, the timing of adult children's individual transitions often conflicted with the demands and needs of aging parents. For example, Hareven and Adams found that aging parents discouraged at least one daughter from leaving the parental home and marrying in order to assume continued caregiving in old age. Dennis Hogan, David Eggebeen, and Sean Snaith demonstrate the interlocking of generational transitions in the later years of life: The death of an aging parent enabled caretaking children who were themselves "old" to begin providing for their own old age and for their adult children or grandchildren.

Another key feature of the life course approach is the cumulative impact of earlier life events on subsequent ones. The "early" or "delayed" timing of certain transitions affects the pace of later ones. Events experienced earlier in life may continue to influence an individual's or a family's life path in different forms throughout their lives. For example, Elder has documented the negative impact the Great Depression had on the cohort of young men and women who encountered it in their transition to adulthood. Delayed timing in education or early commencement of the work life also affected subsequent delays and disorderliness in the careers of the Depression cohort (Elder, 1974).

Historical forces thus play a crucial role in this complex pattern of

individual and familial life trajectories. Such forces have a direct impact
on the life course at the time when individuals or families encounter
them, and continue to affect their lives indirectly through life. Thus, the
social experiences of each cohort are shaped not only by the historical
events and conditions its members encountered at a certain point in life,
but also by the historical processes that shaped their earlier life transitions. The impact of historical events on the life course may continue
over several generations. One generation transmits to the next the ripple
effects of the historical circumstances that shaped its life history. In their
respective studies Elder and Hareven (1992) have found that for the
same age cohorts in two different communities, delays or irregularities
in the parents' timing of their work and family careers, which resulted
from the Great Depression, affected their children's timing of life transitions. The children thus experienced the impact of historical events on
two levels—directly, through their own encounter with these events,
and indirectly, in the transmission of the impact of these events across
the generations.

Cohort experience should not be misconstrued, however, as cohort
determinism. The impact of historical events on the life course is cumulative but not irreversible. This means that the negative impact of
societal forces at one point in one's life could be modified or reversed
later. The life course approach has emphasized an interactive rather than
a determinist process between individuals and historical events. For
example, Elder and Hareven have examined the impact of World War II
on the cohorts of young men in Berkeley, California and in Manchester,
New Hampshire, in answer to the question, "Why did the Great Depression not produce a lost generation?" They found that military service
during World War II had a major role in reversing or mitigating the
negative impact of the Great Depression on the lives of these young men
from disadvantaged backgrounds. There was, however, a significant
difference between the Berkeley and Manchester cohorts. Most of the
Berkeley men who started from a lower middle- and working-class base
were able to advance far into the middle class. However, few members
of the Manchester cohort managed to rise above their class origins.
Rather than propelling them into the next level, military service prevented them from slipping below their parents' working class status.
These differences in the life trajectories of the young men were closely
linked to the differences in the occupational structures in the communities in which these men lived; they were thus the products of the
interaction of time and place. (Elder & Hareven, 1992).

The life-course approach helps clarify the distinction between "generation" and "cohort"—two concepts that have been frequently confused
in the gerontological literature. "Generation" designates kin relation-

ships (for example, parents and children or grandparents and grand-children); it may encompass an age span, often as wide as thirty years. "Cohort" consists of a more specific age group that has shared a common historical experience. Most important, a cohort is defined by its interaction with the historical events that affect the subsequent life-course experiences of that group. A generation may consist of several cohorts, each of whom has encountered different historical experiences that have affected its life course. In Hareven and Adams's comparison of patterns of assistance of two cohorts of adult children to aging parents in a New England community, the distinction between cohort and generation emerges with clarity: In families with large numbers of children, siblings in the same family belonged to two different cohorts, with different historical experiences and attitudes toward generational assistance. As Anne-Marie Guillemard points out, several studies have confused generations and age groups when assessing intergenerational equity. She argues that a true measure of intergenerational equity requires longitudinal analysis that follows contributions from successive generations over the entire life course.

LIFE-COURSE ANTECEDENTS IN SHAPING INTERGENERATIONAL SUPPORTS IN THE LATER YEARS OF LIFE

Generational supports in old age are part of a life course continuum of reciprocal relations between the generations. Kiyomi Morioka identifies specific phases in generational exchanges over the life course. Early in the life course, assistance is extended from parents to their children; in the later phases, the children, especially the inheriting child in the stem family, care for aging parents. Analyzing the role transitions of parents and children over the life course of five cohorts in Japan, Kanji Masaoka and Sumiko Fujimi (1996) document considerable variations among cohorts as well as community differences within the general patterns discussed by Morioka.

How was the caretaking child selected, and how was the caregiving relationship formed? What kind of negotiations and bargaining were involved in this process? Kertzer and Hogan (1996), Josef Ehmer (1996), Fauve-Chamoux (1996), and Stanley Brandes (1996) have provided ample evidence that in nineteenth century Europe, inheritance played a major role in designating the caretaker for aging parents. In societies where a stem family system dominated, as Fauve-Chamoux and Morioka point out respectively for the French Pyrenees and Japan, the main caretaking responsibility for aging parents fell upon the inheriting son, who continued to coreside with his parents after marriage, while the noninheriting children left home and maintained contact only from a distance. In the northern Iberian Peninsula, in areas with impartible inheritance, the inheriting son was also the caretaker for aging parents. In areas with partible inheritance, caretaking with or without coresidence took different forms and in landless societies selection of the caretaking child varied by economic circumstances, life-course antecedents, and cultural prescriptions. In central Europe, caretaking patterns for aging parents differed between landholding families and those who engaged in small commodity production in the household, because of the difference in inheritance practices (Ehmer, 1996).

In all these circumstances, designation of a caretaker for parents in their old age was an important life-course "imperative" that often necessitated advance provisions, such as inheritance contracts or other strategies. In urban society, the selection of the caretaker was contingent on specific arrangements between parents and a caretaking child that were formed over life. Other means to select the caretaking child were, therefore, at work: As Hareven and Adams found, among several ethnic groups in the United States at the turn of the century, the "parent keeper" was designated by the parents earlier in life. Parents often discouraged the youngest daughter from leaving home or marrying because she was designated to be the main "parent-keeper." Similarly, in Sri Lanka, Peter Uhlenberg found a strategy of reciprocity between parents' providing assistance to their children early in life and their receiving supports from their children in old age. These types of strong generational reciprocities are also evident in the patterns discussed in this book by Morioka for Japan, John Knodel and his collaborators for Thailand, and Albert Hermalin and his collaborators for Taiwan.

The forging or dissolving of generational ties that takes place over the life course has important consequences for relations later in life. As Glen Elder and Elizabeth Robertson demonstrate, in twentieth-century rural Iowa the migration of sons from the farm in order to pursue occupational careers in the city put a strain on generational relations. When sons continued in farm careers and resided in the same communities with their fathers, they were more consistently engaged in caring for and supporting their aged parents than those sons who had moved to the city.

One of the persistent questions underlying the chapters in this book involves the impact of demographic factors and the availability of "caregivers" for aging parents. Does higher fertility guarantee a couple or an individual surviving into "old age" availability of a larger number of caregiving children in old age? Or, as is evident in nineteenth-century American society, regardless of how many children a couple had, did only one child carry the major role of parent-keeper (Chudacoff & Hareven, 1978; Smith, 1981)? George Alter, Lisa Cligget, and Alex Urbiel (1996) conclude that in nineteenth-century Belgium, high fertility made a larger number of supporters available to aging parents. Caretaking of aging parents was related not only to the number of available children, but also to inheritance systems, the cultural values governing generational supports, and the importance of gender and birth order of the children in shouldering these responsibilities.

CORESIDENCE

The household arrangements of older people have run as a continuing theme through historical research on the family, as well as in the essays included here. As a large body of scholarship has demonstrated, nuclear household patterns have predominated since the preindustrial period in the United States and western Europe. The modal pattern has been one where the younger generation establishes a separate household. Except for some variation over the life course, elderly couples and aging widows have attempted to maintain separate households for as long as possible. The prevalent residential arrangement of older people and their children has been one of "intimacy from a distance."

This pattern was modified, however, in the later years of life. Coresidence with a child, single or married, was the major solution if aging parents were unable to live separately (Laslett, 1977; Laslett & Wall, 1972; Hareven, 1982). As Alter and his collaborators found, in nineteenth-century Belgium, coresidence with adult children tended to increase in the later years of life. (Alter, Cliggett, & Urbiel, 1996). Similarly, Timothy Guinnane (1996) has found high rates of coresidence of elderly parents with adult children in Ireland. Generally, parents preferred to coreside with an unmarried child. Similarly, Stanley Brandes (1996) has found in northern Spain and Portugal a preference among elderly parents for the autonomy of their households. Coresidence occurred, however, when the parents—especially an aged widow or widower—were too frail to live alone. Under such circumstances, the elderly parent resided in the households of various children through a "rotation" system. In regions with impartible inheritance, the inheriting son coresided with the aging parents and was expected contractually to be their main supporter. Whenever possible, older widows continued to lead their own households by taking related as well as unrelated individuals, such as boarders and lodgers, into the household. Among several ethnic groups in the United States, parents assured themselves in advance of having an unmarried child remain at home, as a security for support in later life. Jane Zachritz and Myron Gutmann (1996), for example, found that in nineteenth-century Texas widowhood in later life was a main determinant in leading elderly women to coreside with their children.

As would be expected, in the Asian countries discussed in this book there was a higher rate of coresidence of elderly parents with adult children than in the West. Coresidence with at least one adult child has been the customary pattern for aged parents in Taiwan, Thailand, and Japan—a pattern typical for East Asia. John Knodel and his collaborators report that in Thailand, the majority of men and women over 65 coreside with one child. There are, however, considerable variations over the life course. Older children move out and set up their own households, but typically one unmarried child coresides with aging parents, especially when they begin to need assistance. This practice is more pronounced for aged widows, for whom coresidence with a child still constitutes the major form of support.

Even within Asia, however, important variations occur: Hermalin and his collaborators found in Taiwan significantly lower rates of coresidence among the mainland Chinese than among the Taiwanese. In Thailand, older children are less likely than younger children to coreside with their parents at the very point in their parents' lives when support from a coresident child was most needed. The needs of elderly parents, especially widowed mothers, are met through coresidence with a younger child.

Both the United States and Japan have seen a decline in the rates of coresidence of aging parents with adult children. Steven Ruggles argues that in the United States, the decline since the turn of the century in the coresidence of people older than 65 with kin may be as significant a change as the earlier major demographic transitions. In Japan, the rates of coresidence are lower than in the other Asian countries discussed here: As Morioka shows, among people older than 65, in Japan, about 60% coreside with a child. Morioka anticipates, however, that this type of generational coresidence will continue to decline in Japan. He found that in Japan the proportion of elderly people over 65 coresiding with an adult child has declined steadily between 1960 and 1980. He attributes this change to the disintegration of the traditional *ie* system following World War II, and to the increasing preference of the younger generation to live separately from their parents. Morioka argues that this change in the traditional patterns of coresidence raises serious questions about the future consistency and continuity of filial supports for the aged.

An examination of coresidence among the generations raises several questions related to household headship and to the nature of generational supports. When a household record in a census lists a parent as being the head of the household and an adult child as residing in the household, who in reality heads the household, and what are the dynamics of flow of assets and assistance within such a household? It is difficult to answer these questions from cross-sectional data; nor can this type of data explain what the dynamics are in this pattern of coresidence. Did the son become the head of the household after his father retired or became too old or frail to support himself and manage the family's affairs? Or did the parents move into the son's household? Under what circumstances did the older generation coreside with adult children or other kin? And conversely, under what circumstances did aging parents reside separately and interact with kin in various forms of assistance outside the household?

Rates of coresidence recorded in cross-sectional data may reflect a life-course pattern in which elderly parents who do not coreside with their children at the time of a census or survey may do so later when they become more dependent. Morioka's data bear out such a hypothesis, since the rates of coresidence with the children of chronically ill or terminally ill elderly are higher than those of the overall group of people older than 65. Similarly, Hogan, Eggebeen, and Snaith noted in their chapter that cross-sectional data may obscure considerable variation in patterns of coresidence over the life course. They found in the National Survey of Families and Households that only seven percent of Americans 55 and older with a surviving parent had the parent living with them at the time when the survey was taken; but by their late fifties, one-quarter of persons had an aging parent living with them at some point.

ASSISTANCE TO AGING PARENTS FROM CHILDREN AND OTHER KIN WHO DO NOT CORESIDE

Related to the designation of children as caretakers is the question of the respective roles of adult children and other kin in carrying such responsibilities in later life. When children served as the primary caretakers, how was their assistance augmented by that of other kin, and, if it was, by what other kin? For example, were older widows more likely to receive assistance from their siblings than from their children? Or did siblings step in only when children were not available? How consistent or continuous the support from nonresident children or other kin to aging parents has been in the United States, is still widely open to future research. Earlier studies have documented visiting patterns and telephone communication rather than regular caretaking (Shanas, 1962). More recent research has emphasized the existence of various supports from adult children to aging parents, even if they were not residing in the same household. (Cantor, 1983; Brody, 1990; Brody, et. al, 1983).

The authors in this volume agree that the most consistent and reliable form of caretaking of aging parents is best achieved if they coreside with an adult child. Several of the authors found that in East Asia supports from coresiding children are more secure than those from children who live separately, even if the latter are in proximity. As Peter Uhlenberg points out, in Sri Lanka coresidence seems the only guarantee that elderly parents will receive support services from adult children. Supports from noncoresident children to aging parents take the form primarily of financial assistance. Knodell and his collaborators found a similar pattern in Thailand. They concluded that the type of supports provided by children who do not coreside depend on the children's proximity to aging parents. Children living closer to their parents are more likely to provide food and clothing, while children living at a greater distance more commonly provide money. Morioka is skeptical as to how reliable and effective the caregiving of aging parents in Japan would be without coresidence. In the region of Emilia Romagna, in Italy, Marzio Barbagli finds that supports to aging parents from adult children who do not coreside are persistently widespread. The relationships are, however, patrilineal rather than matrilineal: The assistance comes from sisters-in-law and daughters-in-law rather than from sisters and daughters. In American black families, as James Jackson, Rukmalie Jayakody and Toni Antonucci point out, the support relations are predominantly matrilineal. These supports are subject, however, to a complex interaction of various factors: income, educational levels, proximity in residence, and the environment. Such complex models have not been applied, however, to the study of the white American population or to European populations.

The role of kin other than children who do not coreside with elderly people in providing assistance awaits systematic investigation. The extent to which kin are available to provide supports to aging relatives is still an open question. Through their modeling of demographic determinants of kin availability to assist aging relatives, Douglas Wolf, Beth Soldo, and Vicki Freedman show that kinship networks are determined not only by demographic factors, but also by the familial characteristics of network members and by their familial position vis-à-vis aging relatives. For example, whether siblings are married or not, and what kind of obligations they carry toward the parents of their spouses, helps determine their availability. The important conclusion reached in their chapter is that generational assistance must be studied in a familial, rather than an individual, context. Configurations of siblings and the marshaling of assistance and division of responsibility among them are significant factors. Since the data used by these authors are demographic, the general question concerning kin availability still needs to be addressed: to what extent is the *presence of kin proof of their actual involvement* in care for the elderly?

Along these lines, John and Matilda Riley emphasize the significance of "latent" kin relations or of surrogate kin networks as a future avenue for generational assistance. Major changes in the timing of life transitions and in what Guillemard calls the "deinstitutionalization of the life course" have also had a significant impact on reciprocal relations among the generations. As Guillemard points out, the erratic timing in exit from the work life, in recent years, and the deinstitutionalization of retirement, have rendered the ability of generations to assist each other less predictable.

THE IMPACT OF SOCIAL CHANGE

What was the role of the welfare state and of charitable or public welfare services and institutions, such as homes for the aged and nursing homes, in influencing generational coresidence and assistance?For Sweden, Lars Göran Tedebrand (1996) attributes the decline in coresidence among generations over the twentieth century to the development of the welfare state. Similarly, Morioka highlights the significance of the Japanese social security policy and social welfare services both in substituting for an earlier intensive kin support system for the aged and in providing "an effective buffer system to keep the coresidence functioning positively," in those cases where coresidence is still surviving. Hareven and Adams demonstrate that in the United States the readiness of elderly people and of their adult children to accept help from the welfare state and external agencies has varied by their ethnic background and their cohort experience. Later cohorts, who are less kin oriented and who have had a greater exposure to bureaucratic agencies over their lives, were more inclined to view public agencies as sources of support than earlier cohorts, who had relied more exclusively on kin assistance over their lives.

In the United States, the transfer of social-welfare functions from the family to public institutions over the past century and a half has not been fully consummated. The family has ceased to be the only available source of support for its dependent members, and the community has ceased to rely on the family as the only agency of welfare and social control. Who actually provides supports for the elderly, and what form those supports take, have been subject to ambiguities. The problems are exacerbated by the expectation from the public sector that family and kin carry the major responsibilities for the care of aged relatives still prevails, without the provision of the necessary social and economic support that would enable kin to discharge such responsibilities (Litwak, 1985).

The increase of women's labor force participation as full-time workers, and the fact that in the aging society the "children" of the "old old" are themselves old, undermines the possibility for kin to be the main caregivers. The decline in instrumental relations among kin and their replacement by an individualistic orientation toward family relations, with sentimentality and intimacy as the major cohesive forces over the past century, has led to the weakening of the role of kin assistance in middle-class families in particular, and to an increasing isolation of the elderly in American society (Hareven, 1994). While in working-class, ethnic, and black families kin still carry a major share of caregiving for elderly relatives, this is achieved at a very high price to the caregiver. It is unrealistic to expect kin to fulfill major responsibilities of caregiving without public supports.

All the issues discussed above need to be interpreted in the larger context of social and economic change. Did industrialization and urbanization lead to the dramatic restructuring of generational relations and mutual assistance? A comparison of the patterns in Europe and the United States with those in East Asia raises important questions about global change: Is the trend toward the residential separation of older people from their children in Asian countries part of a "convergence" process with the West? Are Asian countries recapitulating the historical transitions that have already occurred in Western Europe and the United States at a more rapid pace? Even if this were the case, are similarities between Asian and Western societies on the surface a disguise for much more profound cultural differences? For example, do elderly parents now living in a nuclear household in Japan and Taiwan experience an interaction with adult children similar to that of contemporary Americans living in nuclear families?

Since cultural traditions have played a major role in shaping patterns of generational assistance and the expectations of generations from each other, it is important to compare more systematically these patterns in different societies. For example, in the societies discussed here, what may appear on the surface to be an "isolated" nuclear family by no means suggests that elderly parents are isolated from assistance from their children and other kin. This is precisely an area where comparative research is needed. Such comparisons need, however, to employ the same variables on types of supports and services across several societies. Even such systematic comparisons require sensitivity toward the internal differences within each society and differences in the cultural meaning of family relations and obligations for support across societies. Within Taiwan, for example, Hermalin and his associates found major differences in supports to aged parents between Mainland Chinese and Taiwanese. Within the United States, one needs to examine more systematically such differences among ethnic groups and social classes. When addressing these questions, it is also important to keep in mind that patterns of change that appear on the surface to be similar may not really be the same. It is not sufficient to compare changes in Asia and Western Europe without understanding the difference in the starting points of these changes in the societies examined. This issue in itself provides a future agenda.

Tamara Hareven

REFERENCES

Alter, G., Cliggett, L., & Urbiel, A. (1996). Household patterns of the elderly and the proximity of children in a nineteenth century city: Verviers, Belgium, 1831–1846. In T. K. Hareven (Ed.), *Aging and generational relations over the life course: A historical and cross-cultural perspective*. Berlin: Walter de Gruyter.

Brandes, S. (1996). Kinship and care for the aged in traditional rural Iberia. In T. K. Hareven (Ed.), *Aging and generational relations over the life course: A historical and cross-cultural perspective*. Berlin: Walter de Gruyter.

Brody, E. M. (1990). *Women in the middle: Their parent-care years*. New York: Springer.

Brody, E. M., Johnson, P. T., Fulcomer, M. C., & Lang, A. M. (1983). Women's changing roles and help to elderly parents: Attitudes of three generations of women. *Journal of Gerontology, 38*(5), 597–607.

Cantor, M.H. (1983). Strain among caregivers: A study of experience in the U.S. *Gerontologist, 12*, 597–624.

Chudacoff, H. & Hareven, T. K. (1978). Family transitions to old age. In T. K. Hareven (Ed.), *Transitions: The family and the life course in historical perspective*, (pp. 217–43). New York: Academic Press.

Demos, J. (1978). Old age in early New England. In J. Demos, S. Boocock, (Ed.). Turning Points. *American Journal of Sociology* (Supplemental 84), S248–87.

Ehmer, J. (1996). "The life stairs": Aging, generational relations, and small commodity production in central Europe. In T. K. Hareven (Ed.), *Aging and generational relations over the life course: A historical and cross-cultural perspective*. Berlin: Walter de Gruyter.

Elder, G. H. (1974). *Children of the great depression*. Chicago: University of Chicago Press.

Elder, G. H. & Hareven, T. K. (1992). Rising above life's disadvantages: From the Great Depression to global war. In J. Modell, G. H. Elder, Jr. & R. Parke (Eds.), *Children in time and place*, (pp. 47–72). New York: Cambridge University Press.

Fauve-Chamoux, A. (1996). Aging in a never-empty nest: the elasticity of the stem family. In T. K. Hareven (Ed.), *Aging and generational relations over the life course*. Berlin: Walter de Gruyter.

Guinnane, T. (1996). The family, state support and generational relations in rural Ireland at the turn of the twentieth century. In T. K. Hareven (Ed.), *Aging and generational relations over the life course: A historical and cross-cultural perspective*. Berlin: Walter de Gruyter.

Hareven, T. K. (1978). The historical study of the life course. In T. K. Hareven (Ed.) *Transitions: The family and the life course in historical perspective*. New York: Academic Press.

Hareven, T. K. (1991). The history of the family and the complexity of social change. *American Historical Review, 96*(1), 95–124.

Hareven, T. K. (1982). *Family time and industrial time*. New York: Cambridge University Press.

Hareven, T. K. (1994). Aging and generational relations: A historical and life course perspective. In John Hagan, (Ed.), *Annual Review of Sociology*, (pp. 437–61). Palo Alto, CA: Annual Reviews, Inc.

Hareven, T. K. & Masaoka, K. (1988). Turning points and transitions: Perceptions of the life course. *Journal of Family History, 13*(3), 271–289.

Hareven, T. K. & Uhlenberg, P. (1995). Transition to widowhood and family support systems in the twentieth century, northeast, U.S. In D. I. Kertzer & P. Laslett, (Eds.), *Aging and the past: Society, demography and old age*. Los Angeles, CA: University of California Press.

Hogan, D., Eggebeen, D. & Snaith, S. (1996). The well-being of aging Americans with very old parents. In T. K. Hareven, (Ed.), *Aging and generational relations over the life course: A historial and cross-cultural perspective* Berlin: Walter de Gruyter.

Kertzer, D. (1996). Toward a historical demography of aging. In D. Kertzer & P. Laslett (Eds.), *Aging in the past: Demography, society, and old age*, (pp. 363–383). Berkeley: University of California Press.

Laslett, P. (1977). *Family life and illicit love in earlier generations*. Cambridge: Cambridge University Press.

Laslett, P. & Wall, R. (Eds.) (1972). *Household and family in past time*. Cambridge: Cambridge University Press.

Litwak, E. (1985). *Helping the elderly: The complementary roles of informal networks and formal systems*. New York: Guilford Press.

Masaoka, K. & Fujimi, S. (1996). Some inter- and intracohort comparisons of generational interactions. From the acquisition of parental roles through postparenthood in Japan, 1914–1958. In T. K. Hareven (Ed.), *Aging and generational relations over the life course: A historical and cross-cultural perspective*. Berlin: Walter de Gruyter.

Shanas, E. (1962). *The health of older people: A social survey*. Cambridge, Mass: Harvard University Press.

Smith, D. S. (1981). Historical change in the household structure of the elderly in economically developed societies. In J. G. March, R. W. Fogel, E. Hatfield, S. B. Kiesler, & E. Shanas (Eds.), *Aging: Stability and change in the family*, (pp. 91–111). New York: Academic Press.

Tedebrand, L. G. (1996). Gender, rural-urban and socio-economic differences in coresidence of the elderly with adult children: the case of Sweden 1860–1940. In T. K. Hareven (Ed.), *Aging and generational relations over the life course: A historical and cross-cultural perspective.* Berlin: Walter de Gruyter.

Zachritz, J. & Gutmann, M. (1996). Residence and family support systems for widows in nineteenth- and early twentieth-century Texas. In T. K. Hareven (Ed.), *Aging and generational relations over the life course: A historical and cross-cultural perspective.* Berlin: Walter de Gruyter.

Acknowledgments

The chapters reprinted in this paperback edition are part of a larger volume entitled *Aging and Generational Relations Over the Life Course: A Historical and Cross-Cultural Perspective*. While the paperback reprints only the contemporary essays, the larger volume also contains historical essays on this subject by George Alter, Lisa Cliggett, and Alex Urbiel; Stanley Brandes; Josef Ehmer; Antoinette Fauve-Chamoux; Timothy W. Guinnane; David I. Kertzer and Dennis P. Hogan; Kanji Masaoka and Sumiko Fujimi; Andrejs Plakans; Steven Ruggles; Lars-Göran Tedebrand; and Jane Zachritz and Myron P. Gutmann.

The original volume resulted from the International Conference on Aging and Generational Relations Over the Life Course which I organized and directed at the University of Delaware, in October, 1991, with a grant from the National Institute on Aging (NIA). I would like to express my gratitude both to the NIA for their generous support and to the University of Delaware for hosting the conference. Special appreciation is extended to the Department of Individual and Family Studies for providing various supports for the editing of the volume.

I am grateful to Judy Wilson for the outstanding organizational supports she provided for the conference, to Martha Dimes for copy editing, to Liz Park and Cindy Chuidian for editing and typing in preparation for the paperback and to Linda Granger, Gladys Llewellen, and Catherine Raphael who earlier prepared camera-ready copy for the larger volume. I would also like to thank the authors for their patience with the long editing process; to Andrejs Plakans, Bianka Ralle at Walter deGruyter in Berlin, and Richard Koffler at Aldine de Gruyter in New York, for their continuing support and encouragement; and finally, to Arlene Perazzini at Aldine de Gruyter for her editorial improvement of the paperback edition.

Tamara K. Hareven
Newark, Delaware

I

THE UNITED STATES AND EUROPE

1

The Generation in the Middle
Cohort Comparisons in Assistance to Aging
Parents in an American Community

Tamara K. Hareven and Kathleen Adams

INTRODUCTION

The gerontological literature generally has treated patterns of support from adult children to aging parents from a contemporary perspective and from one that is limited to one point in time (Bengtson, Kasshau, & Ragan, 1985; Bengston & Treas, 1980; Shanas, 1979; Antonucci, 1990; Cicirelli, 1981). Rarely have these studies addressed the question of how the caretaking relationship was formed over the life course. With some exception, contemporary studies of intergenerational assistance have not examined how adult children's support to aging parents changes over time; nor have they considered caretaking children in the context of their social historical times.

In this chapter we approach intergenerational supports from a life-course and historical perspective (Hareven, 1981). By comparing two cohorts of adult children, we aim to identify changes both in the practices of caregiving in aging parents', and in adult children's attitudes toward caregiving. By following a historical and developmental approach, we examine the ways in which patterns of support among generations developed over the life course and were revised or adapted in the later years of life. A life-course perspective provides a way of understanding how relations of mutual support are formed over people's lifetime, and how they are reshaped by historical circumstances such as migration, wars, or the collapse of local economies. The earlier life-course experiences of each cohort—as shaped by historical events—also affect availability of resources for their members, modes of assistance, coping abilities, and expectations. Exploration of these earlier life course experiences enables us to relate patterns of support in the later years of life to the social and cultural conditions that the respective cohorts encountered over their lives (Elder, 1978a; Hareven, 1978; Riley, 1978).

A life-course perspective, therefore, provides a framework for understanding variability in supports as well as changes in the expectations of both recipients and caregivers, who are influenced by their respective social and cultural milieux. Our research examines adult children who were caring for aging parents in the context of the opportunities and experiences characteristic of their respective cohorts at various periods in their lives. We view behavior and expectations for receiving and providing support as part of a continuing process of interaction among parents and children and other kin, over their lives, and as they move through historical time.

Attitudes toward generational assistance in the later years of life are influenced by values and experiences that evolve or are modified over the entire life course. Ethnic values rooted in premigration culture, call for a more exclusive dependence on filial and kin assistance than do the attitudes in the dominant American culture, which relies on supports available from government programs and community agencies.

This study is based on extensive life-history interviews with former textile workers in Manchester, New Hampshire and two cohorts of their adult children. The parent generation on whom *Family Time and Industrial Time* (Hareven, 1982) is based migrated to Manchester in order to work in the Amoskeag Mills between the turn of the century and World War I. Most of them came from Quebec, Poland, and Greece, and in smaller numbers from Scotland, Ireland, and Sweden. During the period of their arrival, the Amoskeag Company—the world's largest textile mill complex—was at the peak of its production. Following World War I, the mills entered a precipitous decline that finally shut down the mills in 1936, a disastrous event that paralyzed the local economy for almost a decade. Since Manchester was a one-industry town, the shutdown's effect on the workers' lives was particularly severe (Hareven, 1982; Hareven & Langenbach, 1978).

In examining the interaction of adult children with their aging parents, we compare the ways in which two cohorts of adult children who belong to the same generation have differed both in caregiving, and in their attitudes towards providing assistance to their parents. We explore the range of life-course paths of adult children who were caregivers for their frail, elderly parents. In doing so, we try to identify the ways in which the caretaking relationship emerged over the life course, and the price that caregiving children paid in this relationship.

The "generation in the middle" on whom this chapter focuses consists of the children of the generation on whom *Family Time and Industrial Time* was based. Most of the children were born in the United States or were brought there in their childhood by their parents. Several characteristics set them apart from their parents. While the parents often moved back and forth between Manchester and their communities of origin or around New England to seek factory work in various communities during business slumps, most of the children grew up in Manchester in the "shadow" of the Amoskeag Mills. These children were too young to have worked in the mills, and were not old enough to have experienced the pre-World War I period of prosperity in Amoskeag's history that had induced their parents to work there. The older members among the children's generation were old enough to have experienced directly the negative effects of the shutdown of the mills and the Great Depression on the families of Manchester. The children were slated by their parents to escape mill work and to fulfill the American dream. The parents' ideal was for sons, especially, to get a high school education and work their way up to middle-class occupations, or to own a grocery store or a restaurant. As one member of this group put it: "My father said to me: 'No mills for you down there.' So my brother was a postal inspector, I was a cost accountant . . . we went to school. In those days there was a very small percentage that went to college or had a high school education."

Most of the children's generation, however, was unable to fulfill their parents' scenario. The shutdown of the Amoskeag Mills amid the Great Depression blocked this means of escape, especially for the older children, who encountered economic crises in their teenage years. The younger children came closer to fulfilling this dream, but only marginally. The children were the first generation in their families to speak English as their first language, and to "Americanize" in any significant way through their schooling. About half of the children's generation had actually married outside their ethnic group, but remained within their faith. They represent a transitional group. While adhering to some of their parents' traditional values, they also accepted American middle class values and aspired to that life-style. In contrast to the parents' erratic migration patterns, most of the children grew up within a single American community.

From a demographic point of view, the children were the first generation to experience their parents' survival beyond their seventies and to encounter the problems of caring for "old-old" parents. Even though most families had large numbers of children, the primary responsibility of caring for an elderly parent usually fell upon one child. Members of this generation were the first, therefore, to experience a "life-cycle squeeze." They had to care for aging parents at a point in their lives when they themselves were approaching old age, and needed to prepare for their own retirement (Cantor, 1983; Brody, 1981). In addition, they needed to launch their own children. The squeeze was intensified especially for women, who had performed the traditional roles of mother and wife while carrying full-time jobs.

For the purpose of life course analysis, we divided the children's generation into two cohorts according to the historical events they encountered as they reached adulthood: Those born between 1910 and 1919 came of age during the Great Depression (earlier cohort), and those born between 1920 and 1929 came of age during World War II (later cohort). This chapter uses the historical data set that Hareven constructed for the parents' cohort, and on which *Family Time and Industrial Time* is based (Hareven, 1982). We linked the historical data with a new set on the children's cohorts, which we generated from intensive life-history interviews during the period 1981–1985, combined with demographic histories, work histories, and migration histories, which are included in the new data set on the children's cohorts.[1]

INTERGENERATIONAL SUPPORTS OVER THE LIFE COURSE

For the ethnic working-class families studied here, the expectation that adult children care for aging parents was embedded in the traditional patterns of kin assistance and family values that the parent generation had brought with them. Immigrants carried over their kinship ties and customs for assistance from their communities of origin and adapted them to the needs and demands of the urban-industrial setting in the United States. Most members of the parents' generation came to Manchester in their teens or as couples with young children. Many of them had left their own parents behind, but maintained consistent kinship ties with their communities of origin. In some instances, parents followed and joined them later. Those who came from Quebec, especially, were enmeshed in kinship networks across the industrial landscape of northern New England and Quebec (Hareven, 1982).

Assistance among the generations stretched across the life course and tended to be mutual, informal, and recurrent under normal circumstances, as well as during critical life situations. In the regime of economic insecurity characteristic of the late nineteenth century and the first part of this century where kin assistance was the only constant source of support, family coping necessarily dictated that individual choices be subordinated to family considerations and needs. Mutual assistance among kin, although involving extensive exchanges, was not calculative. Rather, it expressed an overall principle of reciprocity over the life course and across generations.

Individuals who subordinated their own careers and needs for those of the family as a collective unit did so out of a sense of responsibility, affection, and familial obligation, rather than with the expectation of eventual gain. The sense of obligation toward kin was a manifestation of family "culture"—supported by a commitment to the well-being and self-reliance or survival of the family—which took priority over individual needs and personal happiness. Family autonomy, essential for self-respect and good standing in the neighborhood and community, was one of the most deeply ingrained values (Hareven, 1982).

Various types of assistance to the elderly grew out of the daily exchanges between parents and children over the life course. Children, especially daughters, helped their aging parents by taking them shopping or to the doctor, by doing household chores and providing supplies, and by visiting frequently. Such ongoing assistance set the stage for coping with subsequent crises, such as widowhood, serious or chronic illness of a parent, and dependence. These helping patterns revolved principally around the generational axis of parents and children. Despite the long tradition of kin assistance among these families, there is only scattered evidence that other kin (the aging person's siblings, nieces and nephews, or grandchildren, for example) cared for an elderly relative. Other kin provided sociability and occasional help for an elderly relative, but the major responsibilities for regular care fell primarily on adult children.

Patterns of assistance to parents that were formed early in life generally carried over into old age. Children who had experienced a closer day-to-day interaction with their parents during their own childrearing years were more likely than their siblings to take responsibility for parental assistance in the later years, except when the relationship was disrupted by migration, death, early impairment, or family conflict. Even in cases where children in the later cohort (primarily daughters) had left Manchester, they tended to return to the parental home if they lost their spouses. Some of these daughters left home again after they reconstructed their lives; others stayed on and later took care of their parents or widowed mothers.

Martha Smith McPherson (born 1918) is a classic case of the continuity of kin assistance embedded in several generations and reaching back to the family's origin in Scotland. Her father came from Scotland with his widowed mother, and then arranged for his siblings to join him one by one. Martha's mother, an Irish immigrant, one of ten children, became a lifelong "kin keeper" after she married Martha's father: She took care of a young nephew who came alone to the United States, and also took her own father into the household. Later, Martha's parents took in her father's mother and one of Martha's father's brothers, who was an alcoholic: "Rather than put him any place else, we took him in." Eventually, the responsibility for caring for these dependent kin fell on Martha when both her parents became sick. In order to care for her relatives, Martha dropped out of school. While caring for various relatives over a forty-year period, she hired nurses and continued to work at her job. "I made my own decision, because my folks could have sacrificed more, but I felt they sacrificed enough, because they took my grandmother in, and they took my uncle in. . . and I couldn't see them sacrificing any more, so I made my own [sacrifice]."

In fact, caring for her aged relatives gave Martha a nurturing role as her marriage disintegrated due to her inability to have a child. After her husband fathered a child with her girlfriend, she divorced him and returned to Manchester. She stayed with her parents: "I loved to be with them." After her father and uncle died, Martha sold the family home in order to pay for her father's cancer treatment and her father's and uncle's funeral costs. Her 87-year-old mother moved with her into an apartment, and died shortly thereafter. In retrospect, Martha said her compensation was "peace of mind." "I haven't got a home, but I have got peace of mind . . . because I never wanted my mother to go to a [nursing] home, I never wanted my father to go, or my uncle. I wouldn't put him out on the street." At the time of the interview, Martha expected she might live together with her sister and her sister's husband in the large house that her sister owns. Martha intimated, however, that she and her sister had different life-styles, and that there would need to be some adjustment. Martha figured that they would be most likely to live together in the event that her sister's husband died.

In another case, two sisters, Marie Bouchard (born 1917) and Joan Riley (born 1914), grew up in a close relationship to their mother, rendered more interdependent by their father's death when they were young children. The mother actually placed the two daughters in an orphanage for day care—a pattern quite common among Manchester's working mothers whose husbands were absent, sick, or dead. Following the shutdown of the Amoskeag Mills, their mother was unable to find another job because she was considered "too old" and because her eyes were worn from many years of textile work. The two daughters supported their mother for the rest of her life. Joan left Manchester after her marriage, but Marie brought her husband into the household. Her mother wanted to leave. She said: "Well, I'm going to get a place of my own. You're married now, you have your life to live." But Marie insisted that her mother stay: "We couldn't see it. We just wanted her with us.

You couldn't help it. My husband. . . was closer to my mother than he was to his own mother."

During the 1940s, Marie and her husband left for Connecticut to find work there, and then moved around to various places, including Florida, because of the husband's military career. Meanwhile, Joan returned to Manchester after her husband's death and stayed with her mother. She did not remarry because her mother "was getting along in years then, and I knew darn well that if ever we got married again, she wouldn't mind, but she would feel. . . ." Marie and her husband returned from Connecticut after her husband's brother died, so that they could take care of her husband's father. Following her husband's death, Marie continued to take care of her father-in-law for another decade. Her father-in-law, grateful for Marie's support, left her his house. Joan and Marie, both widowed and childless, lived in separate apartments in the same building at the time of the interview. They had only each other as sources of support.

CORESIDENCE AMONG THE GENERATIONS

In Manchester as in most other American urban communities, the pervasive residential pattern was one of nuclear households. The older generation rarely resided with their married adult children in the same household. Newlywed children or young families occasionally lived in their parents' household for short periods. They tended to find housing nearby and often received assistance from their parents, especially in establishing a new household or in caring for young children (Chudacoff & Hareven, 1979).

For most of the people interviewed, and for the population in general, "intimacy from a distance" seemed to be the preferred formula for married adult children's interaction with their parents. When both parents survived into old age, the children were more likely to try to maintain them in the parental home. When elderly parents were able to cope on their own, the children made an effort to reside nearby—in the same building or the same block—but not in the same household.

In cases of illness or need, daughters visited their parents daily and often stayed over in the parental home, rather than moving their parents into their own household. After the death of one parent, children initially took in the surviving parent temporarily or for recurring visits. If the widowed parent was able to take care of himself or herself, the children tried to move the parent to a nearby apartment. Adult children were often willing to financially maintain their parent's home. In some cases, several siblings contributed jointly to hiring a nurse to take daily care of a frail parent who was still living at home.

The ideal model of residence for aging parents who were still able to care for themselves is represented by the Duchamp family, where Solange Duchamp's mother moved into the upstairs apartment in her husband's (Guy, born 1928) parents' home.

> Course my mother lives alone and I feel that with Mom and Dad C. downstairs, of course, they have always been good friends anyway, and since we've been married it's like she's in the family and when I come home from work, oh, once twice and you know . . . sometimes during the week, I'll drop by and I'll visit upstairs and I'll visit downstairs. Everybody's there all at once, and sometimes I'll come in and my mother will come down, or they'd come upstairs or anything, and talk and it's reassuring so that everybody cares so much for each other in this household, that if anything happens upstairs I know that I don't have to worry that Mom and Dad C. downstairs would call, or vice versa. If anything happened downstairs, my mother would call. So it is a worry-free type of situation.

In cases where the parents could be left alone for part of the time, daughters tried to juggle a career and care for a parent; some commuted considerable distances in order to maintain a balance between their own family and their parents' needs. Some daughters tried to lead double lives in order to fulfill obligations to parents while not diminishing their contribution to their children's advancement.

Especially in the earlier cohort, the most consistent pattern of assistance was that one child assumed the main responsibility for caring for the parents. Usually other children contributed to the effort through financial support, visiting, or taking turns keeping the parent in their home. One child, however, carried the primary responsibility for parental care, and tried to mobilize and coordinate the efforts of the other children as the need arose. This was not always accomplished without strain.

In one case the sibling, who was the back-up to help his father, found that his part in providing assistance jeopardized his own health. Pierre Bergeron (born 1914) explained: "While John [Pierre's brother caring for the father in his home] was working, I lived across the road, and I would have to go over there two or three times and sometimes four or five times. . . . It was getting so that I was getting sick myself." Pierre's own adult children insisted that the burden of worrying about his father, who was not safe alone, was too much for Pierre.

The people studied here transcended or modified the pervasive custom of the residential separation between generations in American society only in cases of dire need, when aging parents experienced chronic illness, handicap, or dementia, and needed help with their daily activities (Chudacoff & Hareven, 1978). In such cases an adult child, most commonly a daughter, took the parent into her home. In some cases, a daughter who was widowed, divorced, separated, or incapacitated moved in with her parents in order to receive other types of assistance, especially for child care. If that daughter continued to stay in the parental home, she subsequently took on the responsibilities of caring for her parents (cf. Matthews, 1987).

While it was a common pattern for daughters to take in a dependent parent, daughters-in-law also often took on the responsibility of caring for a husband's parent, sometimes even after the husband's death. Women provided the same effort for a parent-in-law as for their own parent. The most common pattern, however, was that a mother moved into her daughter's house. In some cases, a daughter-in-law cared for parents-in-law in their home. Occasionally, however, when couples had to care for a parent from each side simultaneously, they established priorities as to which parent to take in, and worked out alternative arrangements with other siblings.

Bringing a frail, chronically ill, or demented parent into the household required considerable readjustment of the household space and of the family's daily routines. In some instances, limited space made it necessary for the couple or the grandchildren to give up their bedrooms. Helena Debski Wojek (born 1913) first commuted from Manchester to Massachusetts General Hospital in Boston to take care of her mother, who was being treated there. (The mother's second husband refused to take care of her.) "I'd go out of work and run right to Boston, because she could not speak English at all." Then her mother lived with her for six months. "We gave up our bed and we slept up in the attic on a couch. And my son gave up his bed." The family had to get up many times during the night to keep the elderly woman from choking.

The greatest problem of adjustment in caring for an aging parent at home fell on the daughter or daughter-in-law, especially when she had a job. With some exceptions, women carried the major burden of daily care, while the men provided primarily financial assistance and sociability. Most women were in the labor force and were caught, therefore, in the squeeze between caring for an aging parent and their own work and family responsibilities. Many of the caretaking women reported conflicts resulting from the need to spend almost the entire day caring for a live-in aging parent and at the same time continue their careers. Some had to work during the day, and take care of the parent at night. Some had to give up their full-time job, or replace it with part-time and less satisfying work. Such changes in the wife's career deprived the family of the supplementary income necessary in order to own a home or provide a better education for their children (cf. Brody, 1981).

Suzanne LaCasse Miller (born 1916) held two jobs while caring for her sick husband and having her mother in the household. She was married in 1941, and had four children. During her childbearing years she had worked intermittently in the smaller textile mills that had opened up just before World War II in the empty buildings of the Amoskeag Mills, and at Dunkin' Donuts. Her husband's illness made her the main supporter of her family. Suzanne's father and her older brother both died in 1955; her younger brother died two years later. After his death, her mother moved in with Suzanne, who was then the only surviving child in Manchester. Suzanne's sister lived in Center Harbor, New Hampshire (one hour's distance by car), but her mother did not want to move: "She wanted to stay here [in Manchester] 'cause her friends were here."

Initially, Suzanne's mother provided childcare after moving in. But in her last years, she was sick, "and I'd have to run home from the job and get her to the hospital, get her into oxygen. She didn't want anybody else." In 1964, the same year her mother became ill, Suzanne's husband, who had been ill for some time, died. In 1966, Suzanne's mother died as well and her last daughter married and left home. Suzanne lived alone for only a short time before she took on the care of an elderly male relative in her parents' generation, and provided extensive babysitting for her grandchildren.

THE MAKING OF A "PARENT KEEPER"

An only child, especially an only daughter, fell naturally into the role of "parent keeper." Ellen Wojek Mitchell's (born 1922) mother had a stroke at age 50; she had two more strokes and died at age 57. Ellen's father remained alone while Ellen was raised by relatives in Vermont. Her father remarried, but when her stepmother died in 1946, Ellen was fetched back by her brother to take care of her father. (Apparently, the brother was not capable of taking on this role himself). "Well, I wasn't married and it was only right that somebody should stay with him," recalled Ellen. She married in 1955, after her husband's mother died. Then Ellen's husband moved in with her and her father. Her father helped babysit his granddaughter while Ellen worked.

A caretaking daughter's intention to marry caused a great deal of tension between the generations, and many couples sometimes waited decades for parents to die before they could marry. Marianne Trudeau Wiznewski (born 1912), the oldest daughter, was 47 when she finally married. Up to that time she was living with her mother. As a young girl she and her sister witnessed an ongoing conflict between their mother and their father, which was intensified by her mother's belief that her husband had fathered an illegitimate son. Marianne became protective of her mother: "I was afraid to leave my mother alone. My father was quite . . . and I was afraid to leave her." (She never explained what the source of fear was.) When Marianne finally decided to get married in middle age, her mother objected. "She didn't like him [the fiancé]. He was a widower and, I don't know, she didn't trust him." Marianne's husband was commuting from Massachusetts, and finally he moved in. Marianne's mother died six months later of diabetes. "And Mama didn't like him. And then she died in December. I felt so bad . . . makes you feel awful."

Even when a daughter tried to make up for lost time by marrying in middle age, she still encountered her mother's protest. Lucille Martineau Grenier (born 1915) was 48 when she married a 62-year-old widower, a father of five married children. Her 68-year-old mother was upset about the marriage "cause her right arm was gone. . . . I was living with her and I provided for her until I got married. She expected to have me for the rest of her life." Lucille put her mother in a nursing home because she was "really sick." Later, when her husband became sick, Lucille requested his children's help to put him in a nursing home as well. Both her mother and husband died shortly after entering the home.

Young women, aware of the cultural expectation that one daughter remain at home to care for aging parents, followed various strategies to escape early. Sister Marie Lemay (born 1926) was warned in her youth that if she was to avoid being saddled with the care of aging parents, she would have to pay attention to her own timing in her desire to become a nun. Her two older sisters, who were getting married, warned her: "If you don't enter [the convent] now, when we're all gone, you'll find it difficult to leave."

> So they told me their plans so that in a way, three of us left in the same year. Father was always saying "we have this French saying that someone stays home to be the support of the elderly parents. . . ." Most of the time it seemed to be the youngest of the family, or the youngest girl. The oldest grew up and got married, and the parents were getting on in age. By the time the youngest grew up, the parents were getting old enough. . . . So, instead of settling down, that one was almost like naturally left to take care of the family.

Anna Douville (born 1907) the youngest in her family, had to compete with her own sisters in order not to be left the last one at home. When

Anna finally announced she was going to get married, her sisters pressured her to cancel her engagement, claiming that her fiancé was a drunkard. Actually, "they were scheming to get me to support my folks until they died. . . . But my mother told me, 'Anna, don't wait too long. What if I die or your father dies? Then you'd insist on staying with me, and you'll lose your boyfriend." She felt guilty, however, for abandoning her parents.

> They [her parents] were on the city welfare . . . even with the hard times I had during my life, I never stopped for sympathy for myself, because I knew about my mother's life. . . . A lot of things go through your head when your folks are gone. . . . You don't realize it when they are living. You want to live your own life; but when your folks are gone and you think of all the good things that you have today, you wish they could share them.

Anna was never quite free of guilt about her perceived neglect of her parents. Daughters who returned to the parental home due to disruptions in their own lives often fell naturally into the role of parent keeper. Joan Riley (born 1914), who returned from Providence, Rhode Island, after her husband's death to live with her mother, explained why she never married again: "I had my mother to take care of. She came first, because she was getting along in years, and she had to have somebody."

In cases where the parent keeper was not already living with the parents, the main factors dictating the selection of a parent keeper were governed by that particular adult child's ability and willingness to take the parent in, by such other responsibilities as a sick child or spouse in the parent keeper's own family, by the consent or support of the parent keeper's spouse, and by the readiness of the parent to accept the plan. If the other children were already too old and needing care themselves, they were unable to take in and cope with an aging parent. Frank Kaminski's (born 1921) 73-year-old sister did not marry because her salary as a shoe factory worker was needed to help the family keep their home during the Great Depression. Long after their father's death, this sister, who was by then frail herself, continued to live and take care of their mother, who was in her late nineties. The family considered new arrangements, but these plans failed: "They were thinking of having my other sister take care of them. In the meantime her sister's husband died, and she was bedridden. So she can't do it anymore. So, you know, that took care of that solution to the problem."

Most parent keepers evolved into that role over their entire life course; others were pushed into it through family crises. Earlier life-course experience was an overwhelming factor in the designation of a parent keeper. The most significant factor was the continued or recurring proximity of residence of a child and the parent, and the corresponding mutual assistance. Daughters who maintained close contact with their parents after marriage fell into the role of parent keepers, especially when the other siblings "bailed out" by marrying early. Sometimes this was accomplished by eloping. The risk of siblings' bailing out increased if the father's early death necessitated a child's support for a widowed mother and the remaining siblings.

The emotional bond between a parent and a certain child often meant that that child was considered the most appropriate one to care for an aging parent. The bonds frequently grew stronger during the parent's last period of chronic illness; some children reported loneliness following a live-in parent's death; some caretaking children remarried or intensified their relations with their own children in order to maintain close family ties Parents expressed their preference about which child to join, even if that child, usually a daughter, resided outside of Manchester. These mothers went a distance because they preferred to live with a particular daughter, rather than with other children in Manchester. When Anna Charboneau Lessard (born 1928) and her family moved to New York City to manage an apartment building, her mother first lived with Anna's sister in Manchester. "Then she came up to me and asked me if she could live with us." The mother moved to New York and took care of Anna's and her husband's four children. Sandra Kazantakis Wall (born 1921), who lived with her second husband in Maryland, brought her mother from Manchester after her father died, even though other siblings lived in Manchester, because her mother insisted, "I want to come and live with you." Sandra's mother lived with her for the last five years of her life. "Dick [her husband] was very good to mother, and she loved him like a son. . . . In fact, she liked him better than some of her children sometimes."

In both cases, the mother's choice of the geographically distant child was related to earlier life experiences. For example, Sandra had been particularly close to her mother. She had eloped with her first husband at age 20; because her husband was in the military, she lived in various places overseas and in the United States, and adopted a son in Germany. She returned home from time to time, usually when she had marital problems. "My mother and father, yes! that was the home, that was my life, and that's where I found the answers, at my mother's and father's." In 1959, after her husband was killed in a plane crash in Alaska, Sandra and her adopted son moved back to Manchester to her parents' home. After this respite, Sandra remarried and again moved with a new husband to Maryland. When her mother became widowed, she went to live with Sandra.

In another case, a son had to accept reluctantly his parents' decision to leave his home in Manchester and move in with his sister in Rhode Island. Jonathan Fournier's (born 1926) parents insisted on making their move even though his father was working for him in Manchester: "Why do you want to go back down there, you have been up here with me for 15 years?" asked Jonathan. His parents replied that they could be better taken care of in Rhode Island. "How the hell are they going to take care of you any better than I have?" But Jonathan's mother insisted on moving. After the move, his father commuted from Rhode Island to Manchester. He continued work with Jonathan and stayed with him from Monday to Thursday, and then returned to Rhode Island.

In summary, parent keepers' careers followed several trajectories: Some children remained as adults with the family in which they grew up, and gradually took over the care of parents. The caretaker usually was the youngest daughter. In other cases, children returned home due to their own disrupted life course or in response to a parent's need for assistance. This was usually a contingency act, provoked by events and needs that had not been anticipated earlier in the life course. The returning adult child was usually single, divorced, or widowed, and could divert his or her own life more easily than could married siblings. More daughters than sons returned home as adults. Another pattern was that some children did not coreside with their parents, but handled the main responsibilities of caretaking. These children usually daughters, shuttled between their own homes and those of their parents, and often carried the burden of a job as well.

In the fourth pattern, the parent moved into the adult child's home in cases of extreme need for personal care. Adult daughters were willing to give care, even to a bed-bound and incontinent parent; they resorted to a nursing home only in cases where total care was required. In some cases where the sick parent's spouse was still alive, the spouse continued to live separately in an independent household or with another child. If both parents needed care, sometimes each was taken into the home of a different sibling—a concept alien to our times but one that is quite common to immigrants. Some families, especially with all members pitching in, were able to accomplish care for an elderly parent in their home. These adult children were squeezed between their obligations toward their parents and their desire to provide for their own children. In other cases, changes in the relations within the family and the women's commitment to work made the expectation of providing care for an incapacitated parent unrealistic.

The struggle of adult children, often approaching old age themselves, to keep a parent in their own home exacted a high price of them. The extra work of caring for frail parents changed daily life and, for some, led to a disrupted life course. Some children's own health declined because of the strain; others suffered tensions in their marriage, or experienced economic loss because of the wife's withdrawal from the labor force; and others were unable to prepare for their own retirement and old age, because of the financial strain and the demands on the wife's time. Some parent keepers worried about limits on the life plans of their own children (cf. Ory, 1985).

It is not surprising, therefore, that all the children interviewed who had taken care of aging parents in their own homes, expressed a strong desire never to have to depend on their own children in their old age. They considered living with their children the greatest obstacle to maintaining their independence. Sarah Butterick, who had taken care of her father in her own home after he had a stroke, said she would never consider living with her own children. "I hope not; I hope I drop dead. . . . [I] hope I just don't wake up some morning." Helena Debski Wojek (born 1913), whose mother lived with her for six months when she was ill, explained why she lived alone (after her husband's death). "Well I try to, because I know what it is to take care of people that are really sick, and I wouldn't want to see my children go through that. . . . I wouldn't want to live with one of my children because they've got lives of their own, and I've got a life of my own."

In some cases, members of the children's cohort did not want to have to live with their own children in the future because of the aspects of parental control they had experienced firsthand. Stephen Livak (born 1911), who had lived for several years with both his mother and his wife's mother, said he would never want to live with his son because, "I knew what I had to go through living tied with the apron strings. I wouldn't want him to be tied to my apron strings. I would want him to be free, and I wouldn't want to be obligated to him."

Yves St. Pierre (born 1910) and Cora Lemay St. Pierre (born 1910) helped care for Yves' father in the first three years of their marriage, after the father was paralyzed from a stroke. "That was a long three years, I'll tell you." Both Yves and Cora rejected the notion of living with their children in the future: "We've always been independent and we'd feel if we lived . . . with our children we wouldn't be independent. I'd rather live with myself as long as I can, and when I can't I'd go into a home." Even though they upheld their own independence, and placed their mentally retarded 34-year-old daughter in an institution, the St. Pierres, when asked what was different about families today, replied: "They're too independent each on their own side." Yvonne Lemay Gagne (born 1916) and Pierre Gagne (born 1916) both agreed that they would rather live in a nursing home than with their children: "I wouldn't be happy anyway. When you know you're in somebody's way, you don't feel right." Yvonne was less definitive at first: "I'd be lonesome in a nursing home first. I'd feel: they don't need the old lady around!" But then she concurred with her husband, the couple proclaimed their preference for a nursing home almost in unison.

When assessing the children's strong pronouncements about their desire for independence in their own old age, one must keep in mind the life stage at which they were interviewed. There is no telling whether their attitude will change when they reach dependent old age. As 52-year-old Raymond Champagne put it: "I think I would till try to make it alone. Then years from now, I might think differently."

THE SHADOW OF THE NURSING HOME

The unsatisfactory alternative to keeping parents at home was placing them in a nursing home. Parents most commonly went to nursing homes in cases of extreme physical sickness, paralysis, or dementia. For example, when parents wandered around, were irrational, impulsive and unpredictable, or could not be managed by the adult child, then children sought another solution. Indeed, in several cases elderly couples faced this dilemma with regard to their own spouses and committed them to nursing homes.

In cases where children lived in another town and were not able to care for a parent on a regular basis, the nursing home was the only solution. Susanne Robert (born 1927) for example, had a close relationship with her parents since childhood. After her marriage in 1950, her husband's father rented a nearby apartment for the new couple. Susanne's parents also helped with a loan to buy a car, and her mother took care of her children once a week. When Susanne's mother became ill, after Susanne and her young family moved to Maine in 1955, her mother entered a nursing home, while her father continued to stay in his own apartment.

> My intentions were to take care of them, but my mom ended up in a nursing home because my dad couldn't take care of her and we were living in Maine at the time. My sister was in California and my youngest was only two months old. . . . So she was paralyzed for weeks and she did end up in a home which kind of broke our hearts, but there she got good care and she was in about three years. Then he [father] died before her. He had one heart attack and that was it.

Almost simultaneously, Susanne encountered other needs for parent care in the family. Susanne's husband placed his father in a nursing home, and tried to place his mother in subsidized housing for the elderly. According to Susanne, the mother, however, followed her own plan.

> Well, my father was the one that got sick first and she [his mother] tried as much as she could to take care of him, but it was too much. So we had to place him in a home. This was done by my mother. She was about eighty years old and she was still living in an apartment. And my brother had connections with politics, to put her in those high rises that were being built in Manchester, and while waiting for one to be built, she went and placed herself in a nursing home on the west side where the old hospital used to be.

Most elderly parents who went to a nursing home did so during the final period of chronic illness, and died shortly thereafter. Children who lived in Manchester regularly visited their parents in nursing homes, often daily. Daughters did laundry, provided haircuts, bought delicacies, and took the elderly parent on "outings." If the children lived in a distant community, the day-to-day care was left to a local sibling. Jonathan Fournier, whose parents, at their own choice, left his house and moved to Rhode Island, lost contact with his mother. After his father's death, Jonathan's sister placed his mother in a nursing home in Rhode Island. Jonathan deferred to the judgment and planning of his sister, who took charge of their mother's care, but felt guilty:

> I am ashamed to tell you. I haven't seen my mother for a year and a half, two years. I feel bad about it. Really, I should get myself up and get there. . . . It's only the last six months its been bothering my conscience about going down there. It isn't because I have no respect or love for her; I got other things turning all the time. . . . I think it's wrong, but the decision was made to put her in a nursing home. I'm not gonna fight over it.

In some cases, the parent's impaired safety awareness resulted in a long period of anxiety among the siblings before seeking another solution to the home environment. Pierre Bergeron (born 1910) described the problems his brother John had in caring for their father at home. "One day John came home and found all the water faucets on full-strength. And another day he came home and found all the burners on the electric stove." Their father decided to take trips using the public buses; on one of these trips he fell and broke his hip. This was the final straw for the children; they decided to send their father to a nursing home. Pierre felt that was not his decision to make: "I said I would not give him [John] any decision because I thought that he took care of them all their lives, and he's the one who should [make the decision]." In other instances, the children believed in a commonly accepted plan that their parents should enter a nursing home when required. Vincent Duchamp (born

1922) explained: "Arrangements have been made already. If something does happen to one or the other [parents], they can't sustain themselves, then they'll be put automatically into a nursing home." But his mother (born 1899), who was caring for her husband and a retarded daughter, had another point of view: "We didn't think of that yet . . . when that times comes, we will see."

Another case of conflicting accounts concerning a parent's entry into a nursing home occurred when we interviewed Alice Robert St. Martin's (born 1925) 87-year-old mother in a nursing home, with Alice present. The interview ended because the mother burst into tears, prompted by her feelings of being abandoned in the nursing home. Alice had maintained in an earlier interview that her mother had been placed into the nursing home at her own request:

> My mother wanted a nursing home and we never knew, she told us when she was going in the next day. She made arrangements with people that worked in the hospital. I guess, I don't know if Donald [son] knew. I know I didn't. She called me and she said, "I hope you won't be mad but I am leaving, you know," she sold her furniture. What could I say. It was the best way, you know, because she couldn't today at 87.

Even though nursing homes had come into common use by the late 1960s, a stigma remained attached to having a parent in a nursing home. Those interviewed, without exception, felt compelled to provide an excuse or justification for having had a parent in a nursing home. The theme that parents had entered a nursing home on their own initiative, presenting their children with a *fait accompli*, recurred in the children's retrospective narratives. Mary Grzwinski Petrowski (born 1918), for example, who had placed her 82-year-old mother in a nursing home after she was unable to live alone, said she had done so "simply because she [her mother] requested it." "She didn't want to live with us; she felt we had our own life to live, and she said, 'Why don't you put me in a nursing home?' And so we did. Her mother stayed in the nursing home for six months until her death. "But it was her choice, because I was going to take a year off [from teaching school]. My mother was very intelligent, she was very independent and she felt 'this is your life and why should you stop working just to sit with me.'" Had Mary stopped working, her and her husband's plans for retirement would have been financially jeopardized (cf. Scharlach, 1987).

Florida St. Honore Rouillard (born 1926) whose mother lives with her youngest brother, expressed the prevalent ambivalence toward the nursing homes: "[In the past] you took care of them, there was no thought of nursing homes, today there is one on every corner. . . . In a way, they are probably getting better [care] but, of course, it's a much

more distant feeling. I visit nursing homes. I know what I'm saying."
Florida expects that she and her husband will end up in a nursing home,
rather than with their children. "Because of the beautiful facilities they
have there now; they did not have that then. They have nurses, the best
care, professionals today."

COHORT LOCATION IN HISTORICAL TIME

The pervasiveness of the children's involvement with the care of their
aging parents was closely related to their earlier life-course patterns,
over which they had different degrees of control, and to the ethnic and
cultural traditions that governed their family relations. A fuller understanding of the differences in their attitudes depends on our identifica-
tion of the changing social and historical contexts that affected the lives
of the respective children's cohorts.

Members of the parent cohort had been the major supporters of their
aging parents. They viewed kin as their almost exclusive source of assistance over the life course. For that very reason, they also expected their
main support in old age to come from their children. They tried to
remain self-reliant as late as possible, however, and viewed all support
from their children as part of the family's self-reliance. As Andrew Proulx
(born 1922) put it:

> Well they didn't have the old folks home those days like they have today.
> In those days, it was the kids that took care of the parents. Today, the old
> folks they place them some place. Get rid of them! Well, the kids want their
> liberty a little bit more, and they don't want to be straddled to the parents
> that are senile or sick or whatever.

The older members of the parent cohort (in their eighties and nineties at
the time of the interview) were especially articulate on this issue. Having
spent the prime of their lives in an era preceding the welfare state, the
very concept of relying on public agencies was alien to their principles
and upbringing. Their belief in the self-sufficiency of the family led them
to view public support as demeaning. These were the values they had
taught to their children. Ranking their preferences for sources of assistance, they saw assistance within the nuclear family as their highest
priority, followed by assistance from extended and more distant kin. As
expected, they cited public welfare as a last resort. The parents proudly
claimed to have avoided public relief even during the Great Depression.
Those who resorted to welfare agencies did so surreptitiously, and later
denied having received help (Hareven, 1982).

The parents' reliance on support from kin rather than from public agencies was also shaped by their ethnic backgrounds. Their ideology of kin assistance was part of their tradition, and formed a survival strategy carried over from their respective premigration cultures. After settling in the United States, the parents modified this ideology to fit the needs, requirements, and constraints imposed by the insecurities of the industrial environment. Their involvement in mutual kin assistance thus represented both the continuation of an earlier practice of family caretaking among the generations, and an ideology that shaped their expectations of each other and of the younger generation.

Both children's cohorts were socialized with expectations and ideologies of kin assistance similar to those of their parents, but they were challenged to implement these norms under different historical and social circumstances. The children were caught in a bind, and were ambivalent toward the obligation to be the almost exclusive caretakers of their aging parents. The coping strategies they worked out were intended to meet the values of kin assistance passed on by their parents, but new pressures, new aspirations, and the emergence of bureaucratic agencies led them to modify these ideals. The desire to meet their parents' expectations and at the same time launch their own children added to their generation's sense of conflict due to their obligations to them. These children prioritized obligations, worked overtime, reframed the meaning of family obligations for caretaking, and did not expect that their life-course squeeze would be repeated in their own children's middle years.

While the parents expected their children to assist them in old age, the children did not expect (or want) to have to rely on their own children for economic support. They prepared for old age through pension plans, savings, and home ownership, and expected to rely on social security and, if needed, on assistance from the welfare state. In cases of illness or disability, they expected to be in a nursing home. The most they expected from their children was emotional support and sociability. This attitude also resulted from their cohort's becoming accustomed to public agency assistance and to interacting with bureaucratic institutions.

Both children's cohorts shared a deep involvement with the care of aging parents. As discussed above, their commitment was rooted in their life-course antecedents and was reinforced by their ethnic traditions and family culture. There were, however, significant variations within this common theme. Members of the earlier children's cohort had resigned themselves to staying within their social class, because of the devastating impact of the Great Depression and the shutdown of the Amoskeag Mills. They assigned the highest priority to recovering from the Depression and to staying afloat economically. In order to achieve this, they pooled resources among kin, doubled up in housing, and moved around among various relatives within Manchester, and sometimes around New England or other parts of the United States. For them, survival of the family as a collective unit remained the highest goal, rather than the pursuit of individual careers. Within that context, children were expected to stretch their resources in order to keep aging parents within the family, and to support them as long as possible.

The later children's cohort, on the other hand, came of age during World War II. Having experienced the Great Depression and the shutdown of the Amoskeag Mills less directly, they were exposed to a lesser degree to the strong interdependence among kin that was dramatized most during the Depression. Obviously, a majority of the later cohort had younger parents; for many, their trial period was yet to come. In this cohort, generational assistance still flowed more commonly from parents to children, than the reverse. Parents helped newlyweds rent nearby housing, loaned them money to purchase a car, and provided child care. In some cases, the younger children's cohort still benefit from parental assistance, which had continued over their lives.

Taking advantage of the economic recovery brought about by World War II and of the career training and educational benefits that the young men had gained in the military service, the children's cohort was devoted to building new lives and improving their housing conditions. They tried to pull themselves out from a depressed, unemployed, working-class situation into a middle-class life-style (Elder & Hareven, 1992). Realizing their limitations, they also assigned a high priority to the educational opportunities for their children. Ironically, the later children's cohort had been coached by their own parents to aspire toward occupational advancement and to develop a middle-class life-style. But as they attained these aspirations, they were also less available to their parents, especially to those who needed assistance in old age. Florida Rouillard (born 1926) explained how her daughter had realized the dream she had been unable to implement for herself: "I never did become a nurse. My daughter did, though. It's funny, how it worked." William Silvers (born 1927) observed, "I'd like all my children to have more than I have, and we parents try to push them that way."

The later cohort had a higher individualistic orientation. They drew firmer boundaries, both between the nuclear family and extended kin, as well as between the younger generation and the old. They valued a more private life for married couples. Their primary energies were directed toward their children and their own future, rather than toward their parents. Members of this cohort expressed ambivalence about carrying economic obligations for aging parents or taking them into their homes when they became unable to care for themselves. At the same time, they helped their parents, principally by providing services rather than regular financial support. They were also less inclined to take a frail, elderly parent into the household than were members of the earlier children's cohorts. The ambivalence of this younger cohort probably resulted from the erosion of mutual interdependence among kin and from an expectation of assistance from the public sector. Although they had been raised with strong values of familial responsibility, the later children's cohort made the transition to a more individualistic mode of thinking, and into a greater acceptance of public welfare as an extension of kin assistance. They expected this change to continue in the lives of their own children.

In some respects, members of the later children's cohort were also more emotionally distant from their parents. Unlike the older cohort, who stayed home until their marriage, those members of the later cohort who stayed on in Manchester tended to leave home before marriage and reside separately, although near their parents. Many children left home because of World War II. Men (and sometimes, women) went into the service; the women often followed husbands who were stationed in other places. Children's departure from the home in early adulthood produced an earlier separation between the generations than in the earlier cohort. Living away from home also increased psychological separation. Alice Robert St. Martin (born 1925) explained that after her marriage, she felt more separate from her parents. "When I went to my mother's and father's it was like I was visiting. I felt that way."

The later children's cohort expressed a clearer preference that the generations live separately: Pierre Gagnou (born 1926) explained, "It wouldn't be a family [rather than a couple's] life if they would have their father or their mother living with them." Thinking of the children, he continued, "If for some reason they would have an argument, it would make it hard for them." Raymond Champagne (born 1926) upheld the need for separate residence of the couple: "I believe that marriage is something very sacred. It should be a husband-wife situation, nobody else . . . and I have listened when I was younger that families who took in the old people, I always felt that those people [taking in elderly parents] were not fully leading a married life. . . . I just wouldn't want to be in their shoes, and I wouldn't want to put my children through it."

Members of the later cohort had far less experience caring for elderly parents in their own home than the older cohort. They were more likely than the older cohort to place their physically or mentally impaired parents in nursing homes or seek institutional help. Those who most commonly took care of an adult parent in their own home were only children, usually daughters. In other cases, the parent was often shuttled from one home to another among children in the later cohort.

These younger adult children were either less willing or less able than the earlier cohort to make a full-time commitment as a parent keeper.

Viewing themselves as separate from their family origins, members of the later cohort upheld their own nuclear family as a separate entity. Some of them contrasted their own life-styles with those of their parents, setting themselves apart from the values of the previous generation. Marlene Bertram Kaminski (born 1925), for example, said that she exercised greater detachment from her own children, as a reaction against her mother's demanding attitude:

> I mean, when I look back, I say, "My gosh, I never had . . . a life, really, of my own." Because I went from my mother bossing me to my husband bossing me, and [laughs] I never knew what it was to really be on my own. And now Marsha [her daughter] has moved to Merrimack, which is not far from here. But I'm not mad or angry that she isn't calling me every day, because I feel that—for me, my mother was so hurt if I didn't call every night and tell her what kind of a day I had, that it got to be sort of a drag that you have to do this. So my—some day, some weeks I don't hear from my daughter all week. And I don't resent it at all. I really don't. And I, I didn't try to tell my children what to wear, and this and that . . .

Marlene did try, however, to manage her mother's life. When her twice-widowed mother wanted to leave Marlene's house and marry again, Marlene warned her against it. "You've gone through so much— two husbands with illnesses and being upset; now you have a reasonably good job, you can support yourself, you can live here. . . . You have a home here." But her mother insisted on her independence: "You have your husband, you have your family, and even though I'm in the house, I don't have anyone that really belongs to me."

Neither the earlier nor the later children's cohort was free, however, of the complexities involved in handling the problems of generational assistance. While the earlier children's cohort had a more clearly defined commitment to collective family values and kin assistance, its members who had actually cared for elderly parents in their own home, or had sacrificed their own marriage for parental care, did not do so without ambivalence, doubt, bitterness, or the specter of a lonely old age for themselves. Their posture had often been one of resignation to familial norms and acceptance of "fate" rather than free choice. Members of the later cohort, on the other hand, who followed a more individualistic course, were not free of guilt over the way in which the support of their aging parents had been worked out.

Both cohorts were, to some degree, transitional between a milieu of a deep involvement in generational assistance reinforced by strong family and ethnic values, and one of individualistic values that emerged after

World War II. In this historical process, the earlier cohort's lives conformed more closely to the script of their traditional familial and ethnic cultures, while the later cohort, as it Americanized, gravitated toward individualistic middle-class values. The transition was by no means completed. Members of the later cohort had not entirely freed themselves of their traditional upbringing. Both cohorts were the middle generation: They still expressed their parents' values, but the later cohort felt less able or inclined to implement them.

Our comparison of the cohorts of the children's generation suggests differences in the practice of caretaking and in the attitudes of each of the two cohorts toward the care of aging parents. Both cohorts were transitional in that they were still strongly bound by their parents' values and expectations that children should serve as the major caretakers. Both cohorts attempted to fulfill this script, often at a high price to their own marriages, to their ability to help their grown children, and to their preparation for their own "old age." The earlier of the two children's cohorts was more inclined to live by their parents' cultural script, despite the fact that its members were more vulnerable as their own "old age" approached. The later cohort was more ambivalent and more conflicted about a commitment to long-term care for a frail or chronically ill parent; its members were especially hesitant about caring for such a parent at home.

The difference between the two cohorts thus reflects a historical process of increasing individualization in family relationships and an increasing reliance on public agencies and bureaucratic institutions for the care of dependent elderly. The historical process is well known, but the detailed analysis of the interviews of the members of these cohorts provides firsthand testimony about how this change was perceived and experienced by the women and men who were caught up in it. These caretakers revealed a commitment to their parents, as well as ambivalence about their roles, inner conflicts, and strategies that have resulted in various compromises as they try to meet their obligations. They were also attempting to redefine their obligations, as assistance from the public sector became more widely used and accepted.

When identifying these differences among the cohorts, we need to keep in mind that these narratives are derived principally from interviews with the parents and the children. Their statements derive from their own subjective reconstruction of their life course and from their perceptions of their current situations.

The very historical circumstances that influenced behavior and attitudes toward caring for aging parents among the later and the earlier children's cohorts also shaped the ways in which they remembered and interpreted these patterns in the course of the interview. The ways in which members of the two cohorts articulated their problems were shaped, therefore, by their own historical experiences over their life course. Thus, not only were the maps of the cohorts' respective life-course patterns charted by their earlier life experiences, but also the coordinates that they superimposed on these maps, in order to make sense of their own lives, were a product of their location in historical time (Hareven, 1986).

ACKNOWLEDGMENTS

"Hareven gratefully acknowledges the support from the National Institute on Aging for the Manchester study "Aging and Generational Relations: Cohort Change" under a Research Career Development Grant #5 K04 AG00026 and with Research Grant #1R01 AG02468."

NOTE

1. By tracing the children of the historical cohorts, their spouses, the siblings of the spouses, and other family members in Manchester, as well as other parts of the United States, we followed relatives along kinship networks as far as possible (Hareven, 1982). We assembled this group of interviewees in a "snowball" method, and interviewed all kin who responded. We interviewed each person three times, using open-ended questions in two- to three-hour sessions. The interview questions covered a broad range of areas pertaining to the interviewee's life history. Many questions focused in great detail on the issues of assistance over the life course and support networks in old age. Wherever possible, we elicited the perceptions of the children and the parents or of several siblings on the same issues covered in the interviews.

In addition to interviews, we also constructed a demographic history, migration history, work history, and family history for each individual. We then linked this sequential information into a "time-life line," reconstructing the individual's life chronologically, in relation to age and historical time. This enabled us to examine in each individual the synchronization of work-life transitions with family transitions, and to relate patterns of timing to the interviewees' subjective accounts of the life course in the interviews. The time-life lines also enabled us to analyze differences within each cohort.

The detailed reconstruction of the life histories and of the migration and work histories of these cohorts enables us to relate earlier life events to later ones and to identify life course patterns as important variables in kin assistance in old age.

A comparison of the two cohorts provides a perspective on changes over historical time and an understanding of the ways in which the patterns of assistance of each cohort were shaped by the historical circumstances and cultural values affecting their lifetimes.

REFERENCES

Adams, B. N. (1970). Isolation, function, and beyond: American kinship in the 1960s. *Journal of Marriage and the Family, 32*, 575–597.

Antonucci, T. C. (1990). Social supports and social relations. In R. H. Binstock, & L. George (Eds.), *Handbook of Aging and the Social Sciences*, 3rd ed. (pp. 105–117) New York: Academic Press, 205–227.

Bengtson, V. L., & Treas, J. (1980). Intergenerational relations and mental health. In J. E. Birren & R. B. Sloore (Eds.), *Handbook of Mental Health and Aging* (pp. 400–428). Englewood Cliffs, NJ: Prentice Hall.

Bengtson, V. L., Kasshau. P. L., & Ragan, P. K. (1985). The impact on social structure on aging individuals. In J. E. Birren & K. W. Schaie (Eds.), *Handbook of the Psychology of Aging* (pp. 327–353), 2nd ed. New York: Van Nostrand.

Brody, E. M. (1981). Women in the middle and family help to older people. The Gerontologist, 21, 471–480.

Cantor, M. H. (1983). Strain among caregivers: A study of experience in the United States. *The Gerontologist, 23*, 597–604.

Chudacoff, H. P., & Hareven, T. K. (1978). Family transitions to old age. In T. K. Hareven (Ed.), *Transitions: The Family and the Life Course in Historical Perspective*. New York: Academic Press.

Chudacoff, H. P., & Hareven, T. K. (1979). From the empty nest to family dissolution: Life course transitions into old age. *Journal of Family History, 4*, 69–83.

Cicirelli, V. G. (1981). *Helping Elderly Parents: The Role of Adult Children*. Boston: Auburn House.

Elder, G. H., Jr. (1978a). Family history and the life course. In T. K. Hareven (Ed.), *Transitions: The Family and the Life Course in Historical Perspective*. New York: Academic Press.

————. (1978b). *Children of the Great Depression*. Chicago: University of Chicago Press.

Elder, G. H., & Hareven, T. K. (1992). Rising above life's disadvantage. In G. H. Elder, R. Parke, & J. Modell (Eds.), *Children in Place and Time*. Cambridge: Cambridge University Press.

Hareven, T. K. (Ed.) (1978). *Transitions: The Family and the Life Course in Historical Perspective*. New York: Academic Press.

————. (1981). Historical Changes in the Timing of Family Transitions: Their

Impact on Generational Relations. *Aging: Stability and Change in the Family.* New York: Academic Press.

———. (1982). *Family Time and Industrial Time.* Cambridge, England: Cambridge University Press.

———. (1986). Historical changes in the social construction of the life course. *Human Development, 29.* 171–180.

Hareven, T. K., & Chudacoff, H. P. (1978). The last years of life and the family cycle. In T. K. Hareven (Ed.), *Transitions: The Family and the Life Course in Historical Perspective.* New York: Academic Press.

Hareven, T. K., & Langenbach, R. (1978). *Amoskeag: Life and Work in an American Factory City.* New York: Pantheon.

Matthews, S. H. (1987). Provision of care to old parents: Division of responsibility among adult children. *Research on Aging, 9,* 45–60.

Ory, M. G. (1985). The burden of care. *Generations, 10,* 14–18.

Riley, M. W. (1978). Aging, social change and the power of ideas. *Daedalus: Generations, 10,* 39–52.

Scharlach, A. E. (1987). Role strain in mother-daughter relationships in later life. *The Gerontologist, 27,* 627–631.

Shanas, E. (1979). Social myth as hypothesis: The case of the family relations of old people. *The Gerontologist, 19,* 3–9.

2

Fathers and Sons in Rural America
Occupational Choice and Intergenerational Ties across the Life Course

Glen H. Elder, Jr., Elizabeth B. Robertson, and Rand D. Conger

The differences between my father and [his son] were the differences between the generation that came out of the Great Depression and the generation of the FFA that came into prominence after World War II. The FFA had educated [his sons] in the holy writs of modern farming—the "Commandments" as my father refers to them: Thou shalt plant rows close together (my father thought this was greedy and counterproductive).

Howard Kohn, *The Last Farmer: An American Memoir* (1988, pp. 68–69)

There is a cyclical rhythm to farm life in the American midwest—the daily round from sunup to sundown, the passing of seasons from spring planting to harvest time and the months of fallow, and life's turning wheel in which the young face decisions on whether to succeed their parents in farming and lifestyle. This type of decision typically involves young men, since gender equality has little voice or reality in farm country. As Deborah Fink (1986:232) points out, in the farm state of Iowa "only men are recognized and supported as farmers." In this chapter we compare the intergenerational experiences of Iowa men who left the farm with those who entered farming during the 1960s and 1970s.

These decades appeared to hold promise for launching and building a farm, though it is now recognized as the expansionary seedbed of the 1980s farm crisis. The fathers of these men typically grew up on farms in the 1920s and 1930s and entered farming as the demand for agricultural products soared during World War II and the postwar era. Many of these men are still farming in later life, but a third of their sons in this study who ever farmed have since left the occupation for other pursuits.

31

In this chapter, we ask what factors distinguish sons who entered farming from those who chose nonfarm careers, and then investigate the consequences of this career choice and the early father-son relationship for the quality of father behavior and the nature of mid-life relations between the men and their aging fathers. Data are based on 246 American men from the north central region of Iowa. All of the men grew up on a farm.

OCCUPATIONAL CHOICE AND INTERGENERATIONAL TIES

A farmer's son's entry into farming depends on many factors, from motivation to opportunity, with opportunity being greatest when the father is a full-time owner-operator of a farm (Lyson, 1984; Molnar & Dunkelberger, 1981; Straus, 1956, 1964). Motivation has much to do with past experience and family influence. In particular, entry into farming is likely to depend on the attractiveness of the father as a career model. Modeling is unlikely when the son experiences the family home as a battlefield between parents or when the father is harsh and erratic. The relative isolation of farm households would intensify the effect of such behavior. Other factors being equal, we assume that men who chose farming did not experience high levels of marital conflict and punitive parenting in childhood, when compared to men who chose other careers.

Another consideration involves the life history that most facilitates intergenerational continuity—the life cycle from father to son on the family farm. This cycle has been likened to a turning wheel: "the old turn over the work to the young and die, and they in turn get old and turn over the work to their children" (Miner, 1939, p. 85). But it is a turning wheel that passes over common ground from one generation to the next. There is much to the context of farm life that remains the same as the generations reproduce and age. Interaction theory (Cottrell, 1969:564) suggests that any self-other relation learned in one setting is likely to be evoked by situations of comparable structure and content, such as the rural farm environment for parent-child interaction.

Consider, for example, a child who takes the role of a punitive, arbitrary father. In doing so, he or she acquires a repertoire of behavior that forms a parental style for subsequent years. Thus the adult son of an authoritarian father is likely to be described by his wife as "extremely harsh and strict" with his young son. With these observations in mind, we expect a high degree of similarity in the parenting behavior of farm fathers and their adult sons, whether nurturant and authoritative or punitive and harsh (Parke, 1981; Rossi & Rossi, 1990; Whitbeck, Simons, & Conger, 1991). This similarity may occur because of social continuity across the generations in occupational rate and in frequency of interaction. By comparison, intergenerational continuity should be relatively weak among men who left the world of farming for other endeavors. They would have less interaction with their fathers and more social discontinuity across the generations. The more dissimilar the setting of the two generations, the weaker their correspondence on family behavior.

Our final point concerns intergenerational continuity as well as social ties between farm fathers and their adult sons. Although farming may appear on the surface to be a solitary enterprise, it involves much cooperation with family members, relatives, and other farmers. Interdependence is enhanced when two generations of the same family farm in close proximity to one another. Shared work and a shared understanding of the problems and constraints associated with that work lead us to expect the bonds between two generations of farmers to be relatively strong—more so at least than the relation between farm fathers and their nonfarm adult sons (see Sweetser, 1966). This difference could reflect positive aspects of the father-son relation and the potentially aversive experience of frequent contact with a demanding and intrusive parent.

Together, these lines of analysis argue that intergenerational ties influence life choices, as in career and residence, and also are shaped by them in various ways. As hypothesized, early family experiences influence the intention to farm or not, as does the success of the farm itself. The career pursued, farm or nonfarm, involves distinctive constraints and options for the father-son relationship. We turn briefly at this point to a description of the sample and measures before pursuing the analysis.

THE SAMPLE AND GENERATIONS

Data for this study come from the Iowa Youth and Families Project, a study of rural families who were recruited from eight agriculturally dependent counties in the north central region of the state. Seven of the eight had poverty rates above the state average of 10.7 in 1989. The first wave of data collection, begun in January 1989, produced a total of 451 two-parent households with a seventh grader and a near sibling— approximately 78% of the eligible families in the region. The second wave of data collection, in the winter and spring of 1990, included 94%

Table 2.1. Historical and Social Characteristics of Two Generations of Iowa Men

	Father ($n = 245$)	Adult Son ($n = 247$)
Birth Year		
Median	1918	1949
Range	1887–1936	1931–1957
Years Farmed, Median	30	—
Currently Farming (%)	50.4	32.0
Family Size		
Median	6	5
Range	3–15	4–9
Education		
% HS grad	49.0	72.5
% College grad	2.8	25.9
Wives		
% Employed	17.9	88.7
% Fathers farmed	—	49.8

of the original families. At least two more waves of data collection are planned. In each year, data have been collected from the four members of the study households; the primary sources include survey forms, interviews, and videotapes of family interaction.

The subsample in this research consists of 246 men who participated in the second wave and reported that they grew up on farms, as well as their fathers and their adolescent sons. Three of five of these men entered farming at some point, compared to less than one percent of the sons of nonfarm fathers. This result is consistent with Carlson and Dillman's (1983) observation that no occupation matches farming on occupational continuity from father to son.

Whether farming or not, these Iowa men were typically born just after the end of World War II and married for the first time in 1970 (Table 2.1). They average three children. Slightly fewer than half of the men served in the military, usually in Vietnam. Most of the farmers began their career in the late 1960s and early 1970s; the same timing applies to the nonfarm men, approximately a third of whom are now located in professional, managerial, and white collar jobs, while the remaining men are skilled and unskilled laborers. Just over a quarter of the men have a college degree (mean 13 years of education), whereas only three percent of their fathers had a college degree (mean 10.4 years of education).

The fathers of these men typically launched their farm careers in the 1940s and 1950s, when land prices were low and farm commodity prices

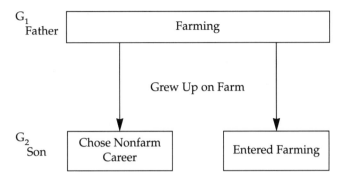

Figure 2.1. Two generations of males in rural America.

were stable and high (Friedberger, 1988; Rhodes, 1989). The farm crisis of the 1980s had little effect on men in the older generation because their land was paid for, their debts were low, and their capital resources were high. The younger generation, however, faced a very different world. A good many of these young men had college degrees in agriculture and training in agribusiness techniques, but they were not immune to the widespread decline in the value of farm land and farm incomes during the 1980s. Several plunged heavily into debt[1] and eventually lost their farms. Indeed, one of three men in the Iowa sample who entered farming had to leave the field by the end of the 1980s.

Figure 2.1 depicts these two generations, fathers and their adult sons (G1 and G2). All of the fathers were in farming; four of five of their sons entered farming, and a third of them did not succeed. The G2 generation divides into two streams at late adolescence, one defined by the pursuit of farming and the other distinguished by the pursuit of nonfarm employment. We asked how the choice of these career paths by the G2 men reflects and affects their relation to fathers who have been and may still be in farming. We asked the G2 men about their fathers during their childhood, and subsequently (1990) asked about social ties and assistance patterns that involve their aged fathers today. The central question here concerns the effects of son's career path on his ties to father within a context of rural economic and demographic decline.

MEASURES

Data used in these analyses, with few exceptions, are based on the adult sons' reports. Approximately a third of the measures involve the recall of such information as events, dates, or description of himself and/or his father and family. These measures are described in Appendix A. The remaining measures are family types or classifications, economic status, fathers' personality and relational style during the adult sons' childhood, qualities of current personalities and relationships between fathers and sons, and adult sons' help and support for aging fathers.

Adult sons of farmers were classified in three ways according to their own farm status. First, men who farmed in 1988 and 1989 were categorized as *farmers* ($n=79$); those who farmed part-time in 1988 and 1989 and those who were displaced farmers in 1989 were categorized as *transitional* farmers ($n=71$); and those who had never farmed were categorized as *nonfarmers* ($n=97$). Second, in examining the choice and consequences of farming as a career, the first two categories were collapsed so that all men who actually had farmed at some time formed one group and those who never had farmed during their adult lives formed the other group. Finally, in assessing intergenerational continuity in behavior and current helping behavior, we compared men who are currently farming with those who never had farmed.

The farm involvement of fathers with sons who now farm full-time and that of sons who have ever farmed were very similar (Table 2.2). By contrast, the farm involvement of fathers with sons who have never farmed was much lower. Not surprisingly, the adult sons who ever had farmed were more likely to have fathers who owned farms than were sons who never had farmed. In addition, the fathers of men who chose farming careers were more likely to be farming currently and to have farmed for more years than fathers of men who chose nonfarm careers.

Adult sons reported the subjective economic well-being of their family of origin with the following question: "As you were growing up, compared to other families in your area, would you say your family's

Table 2.2. Percentage of Farm Involvement of Fathers who ever Farmed by their Adult Son's Current Farm Involvement

	Adult Son's Agricultural Status				
Father's Farm Involvement	Farmers ($n = 78$)	Transitional ($n = 71$)	Nonfarmers ($n = 97$)	Significance Level	
------------------------------	---------	---------	---------	---------	------
Owned farm	84.6	73.2	48.5	$x^2 = 21.3$	.0001
Cash-rented farm	42.3	40.8	32.0	$x^2 = 2.4$	ns
Crop-shared farm	74.4	67.6	55.7	$x^2 = 6.9$	.05
Managed farm for others	12.8	11.3	26.8	$x^2 = 1.0$	ns
Worked as hired hand	9.0	12.7	26.8	$x^2 = 11.1$	.01
Still farming	64.1	59.2	33.0	$x^2 = 19.8$	.0001
Number years farmed ($\bar{X}$)	35.4	31.5	23.6	$F = 17.3$	.0001

standard of living was (1=far below average to 5=far above average). Current *per capita family income* of adult sons was constructed by dividing the 1989 total income (the sum of husband's and wife's wages, net farm income, and income from all other sources, such as dividends and interest, social security, unemployment compensation, sale of property or goods, and so forth) by the number of people residing in the household.

We used two measures to evaluate qualities of the father's personality when the adult son was growing up. *Father's hostility* was assessed with four items from the NEO Personality Inventory (Costa & McCrae, 1985), which concern how often the father was angry at the way people treated him, how violent and physically abusive he was, how often he got into arguments, and how frequently he lost his temper. Adult son's perception of *father's depression* was assessed with three items indicating whether the father was often sad or depressed, felt inferior to others, or was cheerful or high-spirited. Items for both the hostility and depression scales had response categories ranging from 1=strongly disagree to 5=strongly agree. High values indicate greater hostility and depression. Coefficient alphas were .83 for hostility and .64 for depression.

We constructed three measures of the adult son's perceptions of the quality of family relationships during his childhood. *Parents' marital conflict* was assessed using ratings of affection, conflict, and happiness in the parents' marriage (response categories ranged from 1=a lot to 5=hardly any). High scores indicated greater conflict. Coefficient alpha was .77. Adult sons reported their perceptions of *fathers' parental rejection* when they were "about the same age as their seventh grader," using five items concerning the degrees of trust, care, fault-finding, dissatisfaction, and blame they felt. Response categories ranged from 1=strongly agree to 5=strongly disagree, with a high score indicating greater rejection. Coefficient alpha was .71. *Harsh parenting* was measured with four items (Straus, Gelles, & Steinmetz, 1980) concerning father's discipline style when the adult son was about "the same age as his seventh grader." Items assessed the extent to which the father lost his temper, spanked or slapped, hit with an object such as a belt, or told his son to leave the house. Response categories ranged from 1=never to 5=always. Higher scores indicate greater use of harsh disciplinary strategies. Coefficient alpha was .67.

Quality of relations between the adult son and his adolescent son was assessed with a negative parenting measure. We constructed the measure of *adult sons' harsh parenting* with the same items used for fathers' harsh parenting. However, for this index, adult sons reported on their own behavior and the adolescent sons reported on their fathers' behavior. Further, seventh-grade sons responded to a question not included in adult sons' reports on self and father: the extent to which their fathers hit, pushed, grabbed, or shoved them in the past month (1=never to 7=often). The self-report and the seventh grader's report of harsh parenting were transformed to a common scale and then the scores were averaged. Coefficient alpha on the combined measure was .72.

We used two measures of current relations between fathers and adult sons (Bengtson, 1988; Mangen, Bengtson, & Landry, 1988). In each case the adult son reported his perception of the relationship. We measured *demandingness* with a single item: "How often do you feel your father makes too many demands on you?" (1=never to 4=often). The measure of *positive relations* included seven items that represent three dimensions of the current relationship: *support, negativity,* and *satisfaction.* We assessed *support* with three items on how much the adult son could depend on his father, how much concern or understanding his father shows, and how much his father makes him feel appreciated, loved, and cared for. Two items were used to assess *negativity* between father and son: "How much conflict, tension, or disagreement is there between you and your father?" and "How critical of you is your father?" Response categories for the five items that represent support and negativity ranged from 1=not (none) at all to 4=a lot. We evaluated the adult son's *satisfaction* with his relationship with his father by two items, one concerning his happiness with it (from 1=very happy to 4=very unhappy), the other concerning a rating of its quality (1=very poor to 5=excellent). Items for each component were summed and then transformed to a common scale. The three measures were averaged to form a single index (a coefficient alpha of .82).

The remaining measures relate to attitudes toward helping and actual helping behavior. Men responded to six statements concerning *attitudes toward the aging of parents,* including: "I don't know how I will manage if my parent(s) need a lot of help" and "I always have a nagging sense of concern about my parents." Responses were originally on a scale from 1=strongly disagree to 5=strongly agree. We dropped the middle category of neutral/mixed and combined the upper and lower categories into a dichotomy. Four dichotomous questions about actual *helping behavior* were asked: "Do you provide any of the following types of help to your father . . . transportation or shopping, housework or meals, help when he is sick, personal care?" (0=no, 1=yes).

RESULTS: THE PATH CHOSEN

Why did some Iowa men who grew up on a farm enter farming while others pursued nonfarm careers? Prior research on farming careers

Table 2.3. Comparison of Farm and Nonfarm Adult Sons on Family Background

	Farmers (n = 149)	Nonfarm (n = 96)	t
Family Structure			
Number of brothers	1.5	2.0	2.5**
Birth order	2.4	2.5	.6
Standard of living	3.0	2.7	−4.2***
Father-son age difference	31.4	30.5	−1.0
Father—Education & Occupation			
Education	10.6	9.9	−2.3*
Unemployment	1.1	1.3	2.9**
Farm involvement	3.7	3.2	−4.8***
Years farming	33.5	23.6	−5.6***
Father—Early Psychosocial Characteristics			
Marital conflict	1.8	2.3	3.2**
Hostility	2.0	2.1	.5
Depression	2.3	2.4	1.0
Parental rejection	1.9	1.8	−.3
Harsh parenting	2.0	2.1	1.3

* $p \le .05$
** $p \le .01$
*** $p \le .0001$

points to several factors that distinguish young men who enter these diverse pathways (Lyson, 1984; Molnar & Dunkelberger, 1981; Straus, 1956, 1964), such as early family environment and modeling of paternal behavior. We compared means on 13 variables representing aspects of these two factors for adult sons who ever and never went into farming (Table 2.3). Some characteristics of the family of origin and attributes of father's education, occupation, and psychosocial functioning during the adult son's childhood years distinguish the two groups.

Adult sons who went into farming came from families with fewer male children and higher standards of living than did those who chose nonfarm careers. No mean differences were apparent in sons' birth order or in the age difference between fathers and sons in the two groups. These findings suggest that economic advantage is related to attainment of a farming career. Adult sons who farmed came from families with greater financial resources and fewer brothers with whom to compete for those resources. We have no data on inheritance or gifts of farmland or on financial help from parents in getting started in farming, but these observed mean differences suggest that men who successfully attained farming careers received some assistance from their families of origin.

Differences between the two groups also are apparent in father's educational and occupational history. Adult sons who farmed had fathers with higher levels of educational attainment, fewer incidences of unemployment, greater farm involvement, and more years of farming than those who did not farm. Father's educational attainment and unemployment history are probably related to his standard of living and his farm involvement. Men who own and operate farms, instead of leasing or laboring on them, would be expected to have greater financial assets and perhaps better managerial skills. They also would be expected to have a greater personal investment in the farm life style, which would promote longevity in the field.

Family farms typically involve the labor of many family members in maintaining operational efficiency, especially in planting and harvesting times. Boys growing up on owner-operated farms would be more likely to have firsthand experience with farm work than those whose fathers managed or labored on farms others owned. Anticipatory socialization experiences (working on a farm), parental emphasis on son's work role, self value of hard work, and parents' approval of son's farming all have been found related to aspirations to farm (Kaldor, Eldridge, Burchinal, & Arthur, 1962; Straus, 1956, 1964). Taken together, these findings suggest a link between role enactment and the modeling of parental behavior, on one hand, and aspirations and attainment relative to farming careers, on the other.

It seems reasonable to expect that modeling also would depend on the father's psychological well-being and style of relating to family members. We find a mean difference between the two groups of adult sons on only one measure that is relevant to the above. As expected, adult sons who had ever farmed reported lower levels of marital conflict between their parents during the childhood years than did those who never had farmed. However, we find no differences in reports of fathers' depression, hostility, rejection, and harsh parenting when the sons were young.

To determine the magnitude of the relationship between intergenerational factors and adult sons' farm and nonfarm career choices, we employed a discriminant function analysis with eight predictor variables (Table 2.4). Seven of the significant differences between the two groups match the results from the previous analysis. Harsh parenting represents the early relationship between father and son. We calculated one discriminant function ($\chi^2[8]=57.52$, $p<.0001$) and arranged the predictors by order of magnitude of importance in Table 4.

The matrix of correlations between predictor variables and the discriminant function indicates that the primary variables that distinguished between the two career paths were father's involvement and longevity in farming. The ordering of variables suggests that family economic status and modeling are important in attaining a farming career. Only harsh parenting fails to distinguish between the two groups.

Table 2.4. To Farm or Not To Farm—Family Structure and Characteristics of Father as Predictors

Predictor Variables	Correlations of Predictor Variables with Discriminant Function	Univariate F (1,229)	Pooled Within-Group Correlations Among Predictors						
			2	3	4	5	6	7	8
Farm Involvement	.71	33.07	.30	.19	−.28	−.20	−.01	.06	−.09
Years Farmed	.66	28.91		.17	−.21	−.16	.05	−.05	.06
Standard of Living	.51	17.59			−.18	−.22	−.19	.14	−.19
Unemployment	−.40	10.46				.15	.07	.03	.01
Marital Conduct	−.35	8.00					−.01	−.02	.16
No. of Brothers	−.34	7.81						.04	.27
Education	.28	5.24							−.00
Harsh Parenting	−.13	1.05(ns)							
Canonical R	.47								
Eigenvalue	.29								

The model accounts for 22% of the variance in the farm-nonfarm career choice, although it examines only characteristics of the family of origin and does not incorporate personal, social, or educational attributes of the adult son. Considering only the cases from whom the discriminant function was derived, we obtain a 73.5% correct classification rate.

Men who entered farm and nonfarm employment established different life settings for the events of marriage, childbearing, and the parental experience; but their life courses are remarkably similar when measured by the timing of such events. To make such comparisons, we first had to locate the men in their historical time and birth cohort. Some of the adult sons were born during or before World War II and thus faced the disruptions of the Vietnam War in their maturing years. Other sons were born in the postwar era and consequently may have been too young for mobilization into the Vietnam War. We placed all men born before 1949 in the older cohort. These men were more likely than members of the younger cohort to have served in the military (Table 2.5), and they tended to follow a course of more education and later family events—in fact, much later. Military service could account for some of the late family pattern, but we cannot say much about the difference since we do not have representative samples of the two birth cohorts. In any case, the younger men are more likely to be living in town than on the farm, compared to older men, in accord with migration trends.

Within each birth cohort, the choice of farming or a nonfarm career was of little consequence for family or socioeconomic events. Adult sons

Table 2.5. Pattern of Life Events and Achievements by Birth Cohort and Occupational Choice (Farm vs. Nonfarm) in G2 Generation

| Social Factors | Birth Cohort of G2 Men | | | | Birth Cohort | |
| | Older Cohort, < 1949 | | Younger Cohort, 1948 | | | |
	Farm N = 82	Nonfarm N = 42	Farm N = 68	Nonfarm N = 55	Older N = 124	Younger N = 123
Early Events						
Military service % ever	56.0	60.0	25.0	33.0	57.0	28.0
Education X̄ level	13.8	14.3	13.2	13.4	14.0	13.3
Marriage X̄ age at entry	25.0	25.0	21.0	21.0	25.0	21.0
First birth X̄ age at entry	29.0	28.0	23.0	23.0	29.0	23.0
Socioeconomic Status						
Unstable work (%)	12.0	12.0	12.0	13.0	12.0	12.0
Debt-to-asset ratio (X̄)	0.88	0.41	0.52	0.56	0.73	0.54
Per capita income X̄, U.S. $1990	$10,434	$9,025	$9,200	$7,792	$9,955	$8,570
Current Residence (%)						
Farm	67.0	7.0	69.0	2.0	47.0	39.0
Rural area	11.0	11.0	9.0	13.0	13.0	11.0
Town	22.0	76.0	22.0	85.0	40.0	50.0

in the G2 generation who entered farm and nonfarm occupations have much in common on the likelihood of military service, education attainment, and the timing of family events. They also have much in common on socioeconomic indicators, from unstable work to indebtedness and per capita income. The older sons who entered farming do rank much higher on indebtedness, and this difference reflects their misfortune in the farm crisis. Some of these men lost their farms, while others survived but with a large debt. Despite these many similarities, men who entered farming and nonfarm employment are clearly living in different ecological worlds. Most of the men who entered farming are still living on a farm, but only a few nonfarm men reside on a farm. The latter are all displaced farmers, living in a farmhouse but not farming the land.

How do these differences in occupation and residential ecology bear on the resemblance between the parental behavior of the men's fathers, as they remember it, and their own behavior as fathers? Is intergenerational continuity more prominent among the men who entered farming? We turn to this issue now.

FATHERING FROM GENERATION TO GENERATION

In theory, the continuity of careers across the generations should favor continuity in parenting style. Parental behaviors observed in childhood are likely to be reproduced in corresponding situations in adulthood. To test the continuity thesis, we drew on behavioral measures available for the two generations of men. Correlations between harsh parenting and hostility across the generations show that continuity is marked among men who stayed in farming. Fathers who were themselves harsh and hostile are likely to have sons who are in turn harsh and hostile. By comparison, correlations for the nonfarm group are low and generally not reliable (Figure 2.2).

Are the differences in cross-generation correlations (by farm and nonfarm settings) statistically significant? To obtain an answer to this question, we carried out a set of regression analyses (Table 2.6). The farming status of adult sons (0=never farmed, 1=ever farmed) represents our measure of life- course continuity. We assessed behavioral continuity by examining the relationship between the harsh behavior of fathers and that of their adult sons. In these analyses, standard of living of both generations of men was controlled.

The stronger intergenerational continuity among fathers and sons in the farmer lineage is clearly demonstrated. In the first two models, father's harsh parenting behavior and son's lower standard of living are

A. Adult Sons in Farm Careers (N = 67)

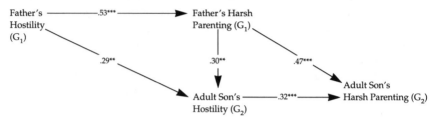

B. Adult Sons in Nonfarm Careers (N = 42)

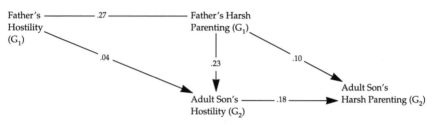

**p < .01
***p < .001

Figure 2.2. Intergenerational patterns of hostility and harsh parenting for adult men (G₂) in farm and nonfarm careers: zero order correlation coefficients.

Table 2.6. Intergenerational Factors in the Harsh Parenting of Iowa Men: Regression Coefficients in Standard Form

| | Harsh Parent Behavior, Adult Son | | |
| | I | II | III |
Factors	beta	beta	beta
Father			
Harsh parenting	.32***	.32***	.08
Standard of living	.07	.05	.08
Adult Son			
Harsh parenting	—	—	—
Per capita income	−.21*	−.22*	−.24**
Farming status	—	.09	−.65*
Interactions			
Father harsh X adult son's farming status	—	—	.80*
Adult son harsh X farming status	—	—	—
R²:	.12***	.12**	.16***

* p ≤ .01
** p ≤ .001
*** p ≤ .0001

associated with the son's harsh parenting behavior. The third model tests the interaction of father's harsh parenting and adult son's farm status, and finds it statistically significant. The interaction value adds significantly to the explained variance ($F[1,109]=4.90$, $p=.05$), an indication that the interaction term is itself significant. Overall, it is clear that life style continuity does play a role in the behavioral continuity of two generations of adult farm men. In addition, the economic well-being of adult sons influences their own parenting behavior; those who are less well-off are more punitive.

A substantial part of these data comes from retrospective reports. Whatever the limits of such data, there is support for the notion that behavioral continuity is enhanced by environmental continuity, a thesis that fits the lineages of farmers. We cannot rule out the possibility that accurate recall is most likely when living conditions remain much the same. However, the observed level of intergenerational continuity on parenting style among fathers and sons in farming cannot be attributed merely to a methodological artifact, because our index of harsh parenting for adult sons combines their self-reports with the reports of their sons.

We conclude that across the generations, persistence in farming sets the stage for greater continuity between the behavior of men and their adult sons than does a nonfarm career. Members of farm families typically share labor. This labor is often divided along gender lines, making it possible for two generations of males living on farms to have more contact with one another than do males living off farms. Under these circumstances, sons are more likely to model the behavior of their fathers. Moreover, prior research suggests that family financial pressures lead to relational stresses, including marital conflict and punitive, rejecting parenting (McLoyd & Flanagan, 1990). Data presented here are consistent with this earlier work.

CURRENT RELATIONS WITH FATHER

In the second year of the panel study (1990), men in the middle generation were approximately 40 years old and most of their surviving fathers had entered the seventh decade of life. Half of the fathers still kept a hand in farming at this age, and possibly in their sons' farm affairs as well. If men who currently farm report more interaction with fathers than do nonfarm sons, this differential contact may be associated with a perception of support from father and a greater sense of his demandingness.

We compared the farm and nonfarm sons on three scales (frequency of interaction, demandingness, and positive quality of current relations) using multiple classification analysis. As described earlier, the positive quality of current relations refers to subscales of support, satisfaction, and negativity (reversed score). We average the scores on each to form a general measure of positive relations. Scores on the three general scales were standardized to compare their deviations from the sample mean. Covariates for the analysis included the harsh parenting and hostile behavior of the fathers of the men, proximity of father and adult son, age differences between the two generations of men, and the adult sons' per capita income.

As expected, men who followed their fathers into farming tended to live closer to them than do nonfarm sons in relation to their own fathers ($\chi^2[1, 175]=13.71$, p=.0001). Virtually all of the sons in farming lived within 25 miles of their fathers, whereas only one of four nonfarm sons lived as close to their fathers. Even when we statistically control for the effects of proximity, as well as for age differences, father's hostility during childhood, and income level, sons in farming score (Figure 2.3) much higher on frequent interaction with father than do nonfarm sons (F[1, 101]=12.17, p=.001). This contact also entails some cost in that sons in farming perceived their fathers to be demanding, especially when compared to the reports of nonfarm men (F[1,101]=7.30, p=.01). Frequent contacts with a demanding father added up to limited freedom of action and scope of control.

Different views on farming may lie at the heart of the demandingness perceived by sons in farming. In example of such intrusiveness, a writer describes his elderly father's evaluation of another son's farming practice. The father had farmed all his life.

> I had gone with my father once to inspect one of Don's cornfields. "See how thick he's planted, way too thick. Defeats his purpose. Guarantee you he'll get a lot of stalk and few cobs. And the air won't get through to dry the cobs that he does get. He'll pay thirty-five cents a bushel at the elevator to gas-dry them and still not have top grade. Field-dried is top; it cracks into chunks. Gas-dried turns powdery. And, planting this thick, you have to pay for extra fertilizer, and you wear out your soil faster." Legitimate points every one of them, although it was true that Don's bushels-per-acre yields were higher than my father's. Through all my father's differences with my generation of farmers—and with my generation, period—ran a single, simple objection: "You guys are in too much of a hurry to get ahead." (Kohn, 1988, p. 69)

Daily living with the intrusive judgments of fathers who "know best" entails some cost in emotional bonds, and we observe a modest, though insignificant, tendency of nonfarm sons to report more positive ties to their fathers than do the sons of farmers (F[1,101]=3.0, p=.09). What about the three component scales of positive ties (support, negativity,

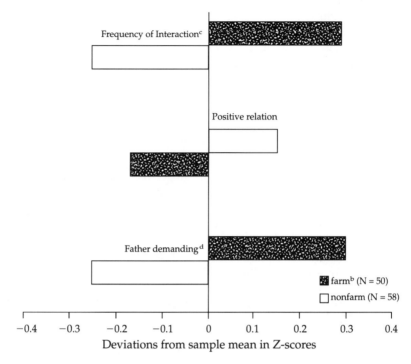

Figure 2.3. Current perception of relations with father by adult sons who had grown up on farms, by their farm or nonfarm status.

[a] Covariates are father's harsh parenting, father's hostility, current proximity of father and son, and son's per capita income, and the difference in fathers' and son's ages.
[b] The farm group for this analysis includes only those men who currently farm.
[c] $p < .001$
[d] $p < .01$

and satisfaction)? Do they show a different picture? Nonfarm sons do report greater "satisfaction" with ties to father than sons in farming (t[1,101]=1.91, p=.06). However, the other scales show no reliable differences.

Recollections of childhood experience with father continue to play a role in shaping the contemporary quality of relations with him. Men who depict their father as hostile and irritable during the son's early years were less likely than other men to report positive relations with him in old age (F[1,101]=3.81, p=.05). Whitbeck, Simons, and Conger (1991) present more details on this relationship history in the Iowa generations. As noted earlier, we included this early experience factor in the analysis. The observed effect is also independent of proximity to father, age difference, and income level.

Considering all aspects of relations with father, the career lines followed by farm-reared sons play an important role in shaping their ties with the father. Sons who followed their fathers into farming live closer to them, have more frequent interaction with them, and experience more demandingness in this relationship than nonfarm sons report. The former also have less rewarding or satisfying contact with their fathers, a finding that undoubtedly reflects the intrusive quality of fathers' interactions when both generations are or have been in farming.

A middle-aged man would be expected to show more interaction and stronger affection toward his father than toward his father-in-law, but are there differences in this dissimilarity between men who chose to follow their father into farming and those who sought their fortunes in other domains? In the realm of social contact, the Iowa men reported much greater interaction with father than with father-in-law, as we expected ($p < .002$), but the difference is twice as great among men who are now farming. The high level of interaction between father and son in farming undoubtedly accounts in part for the higher perceived demandingness and negativity of these fathers, when compared to the nonfarm group. Only in the farm category does the perceived demandingness and negativity of father and father-in-law differ significantly ($p > .0002$). Despite this characterization of fathers in farming, adult sons in farming are just as likely as the nonfarm sons to view father as supportive. And both place their fathers well above their fathers-in-law on supportiveness ($p < .05$). We find no reliable difference on feelings of satisfaction with the relationship.

What about a man's relation to his mother and mother-in law? For the most part, the Iowa men have similar things to say about their ties to mother and father, but especially on sentiment; thus the contrast by farm and nonfarm on relations to mother and mother-in-law is remarkably similar to the above for fathers and fathers-in-law. The major difference reflects the authority roles of men and women in farm families. The demandingness and negativity men attribute to their fathers expresses to some degree the authority of the elder male over his middle-aged son. Mothers on farms do not exercise such authority or sanctioning power and are not perceived in this manner. However, adult sons see mothers as more demanding than mothers-in-law ($p < .05$), regardless of setting.

Whatever men's relationship to parents and in-laws among farm and nonfarm sons, they are most similar among men who chose to stay on the farm. That is, a man's relation to his father corresponds with his relation to his father-in-law. Correlations were computed on demandingness, negativity, satisfaction, and support in relation to father and father-in-law. In all cases, the correlation among farm men is stronger, an average of .14 greater on fathers and fathers-in-law. The very same pattern appears among relationships to mother and mother-in-law.

SONS' CAREER SUCCESS AS A FACTOR

In theory, the son's career success has implications for the quality of father-son relations, which seems most plausible for generations engaged in farming, the same business or occupation. We find no evidence that the earnings level of men has direct consequences for their current relations with fathers, but income could specify circumstances under which career matters most for this relationship. For example, the perceived demandingness of fathers may shift toward nonfarm sons when the latter are relatively unsuccessful.

To explore the role of economic success, we divided the sons into two groups at the median on per capita income, and then compared the farm and nonfarm groups of G2 men on negativity, satisfaction, support, demandingness, and interaction frequency. Each measure was dichotomized (Table 2.7). Economic success did not influence the frequency of interaction. Rather, sons in farming, regardless of economic well-being, are significantly more likely to interact with their fathers once a week or more often than are nonfarm adult sons. Demandingness shows a similar nonsignificant pattern, with farmer's sons tending to perceive fathers as more demanding than do nonfarm sons, regardless of economic status.

Some differences between the income groups appear on negative,

Table 2.7. The Role of Economic Success in Determining the Quality of Father-Son Relations: Farm vs. Nonfarm in Percentages

| | *Per Capita Income of G2 Men, 1990* | | | |
| | *Below Median* | | *Above Median* | |
Perceived Relations to Father	*Farm* *(N = 26)*	*Nonfarm* *(N = 26)*	*Farm* *(N = 24)*	*Nonfarm* *(N = 24)*
Frequency of interaction (once/week or more)	87.5	59.4	88.5	65.4
Father demanding (sometimes/often)	29.2	15.6	26.9	11.5
Father negative (above median)	45.8	31.3	57.7	50.0
Father positive (above median)	58.3	78.1	61.5	57.7
Father supportive (above median)	70.8	71.9	65.4	73.1

Note: No percentage differences are statistically significant. The sample in this analysis includes all 62 men with living fathers who are either in farm or nonfarm employment. The farm group does not include men who once farmed, but are not currently so employed.

supportive, and satisfying relations. For farm and nonfarm men with higher incomes, the perception that relations with fathers are satisfying and supportive is especially common. In addition, more men in these two groups report higher levels of negativity (criticism, harsh judgments) in their relationships with father than do either of the lower-income groups of men. Perhaps fathers of men who are relatively well-off feel freer in expressing criticism and disagreement with their sons than do fathers with adult sons who are struggling financially.

Among men with low income, we see an accentuation of the pattern found in the previous analysis: nonfarm adult sons report less negative and more satisfying relations with their fathers than do adult sons who farm. These differences are not significant, but they suggest that economic well-being interacts with career choice in shaping the relations of men and their adult sons. Interestingly, men who do not follow in their fathers' footsteps appear to benefit most from this interaction.

Clearly, occupational choice matters for ties to father. A son's persistence in farming is related to close proximity, frequent interaction, a perception of father as demanding, and a slight tendency to experience more paternal negativity, such as criticism. Are such relations linked in any way to helping father when such aid is needed?

FATHER CARE IN ATTITUDES AND ASSISTANCE

For many reasons, sons in farming give assistance to fathers than do nonfarm sons—especially in greater proximity and frequency of interaction (Finch, 1989). Such care may have little to do with the quality of emotional ties, for, as Raymond Firth and his colleagues (1970) have put it, kin assistance is often "against the grain behavior." Kin help out because it is expected. To explore such help, we must take the life stage of the G2 generation into account, since care depends on the elderly's functional status.

To answer these questions, we first divided the G2 men into older and younger age groups (born in 1948 or earlier, born later), and then compared the two career groups on agreement with six attitudes about the aging of their parents. The older men in both groups were more likely to be concerned about their parents, than were the younger (Table 2.8). Within the older group, nonfarm sons stand out in their felt inadequacy for the task of caregiving. These men were most likely to wonder whether they could manage "when parents need a lot of help." By comparison, older sons in farming appear to be more in control of such matters and

Table 2.8. Men's Attitudes toward their Parents' Aging by Farm Status and Birth Cohort

Attitudes Toward Aging of Parents	Born 1948 or Earlier		Born 1949 or Later	
	Farm (n = 50)	Nonfarm (n = 33)	Farm (n = 48)	Nonfarm (n = 50)
Don't know how I'll manage if parents need a lot of help	24.0	**35.5**	14.6	18.9
Afraid keeping my parents will take all of my resources	7.0	**24.0**	10.3	9.5
I worry that I'll have to care for my parents	14.0	**25.9**	16.7	20.0
Don't know what I'll do if my parents ask for help	18.0	**23.3**	15.0	17.0
I feel uneasy about being away from parents too long	**50.0**	28.1	36.9	44.0
I have a nagging sense of concern about my parents	58.7	**63.6**	47.7	48.0

Note: The largest percentages in each category are in bold to highlight their clustering on the older nonfarm men. The sample for this analysis includes all 62 men with at least one living parent who are either in farm or nonfarm jobs.

prospects, perhaps because they have had the experience over the years through shared living and work. These men were less concerned with possible inadequacy than with how their parents will manage when the sons are not available.

These observed differences could reflect the economic well-being of the G2 generation as well as parents' age and functional status. For example, the fear that "keeping my parents will take all my resources" clearly speaks to the resource level of the G2 men, and we find that agreement with this statement is significantly related to current income among the men. In a multiple classification analysis based on the four groups and income level, men with low income were most likely to claim they worried about resource depletion through care for parents ($p < .01$). However, this is the only significant effect. The ages of the G1 generation made no difference in the observed results.

Attitudes and sentiments tell us much about relations between father and son, but they do not tell us about actual behavior in helping parents. In closing our analysis, we focused on four types of helping behavior that involved the largest number of G2 fathers: assistance with housework, help with personal care, providing transportation, and help during illness. The last two activities are especially relevant to differences between farm and nonfarm sons. In rural America, transportation of the elderly to stores, medical care, and government agencies must involve kin to a very great extent. Likewise, home care for the ill seldom can involve a nurse; family members have to step in to fill the need. With these considerations in mind, we expected sons in farming to exceed the sample mean on providing transportation and help during illness, with the contrasts most dramatic among older men.

To assess caregiving in these domains, we calculated deviations from the sample mean on transportation and help during illness expressed in z-scores across four age and farm-nonfarm groups—older and younger farmers and nonfarmers. The per capita income of the G2 generation was included in the analysis as a covariate. As expected, caregiving in both domains is linked to age and farm status. Older men are very much involved in providing transportation and help during illnesses, regardless of their occupation, but sons in farming clearly stand out in helping their fathers when compared to other men. Proximity and frequency of interaction are important factors in this assistance, but we find no reliable evidence that aid to father is linked to how his son regards him. Whatever their feelings, adult sons are important sources of assistance for elderly fathers in farm country, and this may be even more true of adult daughters.

This account of caregiving is not informed by the actions of other siblings, and we do not have information on whether sisters or brothers play an important role in providing such assistance. Traditionally, women carry the heaviest burden of kin care, and we might expect this to be the case among the sisters of the men in the study. Indeed, adult men with one or more sisters may be less involved in caring for an aged father than men who have no sister to rely upon. In this sample, over four of five men have at least one living sister. A family of all brothers is too rare to provide a reliable contrast with the mixed household of brothers and sisters. Nevertheless, we carried out the same analysis shown in Figure 2.4 on only the men with sisters, and compared the findings with those obtained in the total sample. Among older men, the differences between the results on farm versus nonfarm sons are almost nonexistent. The presence of an adult sister does not seem to diminish the caregiving of middle-aged farmers in relation to their aged fathers.

Apart from the full picture of sibling contributions in caregiving, another issue affects the accuracy of self-report data and more generally the source of the report itself. Men may not provide the most accurate report of their own contributions to caregiving. Their wives' accounts would be useful in making sense of the men's role. And what would the fathers of the G2 men say about their sons' assistance? Would there be agreement? Disparities in accounts may tell us something about the quality of the father-son relationship. Unfortunately, we have no evidence by which to sort out these complexities.

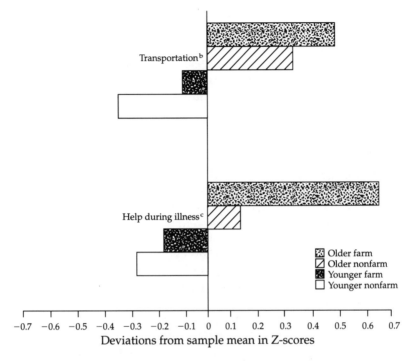

Figure 2.4. Provision of care and support for aging father by adult sons: farm vs. nonfarm.[a]

[a] Covariate is per capita income in multiple classification analysis.
[b] $p < .05$
[d] $p < .01$

SOME HISTORICAL IMPLICATIONS: A CONCLUDING NOTE

This account of family relations among rural generations of older men acquires particular significance within the rapidly aging population of the midwestern farm belt and the relation between urban-industrial change and kinship. Largely because of the farm crisis of the 1980s, Iowa lost more of its population (approximately 300,000) to out-migration during the decade than any other state except one. The north central counties which this study examined suffered losses of up to 15% of their 1980 population. Some of the loss involves the displacement of farmers from the land, in addition to the out-migration of youth to more prosperous regions. If trends continue, half of all Iowans will be older than 35 by the year 2000. This figure is projected to increase to 40 years by 2010, a change certain to be far more dramatic in rural sectors of the state.

The Iowa fathers in this study launched their careers in farming over a 30-year period, the 1920s to the 1950s, from an initial period of great hardship through the prosperous postwar years. Over this period the farm economy grew appreciably and price supports for farm commodities became the norm. Most of the men had sons who chose to go into farming, though only two-thirds remained in the field, owing perhaps to the economic crisis of the 1980s. The lessons of this era left their imprint on the third generation, the grandsons. Only 16 of the study boys in this generation expressed an interest in farming as a career.

Men in the G2 generation who left farming for nonfarm opportunities established different relationships with their fathers than did men who entered farming as a career. Consistent with the continuity of their life, sons in farming more closely replicate the parenting style of their own fathers than do nonfarm sons. They live closer to them, interact more frequently with them, feel the father is more demanding, and report providing more care in areas of transportation and health. They feel slightly less supported emotionally by father than nonfarm sons do in relation to their fathers, and report more incidents of criticism. Nevertheless, fathers and sons in farming are mutually significant figures.

This study of men in the G2 generation, and of their relation to fathers in farming and to their young adolescent sons, provides some intimations of a historic family dynamic in which intergenerational continuities and change in occupational life gave shape to different family forms. Industrialization is one of the master transformations of this kind, and the decline of agricultural employment represents a specific aspect of the change. This study has relevance to depopulation and out-migration, a process that has been underway in the American farm belt since World War I. The abrupt decline of land values in the region during the early 1980s accelerated the population decline.

The story of rural out-migration to urban employment opportunities has been told in numerous studies of American communities in the twentieth century, including Schwarzweller and associates' (1971) study of Beech Creek migrants to Ohio during World War II and Hareven's (1982) study of the Amoskeag Mill families (c. 1900–1935) in Manchester, New Hampshire. Both analyses depict migration within a kinship-based system for matching people to job opportunities. Hareven's research reflects this process from the vantage point of the family's priority in maximizing its well-being. Thus members of a family migrated to employment opportunities in different industries to minimize the economic risk for family support. Hard times did not occur evenly across all industries in early twentieth century New England.

This holistic perspective on the family, life course, and aging highlights future research steps and identifies some important limitations of our inquiry. By focusing mainly on fathers and sons, we do not capture the role of other family members (e.g., siblings) within the context of family life. The meaning of a son's relation to his father acquires important details from knowledge of the father's relation to other siblings. What careers did other members of each sibling set pursue and how did they affect interaction, caregiving, and sentiments involving father and mother? Some farmers in the G1 generation may have had as many as two sons follow in their occupational footsteps, while other farmers lost all of their offspring to nonfarm employment—sons as well as daughters. Such differing family patterns undoubtedly had some effect on the caregiving role of sons who moved out of farming.

Gender is another consideration. Whatever the career choice, in or out of farming, the central role of women in kinship suggests that daughters may compensate for their brothers' emotional distance or unresponsiveness to parent needs. Since farming was not a career option for Iowa women in the postwar era, their opportunities centered on marriage to a man in farming or in nonfarm pursuits. Neither type of marriage would match a brother's proximity to farm parents if he runs the farm.

Whether a son or daughter of farm parents, the divergent careers (farm versus nonfarm) they pursued in marriage and work have consequences for their own relationship as siblings, as well as for their ties to parents. Differences in subjective orientation, in disdain, value conflicts, or attitudinal clashes can arise between siblings who pursue different occupational careers (Adams, 1967), but they appear to have little bearing upon frequency of interaction. Obligation and proximity have much to do with frequency of contacts. This finding based on an urban population may apply to siblings in farming and their relation to brothers and sisters who have made their way out of agriculture. The consequences of occupational differences for sibling bonds warrant more attention than they have received in studies of kinship, family support, and aging.

In closing, we note that the empirical study of work and family has come a long way since Lee Rainwater (1974, p. xiv) noted in the early 1970s that studies of each topic have tended to "proceed along their separate narrow ways, barely acknowledging the existence of each other." This observation and others like it encouraged studies of the interplay of work and family. Indeed, the field has literally exploded since then with empirical facts and a deeper theoretical understanding that draws on history and comparative studies. However, the advance has not made sufficient headway in the study of multiple generations across the life course, despite the relevance of changes in work and family for intergenerational patterns. This study represents an initial effort in this direction on rural generations and aging.

ACKNOWLEDGMENTS

Originally prepared for the Conference on Family and Intergenerational Relations, University of Delaware, Newark, October 9–10, 1991, this chapter is based on collaborative research involving the Iowa Youth and Families Project at Iowa State University-Ames and the Social Change Project at The University of North Carolina at Chapel Hill. The combined research effort is currently supported by the National Institute of Mental Health (MH43270), the National Institute on Drug Abuse (DA05347), the John D. and Catherine T. MacArthur Foundation Program for Successful Adolescent Development Among Youth in High-Risk Settings, the Bureau of Maternal and Child Health (MCJ-109572), and a Research Scientist Award (MH00567).

NOTE

1.   The mean debt-to-asset ratio (total of all farm, business, personal property, and consumer debt divided by the sum of all farm, business, and personal property assets) of adult sons who currently farm is .44, of transitional (part-time and displaced) farmers is 1.03, and of nonfarmers is .49.

REFERENCES

Adams, B. N. (1967). Occupational position, mobility, and the kin of orientation. *American Sociological Review, 32,* 364–377.
Bengtson, V. L. (1988). *The Longitudinal Study of Three Generation Families.* Los Angeles: Andrus Gerontology Center, University of Southern California.
Carlson, J. E., & Dillman, D. A. (1983). Influence of kinship arrangements on farmer innovativeness. *Rural Sociology, 48,* 183–200.
Costa, P. T., & McCrae, R. R. (1985). *The NEO Personality Inventory Manual.* Odessa, FL: Psychological Assessment Resources.
Cottrell, L. S., Jr. (1969). Interpersonal interaction and the development of the self. In Goslin, D. A. (Ed.), *Handbook of Socialization Theory and Research* (pp. 543–570). Chicago: Rand McNally.
Finch, J. (1989). *Family Obligation and Social Change.* London: Polity Press.
Fink, D. (1986). *Open Country, Iowa: Rural Women, Tradition and Change.* Albany: State University of New York Press.
Firth, R. W., Hubert, J., Forge, A., & Team of the "London Kinship Project." (1970). *Families and Their Relatives: Kinship in a Middle-Class Sector of London: An Anthropological Study.* New York: Humanities Press.

Friedberger, M. (1988). *Farm Families and Change in Twentieth-Century America.* Lexington: University Press of Kentucky.

Hareven, T. K. (1982). *Family Time and Industrial Time: The Relationship Between the Family and Work in a New England Industrial Community.* New York: Cambridge University Press.

Kaldor, D. R., Eldridge, E., Burchinal, L. G., & Arthur, I. W. (1962). *Occupational plans of Iowa farm boys.* Ames: Iowa Agricultural Experiment Station, Bulletin 508.

Kohn, H. (1988). *The Last Farmer: An American Memoir.* New York: Summit Books.

Lyson, T. A. (1984). Pathways into production agriculture: The structuring of farm recruitment in the United States. In H. K. Schwarzweller (Ed.), *Research in Rural Sociology and Development.* Vol. 1, Focus on Agriculture (pp. 79–104). Greenwich, CT: JAI Press.

Mangen, D. J., Bengtson, V. L., & Landry, P. H., Jr. (1988). *Measurement of Intergenerational Relations.* Newbury Park, CA: Sage.

McLoyd, V. C., & Flanagan, C. A. (Eds.). (1990). *Economic Stress: Effects on Family Life and Child Development.* San Francisco: Jossey-Bass.

Miner, H. M. (1939). *St. Denis: A French-Canadian Parish.* Chicago: University of Chicago Press.

Molnar, J. J., & Dunkelberger, J. E. (1981). The expectation to farm: An interaction of background and experience. *Rural Sociology, 46,* 62–84.

Parke, R. D. (1981). *Fathers.* Cambridge, MA: Harvard University Press.

Rainwater, L. (1974). Foreword. In M. D. Young & P. Wilmott (Eds.), *The Symmetrical Family* (pp. ix-xix). New York: Pantheon.

Rhodes, R. (1989). *Farm: A Year in the Life of an American Farmer.* New York: Simon & Schuster.

Rossi, A. S., & Rossi, P. H. (1990). *Of Human Bonding: Parent-Child Relations Across the Life Course.* New York: Aldine de Gruyter.

Schwarzweller, H. K., Brown, J. S., & Mangalam, J. J. (1971). *Mountain Families in Transition: A Case Study of Appalachian Migration.* University Park: Pennsylvania State University Press.

Straus, M. A. (1956). Personal characteristics and functional needs in the choice of farming as an occupation. *Rural Sociology, 21,* 257–266.

———. (1964). Societal needs and personal characteristics in the choice of farm, blue collar, and white collar occupations of farmers' sons. *Rural Sociology, 29,* 408–425.

Straus, M. A., Gelles, R. J., & Steinmetz, S. K. (1980). *Behind Closed Doors: Violence in the American Family.* Garden City, NY: Anchor Press/Doubleday.

Sweetser, D. A. (1966). The effect of industrialization on intergenerational solidarity. *Rural Sociology, 31,* 156–170.

Whitbeck, L. B., Simons, R. L., & Conger, R. D. (1991). The effects of early family relationships on contemporary relationships and assistance patterns between adult children and their parents. *Journal of Gerontology, 46,* 330–337.

Appendix A. Objective measures

Measure	Response set or Range	$\bar{x}$	sd	Item
Father:				
Birth year	1887–1936	1916.7	8.7	Year your father was born.
Education	3–16	10.4	2.4	What was the highest grade of regular school your father completed?
Family size	3–15	6.2	2.0	Total no. of siblings, parents in household when adult son was growing up.
Unemployment	1 = never 4 = often	1.2	.5	Think of the times when you were growing up that your father was out of work or unemployed even though he wanted a job. Would you say that he was (unemployed)?
Years farming	1–67	28.9	13.4	While you were growing up, in what years was your father involved in farming? (Ending year minus beginning year).
Currently farming	1 = yes 2 = no			Is your father currently involved in farming?
Type of farmer	1 = yes 2 = no			While you were growing up did your father ever (5 = separate items) . . . own a cash rent a farm? crop share? manage a farm for someone? work as a hired hand?
Farm involvement	1 = owner 2 = tenant only 3 = tenant and laborer 4 = laborer only	3.5	.8	Constructed from type of farm items
Mother's employment	1 = yes 2 = no			When you were growing up did your mother ever work for pay on a continual basis (6 months or longer) either part- or full-time?

Adult Son:

	Range/Coding	Mean	SD	Question
Birth year	1931–1957	1947.8	4.6	What year were you born?
Education	8–20	13.7	2.1	What is the highest grade of education you completed or are enrolled in currently?
Family size	4–9	4.9	.9	Sum of number of household members.
No. of brothers	0–7	1.7	1.4	How many brothers did you have when you were growing up (including step or adopted brothers)?
Birth order	1–11	2.4	1.4	What is your birth order? That is, were you the first child, the second child, or what?
Wife's self-reported employment	1 = yes 0 = no			What is your current employment occupational status? Coded, yes employed if reported: employed by other, self-employed, temporarily laid off, on maternity leave, disabled but work seasonally.
Residence	1 = on a farm 2 = in rural area 3 = town or city			Does your family live . . . ?
Father proximity	1 = live together 7 = over 250 miles	3.0	1.3	How far do you live from your father?
No. of relatives within 100 miles	0–98	35.9	31.2	How many of your or your spouse's relatives live less than 100 miles from your home?
Difference in father and adult son's ages	15–50	31.0	6.7	Son's birth year minus father's birth year.

3

The Well-Being of Aging Americans
with Very Old Parents

Dennis P. Hogan, David J. Eggebeen, and Sean M. Snaith

INTRODUCTION

Several age-graded events during mid-life are life course—defining events that transform the nature of intergenerational relations. The elements that make up this transition, the differentials in their occurrence and timing, and the consequences of the transition have been neglected by life course researchers. In this chapter, we concentrate on parental death, one of the key events in the transition in intergenerational relations. First we summarize what is known about the timing of parental death and other events that constitute the transition in intergenerational relations. Using nationally representative sample survey data, we then describe sociodemographic differentials in the likelihood that parental death occurs relatively late in the life course, and investigate the social, psychological and economic correlates of being at various stages in this transition.

THE TRANSITION IN INTERGENERATIONAL RELATIONS

Sociological studies of the life course largely have concentrated on those early life transitions that mark the passage to adulthood (school completion, labor force entry, marriage, parenthood) and on those late life transitions that mark the passage to old age (retirement, widowhood). These are the transitions to which our society is most attuned; probably not coincidentally, they are the transitions whose occurrence is most predictable because of sharp age-grading (Brim & Ryff, 1980). Although these receive less attention, it is possible to distinguish a set of transitions (the last child leaves home, grandparenthood, and the death of the last surviving parent) that occur about two-thirds of the way through the life span (Winsborough, Bumpass & Aquilino, 1991). More than any others, these transitions transform the nature of intergenerational relations.

Winsborough, Bumpass, and Aquilino (1991) have described the timing of the events that mark the transition in intergenerational relations in the contemporary United States. By their early forties, one-half of all Americans have lost one parent, but fewer than one-fifth have had their last child leave home or are grandparents. One-half become grandparents by age 50. By their mid-fifties, half have lost both parents, no longer have children living at home, and nearly three-quarters are grandparents. For these people, the transition in intergenerational relations is complete.

The events that mark the transition in intergenerational relations are gradually age-graded, and the overall transition is composed of several distinct, unrelated events. Thus, the overall transition for a cohort is not at all compact, but occupies roughly the entire middle third of the life span. The work by Winsborough and his associates (1991) represents a first pass at describing the family sociology of this portion of the life span. The next step in their research will be to investigate socio-demographic differentials in the transition in intergenerational relations, as well as the intercohort trends in this transition.

DESCRIPTION OF OLDER PERSONS AND THEIR PARENTS

Here we address a more specific question: What kinds of persons have parents survive beyond the usual age at parental death, prolonging the transition in intergenerational relations? To answer this question, we analyzed data from the 1987/88 National Survey of Families and House-holds (described below), limiting our attention to Americans 55 and older. Of all these older persons, 17.6% have one (15.8%) or both (1.8%) of their parents still living.[1]

Table 3.1 provides some information about the characteristics of persons 55 and older with and without a living parent. Those with a living parent are predominantly relatively young: half are 55–59 and almost one-third are 60–64. Somewhat more than half are female, but this difference corresponds to the proportion of females in the elderly population. Older persons with a living parent are more likely to be currently married (77 vs. 62%) and less likely to be widowed (10 vs. 26%). Only 9%

Table 3.1. Characteristics of American Adults 55 and Older with and without Living Parents (%)

	No Living Parent	Living Parent
Age		
55–59	16.3	49.4
60–64	20.0	30.1
65–69	20.8	15.7
70–74	17.8	03.7
75–79	13.9	01.2
80+	11.2	00.0
Gender		
Male	44.4	45.2
Female	55.6	54.8
Parental status		
No children	14.6	09.3
Children <18 only	02.4	01.1
Children >18 and 19+	07.4	06.0
Children 19+ only	75.6	83.6
Level of Education		
Less than high school	41.2	27.9
High school diploma	36.5	39.9
Some college	10.4	12.2
College degree or more	11.9	20.1
Marital Status		
Married	62.3	76.9
Separated/divorced	07.4	10.4
Widowed	26.1	10.3
Never married	04.1	02.4
N	2,696	513

of those with a surviving parent have no children, and only 7% have a dependent-age child; 84% have only adult children. Older persons without a living parent are somewhat more likely (15 vs. 9%) to report they are childless. About one-fifth of those with surviving parents have a college degree, compared to 12% of those without a living parent.

But many of these apparent correlates of parental survival may result from the concentration in the early years of old age of those people with surviving parents.[2] To determine the extent to which this was the case, we estimated a logistic regression model that predicted whether a parent was alive using the independent variables shown in Table 3.1. This model indicates that when age is taken into account, there are no significant gender, parental status, or marital status differences between these two groups. Education differences in parent survival do persist, controlling for these other variables, with respondents who have a college degree significantly more likely than respondents who are high school dropouts to have a living parent.

For most (86%) of these older persons with one or more surviving parents, it is the mother who survives. One-half of these surviving parents are 85 or older. Fifty-two percent have only an elementary school education. Just over one-quarter (27%) of the parents are in poor or very poor health, and another 37% are reported as being in only fair health. The surviving parents of older persons tend to live nearby (7.4% are coresident, and another 25.3% live within five miles; but one-third live more than 100 miles away). Contact between the older persons and their surviving parent are frequent, with 64.3% reporting contact at least weekly.[3]

GIVING AND RECEIVING BETWEEN ADULTS AND THEIR PARENTS

Over much of the life span, parents provide more support to their children than is reciprocated. But as their parents age, are widowed, and become infirm, many of these adult children do reciprocate the lifelong support of their parents. This support most often consists of emotional support and advice or assistance around the house; financial assistance is rare (Eggebeen & Hogan, 1990; Hogan, Eggebeen, & Clogg, 1993).

Such support of elderly parents is observed particularly among persons reaching old age who have very old surviving parents. For example, one-fifth of persons in their fifties provided care to an ill parent during the past year, and more than one-third have given their parents emotional or moral support or help around the house (Winsborough, Bumpass, & Aquilino, 1991). More burdensome kinds of support are less commonly observed at any time, because typically it is short-lived. For example, Bumpass (1990) reports that one-quarter of persons have had at least one episode of an aging parent live with them by the time they have reached their late fifties. However, we find that only seven percent of respondents age 55 or older currently have a surviving parent co-residing with them.

One of the reasons the prevalence of providing coresidence to an aging parent is much higher than its incidence is because a sick parent typically is coresident less than a year. The parent's health usually deteriorates and he or she either enters a nursing home or dies.

The transition in intergenerational relations marks the completion of this responsibility for one's parents. With this transition, intergenerational attention focuses down the lineage. Throughout the remainder of their lives, these parents will provide considerable support to their adult children, especially to those children who have borne them grandchildren. While this support is sometimes reciprocated, the balance of assistance will favor the younger generation at least until these persons suffer the infirmities of very old age, as their parents did years earlier (Eggebeen, 1992; Eggebeen & Hogan, 1990; Hogan et al., 1993).

PARENTAL SURVIVAL AND ITS CONSEQUENCES

The transition in intergenerational relations therefore brings to a close a period of the life course in which many individuals have had considerable demands placed on their time and financial resources. Typically, the transition will have begun with the residential independence of one's children and by grandparenthood. Children often need advice and tangible assistance (financial support, child care, help around the house) as they are launched as independent adults. This may be an erratic process, with adult children returning home during a career interruption or marital crisis. The death of one's father and widowhood of one's mother often occurs during this time. Widowed mothers typically get little support from their adult children, even as they reach advanced old age. Support is often, though not always, provided when it is needed—most commonly when their health fails (Hogan et al., 1993; Hogan & Eggebeen, 1991).

If the time of need of an elderly parent coincides with the greatest needs of adult children, a particular squeeze on parental time, financial, and emotional resources of the middle generation person may result. This phenomenon has produced popular interest in the "sandwich" generation (Brody, 1981). While this crisis period of the life course is likely to be short-lived for most persons, it is especially common among persons 55 and older with a surviving parent; most of these, as we have seen, have children and a very old widowed parent with few socioeconomic resources and who is in poor or fair health. This potentially difficult period will continue until the elderly parent dies and the transition in intergenerational relations is complete.

An important issue in understanding the transition in intergenerational relations, then, is to understand the way in which this transition and its component events affect the social, economic, and psychological well-being of middle-aged Americans. Family sociologists and psychologists have intensively investigated the consequences of the last child leaving home (the "empty nest") and the nature of grandparenthood (Cherlin & Furstenberg, 1986). But the defining element in the transition in intergenerational relations—the circumstances surrounding the decline and death of the last parent—have not been studied extensively. Our study begins to address this issue.

DESIGN, DATA, AND METHOD: DESIGN

Ideally, the design of such a study requires longitudinal data on a representative cohort of individuals as they pass through mid-life, tracking information on their parents survival, health status, and need for assistance. The study would track changes in individual well-being as the person moves from having two healthy parents, to the death of the first parent, and finally, to the decline in health, and ultimately the death of the second parent. The study would need to control for factors known to be associated with individual well-being that also influenced parental survival and health (age and education), as well as other events (relating to children) in the transition in intergenerational relations. To our knowledge, the data to conduct such a study is not available now, and given the inattention to this period of the life course, is not likely to be available for analysis in the foreseeable future.

As a first step in investigating the personal consequences of the parental mortality component of the transition in intergenerational relations, we analyze cross sectional data that compares individuals at different points in the transition. Specifically, we compare persons whose parents are both deceased, persons with one or more surviving parents in good health, and persons with one or more surviving parents, at least one of whom is ill. By restricting attention to persons 55 and older, we focus on the consequences of parental survival and health for the social, psychological, and economic well-being of persons who are relatively late in this transition. Ordinarily, they will have completed many of the other child-linked events in the transition in intergenerational relations, and be especially prone to the resource demands and stresses thought attendant on membership in the "sandwich" generation.

Prior research on children of the ill and institutionalized aged suggests that caregivers (especially daughters) are more likely to be in poor health and depressed to the extent that they face competing demands on their time. If they are able to provide some continued assistance to their institutionalized parents, these consequences are lessened (Brody, Dempsey, & Pruchno, 1990). However, financial support for an aging parent remains rare: Only 13% of sons 65 and older contribute financially to the support of their very old parents (Seccombe, 1988). The constriction of social and personal activities is one of the most frequently noted consequences of caring for a frail parent, especially for daughters. This seems to result as much from the perception that caregiving is an all-encompassing burden as from actual time and energy demands (Miller & Montgomery, 1990). In fact, when generational status and family structure are taken into account, the nature of impairment of the elder seems to have little impact on the caregiver's health and psychosocial functioning (Cattanach & Tebes 1991).

DATA

The data for this chapter was drawn from the 1987/88 National Survey of Families and Households (National Survey of Families and Households, 1990). The NSFH included interviews with a representative national sample of 13,017 Americans age 19 and older. The respondents consisted of a main sample of 9,643 individuals plus double samples of minorities (blacks and Hispanics), single-parent families, families with stepchildren, cohabitating couples, and recently-married couples. Of these, 3,209 are 55 and older, 513 of whom had at least one surviving parent.

The NSFH used personal interviews and supplemental self-administered questionnaires to gather detailed information on respondents' past and current family characteristics, social and economic characteristics, and kinship and social networks. Particularly relevant for this study, information was gathered on the survival and health of parents, and the respondents' interactions and exchanges of support with them.

Data on broader social network support for these persons and their levels of assistance to others enabled us to investigate the extent to which care for an elderly parent may limit or expand participation in a broader social network. Ideal for this purpose is NSFH data on exchanges of support (money, household assistance, emotional support or advice, and personal care with children, siblings, other relatives, and friends and neighbors). Data on marital stress, marital conflict over in-laws, and sibling relations permitted us to investigate the effects of parental survival and health on family relations. We used NSFH data on labor force participation and hours worked and on participation in social interactions and group activities to assess the effects of the time demands of this phase of the transition in intergenerational relations on social integration. Inventories of income, wealth, possessions, and debts provided a handle on the financial aspects of this transition. We used a global measure of well-being, a scale of depression, and a self-report of the respondent's overall health to examine the overall effect of these specific life course domains on individual well-being. Specific question-naire items used to construct each of these measures, scaling proce-dures, and descriptive statistics are provided in Appendix A.

METHOD

Many of the variables we associate with the likelihood that a parent survives also effect these measures of social, psychological, and financial well-being. To remove spurious associations between these outcomes and parental survival and health, we used a matched sample design.

For every respondent age 55 and older who has a living parent, we included a randomly selected (without replacement) respondent who did not have a living parent, but had the same combination of age, gender, parental status, level of education, and marital status charac-teristics.[4] These procedures produced a nationally representative sam-ple of 492 respondents 55 and older with a living parent, plus a matched sample of 492 respondents without a living parent.[5]

In order to assess the extent to which a surviving parent was likely to need assistance, we distinguished respondents whose parents were re-ported to be in poor or very poor health from those whose parents were in fair health or better.[6]

RESULTS

Table 3.2 reports differences in the social and psychological situations of older Americans with both parents deceased, with one or both par-ents well, and with one or more parents who are ill. The first three columns contain the mean scores of each group for each of the indica-tors. The fourth column gives the overall F statistic for an analysis of variance test. The last three columns display paired T-tests for signifi-cant differences between groups.

Persons with a sick parent have an overall level of exchange of social support with their children that is significantly lower than that of per-sons with a well parent or of those whose parents are deceased. Those persons with a sick parent provide less support to their children, espe-cially less advice and emotional support. Children do not provide more types of social support to their parents if those parents have a surviving or a sick elderly parent. Nor are the overall levels of assistance from any

Table 3.2. Mean Differences in Family Relations, Social Support, Social Integration, and Well-Being

	No Parent	Well Parent	Sick Parent	F	T-Tests I/II	T-Tests I/III	T-Tests II/III
Social Support							
Total volume of exchange with children	2.00	2.01	1.61	3.19**		**	**
Total volume of exchange with siblings	0.40	0.29	0.30	0.27			
Total volume of exchange with other relatives	0.36	0.34	0.35	0.03			
Total volume of exchange with friends	1.27	1.11	1.04	1.06			
Total volume of giving to children	1.50	1.50	1.17	3.83*		**	**
Total volume of giving to siblings	0.27	0.18	0.20	0.29			
Total volume of giving to other relatives	0.24	0.21	0.24	0.13			
Total volume of giving to friends	0.79	0.69	0.67	0.67			
Total volume of receiving from children	0.51	0.51	0.48	0.41			
Total volume of receiving from siblings	0.14	0.11	0.10	0.35			
Total volume of receiving from other relatives	0.12	0.13	0.11	0.09			
Total volume of receiving from friends	0.48	0.41	0.41	0.97			
Total volume of giving money	0.48	0.45	0.49	0.04			
Total volume of giving household assistance	0.78	0.69	0.60	1.26			
Total volume of giving advice or emotional support	1.07	1.05	0.84	2.65*		**	**
Total volume of giving care	0.09	0.07	0.09	0.32			
Total volume of giving any assistance	2.44	2.28	2.03	1.36			
Total volume of receiving money	0.07	0.07	0.05	0.03			
Total volume of receiving household assistance	0.48	0.44	0.51	0.67			
Total volume of receiving advice	0.66	0.62	0.60	0.57			
Total volume of receiving care	0.03	0.01	0.03	3.56**	**		
Total volume of receiving any assistance	1.23	1.12	1.10	1.28			

(continued)

Table 3.2. (Continued)

	No Parent	Well Parent	Sick Parent	F	T-Tests		
					I/II	I/III	II/III
Family Relations							
Marital stress	6.14	6.06	6.17	0.38			
Marital conflict over in-laws	1.18	1.24	1.41	3.99**		**	**
Sibling relations	1.07	1.04	1.08	1.42			
Social Integration							
How often spend social evening with someone?	7.61	7.31	6.59	2.45*		**	
How often participate in group activity?	3.55	3.52	2.78	1.77			
# of hours usually worked	16.4	20.4	14.8	6.79***	**		**
Well-Being							
How are things?	5.48	5.66	5.18	5.68***		**	**
Depression score	1.02	0.91	1.64	12.91***		**	**
Self reported health	3.83	3.94	3.53	8.52***	**	**	**

Significance Levels: * .10 ** .05 *** .01

70

source higher on any of the dimensions of support for persons with sick parents.

The low levels of assistance received by all persons 55 and older, including those persons with an ill parent, are noteworthy. Of four possible sources of support, persons with ill parents receive only money from just .05 sources, household assistance from .51 sources, and advice from .60 sources. Of a possible 16 points on the "total volume of receiving any assistance" scale (one point for each type of support from each source), persons with an ill parent score only 1.10 points.

In sum, it appears that persons 55 and older receive only limited social support. Those who must provide assistance to an aging, or even an ill, parent do not draw upon a larger network of social support to ease the burden. Neither their children, other kin, nor friends, increase support for those facing these pressures. Surprisingly, this is as true for advice and emotional support as it is for material assistance. Persons 55 and older who undertake the challenges posed by care for by a very old, ill parent largely do so alone.[7] Until this challenge is ended by the death of the parent and they complete the transition in intergenerational relations, these persons will provide less assistance to their children.

Persons 55 and older with an ill parent report more frequent conflict with their spouse over in-laws, although the overall frequency of such conflict remains rare. The unassisted challenge posed by an ill parent does not seem to place stress on overall family relationships. Marital stress and sibling relations are equally good whether one's parents are deceased, well, or ill.

While it is not always statistically significant, there is a consistently lower level of participation in work, voluntary organizations, and informal socializing that occurs among persons with an ill parent. Persons whose parents are deceased do not differ systematically from those who have one or more living parents in fair or good health.

What are the overall consequences of having an elderly sick parent in need of support, with little social support from others, increased conflict with the spouse, and lower social integration for individual well-being? Consistently negative. Persons with an ill parent report that they are in somewhat poorer health, more often depressed, and less often happy than those elderly whose parents are still alive and well or those whose parents are deceased. Persons with a surviving parent who is well are as well off on these measures of well-being as are those whose parents have died. It is not so much a delay in the completion of the transition in intergenerational relations that is problematic, then, as it is the transitory period of illness that may precede the parent's death.[8]

In sum, having a very old parent does not in and of itself create burdens for aging adult children. In fact, children with a healthy parent actually appear better off on a number of indicators than children with no living parent. Having a parent who is in poor health is another issue. These respondents tend to have accumulated less wealth, have greater conflicts over in-laws, engage in fewer social activities, work less, and be in poorer physical and emotional health. What is remarkable is that the greater vulnerability of aging adult children with needy parents has apparently not provoked higher levels of support from others. In fact, aside from their nonsignificance, the mean levels of support received by respondents with a sick parent are in most cases *lower* than the levels received by respondents in the other two groups. Families may very well be the major source of help to dependent elderly. However, those who are likely to have primary responsibility for the care of these elderly appear to have little support, familial or otherwise, for themselves.

Table 3.3 displays the distributions of respondents across net wealth quintiles.[9] Adults with a parent in poor health are disproportionately likely to be in the lowest wealth category, compared to adults with a healthy parent (12%) or those with no parent alive (17%). Furthermore, only 20% of them are in the top income group, compared to 25% of those with a healthy parent and 23% of those without a parent.

Analyses of the components of this net wealth variable showed fairly consistent differences among the three groups. Respondents with a sick parent had significantly lower equity in their homes. They also had substantially smaller savings and investments than did respondents whose parents were healthy or had both died. The measure of "other assets" (a combination of net worth of other real estate, farm or business, and motor vehicles) shows that persons with a parent in poor health were most likely to have no assets and least likely to have the highest level of assets. Persons with healthy parents were least likely to have zero or negative assets, and were most likely to be in the top category. Those whose parents were deceased were in an intermediate situation.[10]

This data, then provides evidence that having a parent in poor health negatively affects financial well-being.[11] Unfortunately, with the cross-sectional data available to us we cannot tell the dynamics of financial transactions that produce these differences in income and wealth. Do sick parents create a financial drain on their children? Why do individuals who, at some point in the past, experienced the death of a parent appear to differ little from those with healthy parents? How much of their current financial status is a function of inheritance?[12] The answer to these questions must await the collection and analysis of appropriate longitudinal data.

Table 3.3. Wealth by Parental Status (%)

	Sick Parent	Well Parent	No Parent
Net Wealth			
< = $19,100	28.9	12.3	16.9
$19,199–56,564	22.7	16.2	17.3
$56,565–102,671	19.9	21.3	15.5
$102,672–189,900	09.1	24.6	27.5
$189,901+	19.5	25.5	22.8
Home Equity			
< = 0	26.1	13.9	17.9
$1–45,999	34.3	28.7	22.7
$46,000–74,999	23.6	28.1	26.1
$75,000+	16.0	29.3	33.3
Other Assets			
< = 0	14.0	06.2	10.6
$1–4,899	34.2	23.7	30.5
$4,900–13,999	30.3	28.6	27.1
$14,000+	21.5	41.5	31.8
Total Savings			
0	36.6	17.1	26.2
$1–9,999	26.6	27.7	24.1
$10,000–49,999	19.5	34.2	28.3
$50,000+	17.3	21.0	21.4
Total Investments			
0	68.4	50.1	58.4
$1–9,999	07.5	19.5	14.7
$10,000–49,999	10.5	14.3	13.9
$50,000	13.7	16.0	13.0
Total Debts			
0	62.9	60.2	62.5
$50–675	11.6	15.5	14.3
$676–1,900	11.7	09.9	06.9
$1,901+	13.9	14.4	16.3

DISCUSSION

During the middle third of their life course, Americans typically experience their parents' decline and death and their children coming of age. These events mark the transition in intergenerational relations that draws to a close their own lives as children and directs their full attention to their roles as parents and grandparents. Delays in this transition because of the survival of a parent to advanced old age, have little social consequence as long as that parent is well. But the declining health of the aging parent initiates a stressful time in the life course, with more serious consequences for the well-being of the individuals involved and their relations with their children.

A person who is on the eve of old age and is responsible for a sick parent faces this challenge largely alone. Such persons experience reduced social integration, more often find themselves in conflict with their spouse, and more often experience financial stress. They feel in poorer health and more often are depressed, reporting a lower level of overall happiness. But the effects of these negative sequelae are modest, and they disappear after the death of the parents. At that time the transition in intergenerational relations is complete, as signified in increased assistance to the next generation.

Longitudinal data is necessary to fully trace out the development of this process over the life course. Our data is consistent with the hypothesis that this negative situation arises in the life course when the parent becomes ill, and disappears after the parent's death. But the degree of parental need that is problematic—whether some individuals are buffered from the negative consequences by social support or by relying on a sibling to carry the burden alone—and the recovery time needed to redirect attention to the younger generation after the death of the parent will remain unknown until longitudinal data permit this process to be followed over the life course.

These findings suggest that medical advances that prolong life will increasingly delay the transition in intergenerational relations for future cohorts of Americans. The consequences will not be problematic, as long as that prolongation of life is accompanied by improved health in old age. If, as seems likely, current medical advances do more to prolong life in poor health than to lengthen the years of healthy life (Olshansky et al., 1990), the resultant delays in the transition in intergenerational relations are likely to be problematic for the individuals involved and for their children and grandchildren.

ACKNOWLEDGMENTS

An earlier version of this paper was presented at a Conference on Aging and Generational Relations, Newark, Delaware, November 1991. Support for this research was provided by NICHD Grant 1 R01 HD26070 and from core support (P30 HD28263–01) provided by the National Institute of Child Health and Human Development to the Population Research Institute, Pennsylvania State University. Computational support was provided by the Penn State University Intercollege Research Programs. The programming assistance of Henk Meij is gratefully acknowledged.

NOTES

1.   The sample sizes shown in Table 3.1 are the number of unweighted cases. The percentage of older adults with a surviving parent and the descriptive statistics in Table 1 are based on data weighted to represent the national population.

2.   The relatively high fertility of the birth cohorts who were in the early years of old age at the time of this survey is a related confounding factor.

3.   In those few cases where both parents survive, these descriptive data are based on the age of the oldest parent, the health status of the parent in poorest health, the level of education of the best-educated parent, and the distance lived from the closest parent.

4.   For purposes of this matching, we categorized these variables as shown in Table 3.1. There were 640 possible combinations of age, education, marital status, parental status, and gender. Respondents with missing information on any of these demographic characteristics were dropped from the study. For most combinations that had at least one respondent with a living parent, there were at least an equal or greater number of respondents with no living parent. Where the number respondents without a living parent was greater, we used a random sample generating subroutine in SAS to draw a sample (without replacement) equal to the number of the respondents with a living parent in that combination. Where the number of persons with and without a surviving parent were equal, all cases were selected.

There were two exceptions to this matching strategy. First, for 13 combinations there were fewer respondents without a living parent than there were respondents with a living parent. In these instances, we used sampling with replacement. As a result, 13 cases were used as matches two or more times. A total of 17 matched sample cases are such replications. Second, there were 18 combinations where one respondent had a living parent, but no matching respondent without a living parent. Lacking any suitable comparison category, we dropped all 18 of these persons (3.5% of the total sample of persons with a living parent) from our analysis.

5.   Note that the matched respondents without a living parent do *not* represent any real population of persons, but are simply a subsample of adults 55 and older with no living parent selected so as to have the same age, education, marital status, gender, and parental status composition as the population of persons with a surviving parent.

6.   In the cases where two parents survived, the health status of the parent in poorer health was used. We had hoped to further distinguish respondents with a sick parent by those whose parents were coresident and those who were not. However, only 30 respondents reported a coresident parent, too few for reliable analysis.

7.   These older adults are less likely to be receiving child care assistance from other children, siblings, other kin, or friends if their parents are alive and well. Presumably, the child care is provided by their elderly parents.

8.   Given the advanced age of the parents, it is unlikely that those who are

now in poor health will subsequently improve to a situation of fair or good health.

9.   The quintile cutpoints derived from the distribution of net wealth of the entire NSFH sample of respondents age 55 and older.

10.   Total debts (excluding debts represented in the net worth categories already discussed) did not vary significantly among the three groups.

11.   Data on total earnings from employment were not wholly consistent with this conclusion, but provided no consistently negative evidence either. Log earnings varied significantly by group, respondents with a sick parent averaging significantly lower earnings than those whose parents were not in poor health.However, there were no differences between respondents with a sick parent and those with no parent. Further analyses that looked at age and gender differences showed that females under 62 with a sick parent had significantly *higher* earnings than similar females with no parent. In contrast, the earnings of males under 62 averaged about $9,000 less than males with no parent, and $13,800 less than males with a healthy parent. Unfortunately, these more refined analyses were based on small groups of respondents—there were only 47 females under 62 with a sick parent, for example.

12.   Thirty percent of middle-aged Americans whose parents are deceased report they received an inheritance (Winsborough, Bumpass, & Aquilino, 1991).

REFERENCES

Brim, O. G., Jr., & Ryff, C. D. (1980). On the properties of life events. In P. B. Baltes & O. G. Brim, Jr. (Eds.), *Life span development and behavior:* Vol. 3 (pp. 368–388). New York: Academic Press.

Brody, E. (1981). Women in the middle and family help to older people. *The Gerontologist, 21,* 471–480.

Brody, E. M., Dempsey, N. P., & Pruchno, R. A. (1990). Mental health of sons and daughters of the institutionalized aged. *The Gerontologist, 30,* 212–219.

Bumpass, L. L. (1990). What's happening to the family? Interactions between demographic and institutional change. *Demography, 27,* 483–498.

Cattanach, L., & Tebes, J. K. (1991). The nature of elder impairment and its impact on family caregivers' health and psychological functioning. *The Gerontologist, 31,* 246–255.

Cherlin, A., & Furstenberg, F. (1986). *The new American grandparent.* New York: Basic Books.

Eggebeen, D. J. (1992). Family structure and intergenerational exchanges. *Research on Aging, 14,* 427–447.

Eggebeen, D. J., & Hogan, D. P. (1990). Giving between generations in American families. *Human Nature, 1,* 211–232.

Hogan, D. P., & Eggebeen, D. J. (1991, August). *Sources of aid and assistance in old age.* Presented at the annual meeting of the American Sociological Association, Cincinnati, OH.

Hogan, D. P., & Eggebeen, D. J., & Clogg, C. C. (1993). The structure of inter-generational exchanges in American families. *American Journal of Sociology, 98,* 1428–58.

Miller, B., & Montgomery, A. (1990). Family caregivers and limitations in social activities. *Research on Aging, 12,* 72–93.

National Survey of Families and Households (1990). Machine readable data file. Madison: Center for Demography and Ecology, University of Wisconsin.

Olshansky, J. S., Carnes, B. A., & Cassel, C. (1990). In search of Methuselah: Estimating upper limits to human longevity. *Science, 250,* 634–640.

Seccombe, K. (1988). Financial assistance from elderly retirement-age sons to their aging parents. *Research on Aging, 10,* 102–118.

Winsborough, H. H., Bumpass, L. L., & Aquilino, W. S. (1991). *The death of parents and the transition to old age.* Madison: Center for Demography and Ecology, University of Wisconsin. NSFH Working Paper 39.

Appendix A

Variable	Definition	Mean	SD
Financial Status			
Net wealth	Summary variable calculated by adding together net worth of respondent's home, other real estate, business or farm, and motor vehicle, and total value of savings and investments, and then subtracting total amount of debts.	$168,017	$522,563
Net worth of home	Calculated by subtracting the respondent's estimate of the amount owed on their home from their estimate of its sale value.	$ 68,719	$180,860
Net worth of other real estate	Calculated by subtracting the respondent's estimate of amount owed on other real estate from their estimate of its sale value.	$ 19,341	$110,968
Net worth of business or farm	Calculated by subtracting the respondent's estimate of amount owed on their business or farm from their estimate of its sale value.	$ 29,297	$294,574
Net worth of motor vehicles	Calculated by subtracting the respondent's estimate of amount owed on their automobiles from their estimate of the sale value.	$ 7,677	$ 9,292
Debts	Total amount respondent reported they owed on credit cards or charge accounts, installment loans, education loans, personal loans from banks, friends or relatives, home improvement loans, and other bills owed more than 2 months.	$ 1,479	$ 5,563
Savings	Approximate total value of savings. Including saving accounts, savings bonds, IRAs, money market shares, and CDs.	$ 26,402	$ 36,146
Investments	Approximate total value of investments, including stocks, bonds, shares in mutual funds, or other investments.	$ 16,634	$ 34,248

Social Support		
Total volume of exchange with children	Sum of the number of dimensions on which giving and receiving occurred with noncoresidential adult children. Range: 0–8	1.95	1.83
Total volume of exchange with siblings	Sum of the number of dimensions on which giving and receiving occurred with siblings. Range: 0–8	0.35	0.85
Total volume of exchange with other relatives	Sum of the number of dimensions on which giving and receiving occurred with other relatives. Range: 0–8	0.35	0.85
Total volume of exchange with friends	Sum of the number of dimensions on which giving and receiving occurred with friends. Range: 0–8	1.18	1.50
Total volume of giving to children	Sum of the number of dimensions on which giving occurred with children. Range: 0–4	1.46	1.38
Total volume of giving to siblings	Sum of the number of dimensions on which giving occurred with siblings. Range: 0–4	0.23	0.58
Total volume of giving to other relatives	Sum of the number of dimensions on which giving occurred with other relatives. Range: 0–4	0.23	0.60
Total volume of giving to friends	Sum of the number of dimensions on which giving occurred with friends. Range: 0–4	0.74	0.97
Total volume of receiving from children	Sum of the number of dimensions on which receiving from children occurred. Range: 0–4	0.51	0.84
Total volume of receiving from siblings	Sum of the number of dimensions on which receiving from siblings occurred. Range: 0–4	0.12	0.41
Total volume of receiving from other relatives	Sum of the number of dimensions on which receiving from other relatives occurred. Range: 0–4	0.12	0.44
Total volume of receiving from friends	Sum of the number of dimensions on which receiving from friends occurred. Range: 0–4	0.45	0.76
Total volume of giving money	Sum of the number of individuals to whom respondent gave or loaned money in the past five years. Range: 0–4	0.47	0.70
Total volume of giving household assistance	Sum of the number of individuals to whom respondent gave help with transportation, repairs to house or car, or work around the house in past month. Range: 0–4	0.73	0.82

(continued)

79

Appendix A (Continued)

Variable	Definition	Mean	SD
Total volume of giving advice	Sum of the number of individuals to whom respondent gave advice, encouragement, or moral or emotional support in past month. Range: 0–4	1.03	1.02
Total volume of giving care	Sum of the number of individuals to whom respondent gave help with child care for preschool child in past week or babysitting of any age child in past month. Range: 0–4	0.08	0.33
Total volume of giving any assistance	Sum of the number of individuals to whom respondent gave any form of help in past month. Range: 0–16	2.33	1.90
Total volume of receiving money	Sum of the number of individuals from whom respondent received money in the past five years. Range: 0–4	0.07	0.32
Total volume of receiving household assistance	Sum of the number of individuals from whom respondent received help with transportation, repairs to house or car, or work around the house in past month. Range: 0–4	0.47	0.69
Total volume of giving advice	Sum of the number of individuals to whom respondent gave advice, encouragement, or moral or emotional support in past month. Range: 0–4	1.03	1.02
Total volume of receiving care	Sum of the number of individuals from whom respondent received help with child care for preschool child in past week or babysitting of any age child in past month. Range: 0–4	0.02	0.17
Total volume of receiving any assistance	Sum of the number of individuals from whom respondent received any form of help in past month. Range: 0–16	1.17	1.40
Family Relations			
Marital stress	Taking things all together, how would you describe your marriage? 1 = very unhappy—7 = very happy	6.11	1.57

Variable	Description		
Marital conflict over in-laws	How often, if at all, in the past year have you had open disagreements about in-laws? 1 = never—6 = almost every day	1.23	0.85
Sibling relations	Do you get along well with all of your brothers and sisters? 1 = yes; 2 = no	1.06	0.26
Social Integration			
How often spend a social evening with someone?	How often do you spend a social evening with relatives, a neighbor, co-workers, friends? How often do you attend a social event at church or synagogue? Go to a bar or tavern? Participate in a group recreational activity such as bowling, golf, square dancing, etc.? Range: 0–28	7.38	4.36
How often participate in group activities?	How often do you participate in each of the following organizations: fraternal groups, service clubs, veteran's groups, political groups, labor unions, sports groups, youth groups, school related groups, hobby or garden clubs, school fraternities or sororities, nationality groups, farm organizations, literary/art/study or discussion groups, professional or academic societies, and church-affiliated groups? Range: 0–60	3.44	4.17
Number of hours usually worked	How many hours a week do you usually work?	17.60	23.57
Well-Being			
How are things?	Taking things all together, how would you say things are these days? Range: 1 = very unhappy—7 = very happy	5.51	1.60
Depression score	Scale which is the average of 12 questions asking about depression-like symptoms. Range: 0 = no symptoms—7 = all the symptoms	1.06	1.55
Self-reported health	Self-reported health status of respondent. Range: 1 = very poor—5 = excellent	2.81	1.07

4

Exchanges within Black American Three-Generation Families
The Family Environment Context Model

James S. Jackson, Rukmalie Jayakody, and Toni C. Antonucci

INTRODUCTION

This chapter explores the influences of sociodemographic and family processes factors on tangible exchanges within three-generation black family lineages. Building on the work of Zajonc (1976) and others (e.g., Bronfenbrenner, 1986), we hypothesize that due to structural arrangements and social interactions, multigenerational families form distinct social, psychological, and physical environments. Features of these family environments are reciprocally related and affect the functioning of individual family members within these lineage structures. We term this framework the Family Environment Context Model (FECM).

We concentrate on the interrelationships among different features of family environments among black three-generation lineages (Burton & Dilworth-Anderson, 1991). Notably, we are concerned with how family-context factors, such as family proximity, contact, satisfaction, and closeness, influence exchange environments.

Analyses are based on the 510 complete three-generation lineage triads ($N = 1,530$ respondents) from the Michigan Three-Generation Family Study (Jackson & Hatchett, 1986). Each complete family unit is composed of three family members, each representing a distinct lineage. Family environment features are conceptualized and operationalized as the average scores on each of the variables of interest within the 510 probability-selected family lineages (Zajonc, 1976; 1983; Zajonc & Markus, 1975). For example, a family-proximity triad measure is created by taking the score for each lineage (based upon the responses of each family member to questions about proximity to relatives) and averaging across these three lineage members to obtain a single measure. Essentially, this triad score is the mean for a family lineage. Perceived family closeness, satisfaction, contact, and tangible exchange measures are formed in a similar manner. Because the triads were obtained through probability selection procedures (Jackson & Hatchett, 1986), we assume that each triad represents a random sample of all possible three-generation lineages for each family. Thus, on average, we assume that the scores provide fairly good estimates of the reports on the family environments that would be obtained if all members in each generational position of the multigeneration lineage had been questioned. In the analyses, we employed nested hierarchial linear regression models using ordinary least squares (OLS) estimation to ascertain the individual and joint contributions of selected structural, social, and psychological family environmental features to the family exchange environment dimensions.

BACKGROUND

In earlier historical periods, much of women's time was spent providing care for the young, the old, and the infirm. Many feel this unpaid labor provided a major source of cohesion in family life and intergenerational relations. Changes in family structure of the general population over the last generation—particularly the movement of married women into the labor force and the development of the two-earner family as a growing proportion of family types—hold profound implications for ways in which generational lineage members within families relate to each other. We should also note that black women have participated in the American labor force for a longer time and in larger numbers than have white women. Thus, this transformation in the general population follows several generations of such two-earner black American families.

Also important is the increasing diversity in family structures. Single-person households, single-parent families, families consisting of many "step" relationships, and blended families resulting from divorce and remarriage are becoming increasingly common. Changes in mortality have significantly changed the composition of families: For example, the "beanpole" family structure refers to family configurations that contain several different generations (grandparent, parent, child), but with fewer members within each generation. The fall in fertility results in a reduction in the proportion of families consisting of collateral kin (e.g., sisters, brothers, and cousins), while the fall in mortality leads to an increase in the proportion of family composed of parents, grandparents, and even great-grandparents (Goldman, 1986). Ryder (1974) demonstrated that a low-fertility/low-mortality society results in an increase in the average person years that each child spends in the household with parents, and a slight decrease in the time spent with siblings. The potential social, psychological, and economic implications of changing kinship structures are innumerable. Changes in the number and types of kin could have a substantial impact on the transfers of wealth and intergenerational exchange (Goldman, 1986). Tracing these changes and their implications for intergenerational family relations is a critical and complicated facet of studying both individual and family well-being, highlighting the importance of understanding intergenerational relations.

Intergenerational research in the tradition of Hill (1970a,b), Bengtson, Rosenthal, and Burton (1990), Markides and Cole, (1984), and Hagestad (1990) offers a firm basis for social relationships in an intergenerational family context. Hagestad (1990) noted the unique opportunity for contact, support, and influence across age groups and cohorts within the family. These ties are of lifelong duration, creating the potential for continuity and stability based on shared experiences and long-term reciprocities. Families are themselves cultural units that bring together different cohorts in their own unique combinations. However, family members are also changing individuals who have different life and historical experiences. Family members vary by generation, but cross-family same-generation members may be from different cohorts, highlighting the difficulty in separating generation, age, and cohort effects (Thornton & Rodgers, 1987).

The major theoretical framework used in this chapter argues that social relationships develop over the life course within families and are influenced by specific racial and ethnic factors, as well as socioeconomic and cultural factors (Jackson, Antonucci, & Gibson, 1990). Specifically, we suggest that there are continuities in social and personal relationships which develop out of early attachment relationships (Antonucci, 1990; Antonucci & Jackson, 1990). The family provides the important socialization and learning crucible for the development of personal and social skills that spread in ever widening circles as children develop and enter new environments. The nature of these socialization experiences and the Bengtson social and physical environments in which they occur is dictated by socioeconomic status, ethnicity/race, family structure, and the cultural beliefs and behaviors of the individual family group (Jackson, Antonucci, & Gibson, 1990). Since these are all mutable factors that change as a function of cohort and period events, they must be assessed continually over the individual and family life course. As we have suggested elsewhere (Jackson & Antonucci, 1994), these social relationships can be best studied methodologically by employing a combination of cross-sectional, cohort, longitudinal, and particularly, multigenerational lineage research designs.

INTERGENERATIONAL FAMILY VALUES AND NORMS

Over the last few decades, families have been increasingly confronted with early pregnancy and childbirth outside of marriage. These changes in family-related events have lead to "value" confrontations across the generations. Similar value issues have been raised by cohabitating, widowed, or divorced parents. For example, comparisons of the 1957 and 1976 Americans View Their Mental Health data found both change and stability in views about marriage and parenthood (Veroff, Kulka, & Douvan, 1981). While little change occurred in the national population on views toward marriage and parenthood (most people highly valued these family roles), there was a notable shift in the attitudes toward family roles. In 1957, family roles were considered the cornerstones of an adequate adult life; by 1976, marriage and parenthood were viewed as choices or options among many others. In addition to the fact that attitudes and values may have simply shifted to keep pace with these behaviors, there are two opposing theories of intergenerational transmission: Solidarity within family or continuity is implicitly assumed; and norms and values of the parent generation spawn opposition (and contrary norms) in the young [see, for example, Markides, Boldt, and Ray (1986); Roberts and Bengtson (1990); and Bengtson, Cutler, Mengen, and Marshall (1985) for discussion of these points]. An alternative theory might assume a life-course progression, with the younger generation rebelling and holding values and attitudes different from their parents until they themselves have children. This individual life-cycle and role-position perspective also requires a consideration of the family life course, with an understanding that the younger generation's attitudes and behaviors affect their parents and even their grandparents (Glass, Bengston, & Dunham, 1986).

Historians and sociologists draw connections between the larger society and the family (Demos, 1970) and assume a close relationship (Lasch, 1977). For example, to determine whether technological development is necessarily accompanied by shifts in the authority structure and relationships in the family, we also need to examine cohort effects on family values and norms which are independent of generation effects.

INTERGENERATIONAL FAMILY EXCHANGES, RECIPROCITIES, AND HEALTH AND WELL-BEING

Social relationships can be viewed as a series of exchanges of various resources (money, goods, services, information, status, and affection) with other individuals (Foa & Foa, 1974). Intergenerational family relations can be characterized in terms of the duration, frequency, and the types of resources involved in the exchanges among family members. Despite the large number of studies on intergenerational aid (see Bengtson et al., 1985, 1990; Hagestad, 1981, 1990, for reviews), the nature of family resource exchanges over the life course is not clearly understood. Conflicting theories and hypotheses have been advanced concerning patterns and rules of resource exchanges within the family (Antonucci & Jackson, 1990). For example, two models—linear relationships and curvilinear relationships between age (or different points in the life course) and intergenerational resource transactions—have existed simultaneously in the family literature for nearly two decades (Cheal, 1983). The linear model indicates the principle of serial transfers in which each generation transfers resources to its successors, while the curvilinear model indicates the principle of lifelong reciprocity, with the middle-aged being net providers for the young and the elderly. Conflicting hypotheses concerning the rules underlying family exchanges have been proposed, such as the communal rule (Clark, 1984), life-course reciprocity (Antonucci, 1990), and the rule of "beneficence" applied to people with limited resources (Dowd, 1984). Further, cross-cultural research reveals important differences in family exchanges of whites and blacks (Dowd & Bengtson, 1978; Mutran, 1985; Taylor, 1988) and Hispanics (Dowd & Bengtson, 1978; Markides & Krause, 1985). Understanding the rules of family exchanges and the exceptions exhibited among the relatively resourceless (e.g., the poor) in particular cultures or subcultures could result in generalizable scientific findings, and also could have important policy implications.

Research has firmly established the positive results of family relations. Family relations have been shown to inhibit mortality and morbidity (Berkman & Syme, 1979; House, Robbins, & Metzner, 1982; Blazer, 1982; Schoenbach, Kaplan, Fredman, & Kleinbaum, 1986; Orth-Gomer & Johnson, 1987) and lead to other positive health outcomes (Antonucci & Akiyama, 1987; House, Landis, & Umberson, 1988; Cohen & Syme, 1985). However, not all influences of family relations are positive. For example, Medalie and Goldbourt (1976) showed that family problems play a major role in the development of heart disease. Additionally, perception of nonreciprocity, (i.e., a lack of balance between support provided and received) is also associated with detrimental outcomes (Belle, 1982; Ingersoll-Dayton & Antonucci, 1988; Antonucci & Jackson, 1990). Lee (1988) has noted that among the current cohort of older Americans for whom independence is a primary value the need for assistance has a much smaller negative effect on morale than does the inability to reciprocate. Reliance on children can be an insidious form of dependence because it involves a reversal of the normative parent/ child roles.

SUBSTANTIVE AND METHODOLOGICAL CONSIDERATIONS

In this chapter, we explore the degree of intergenerational solidarity (proximity, contact, satisfaction, and closeness) in family relations and the perceptions of exchanges among family members. Also of interest is how these vary by sociodemographic factors and sociocultural influences, although here we restrict our analyses to Americans of African descent. We believe that much research on intergenerational relationships has been limited by previous approaches that have not considered important sources of influence. We focus our attention on intergenerational exchanges among black families, using an ecological, family-level, social-environment-analysis framework. Before turning to a theoretical and methodological rationale for this approach, we provide a brief review of methodological and substantive issues involved in research on the black family more generally.

Much literature exists regarding the strengths and weaknesses of different research methods in the study of the family (e.g., Huston & Robins, 1982; Jackson, Tucker, & Bowman, 1982; Kitson, Sussman, Williams, et al., 1982; LaRossa & Wolf, 1985). Particularly relevant to research on black families have been the divergent perspectives on the relative merits of qualitative versus quantitative empirical approaches (LaRossa & Wolf, 1985). Regardless of the specific research procedure employed, a number of conceptual and methodological issues have direct substantive implications in the study of black families (Allen, 1979; Billingsley, 1968; Staples & Mirande, 1980; Taylor, Chatters, Tucker, & Lewis, 1990). Among these issues are the appropriate role of race-comparative research; the need for adequate black family samples in quantitative research; appropriate conceptions of the normative role of the family; meaningful conceptualization, definition, and measurement of systemic environmental factors and contextual variables; and the appropriate unit of analysis.

ROLE OF RACE COMPARATIVE RESEARCH

Historically, many investigations of black families have lacked clearly articulated theoretical orientations (Allen, 1978; Dodson, 1981; Hill, 1981a; Staples & Mirande, 1980; Taylor et al., 1990). Much of the research has been problem-focused, related to particular policy concerns (Moynihan, 1965; Murray, 1985). While both problems and policies are important, the lack of strong theoretical orientations to research has resulted in a "hodge-podge" of findings that are difficult to interpret within a larger conceptual context (Taylor, 1986; Taylor et al., 1990). Similarly, the appropriate role of comparative research on blacks and whites is a major methodological and substantive issue in studies of black families. Investigations have been conducted predominantly in the context of comparisons to the status of white families. This has both positive and negative consequences. Positively, the study of black and white families can contribute to an understanding of how systemic factors may differentially affect family units with nonequal economic and social resources. Race-comparative research may also enhance our understanding of potential new public policies.

However, race-comparative research also may have negative consequences. For example, the fact that approximately 50% of black families are female-headed is a critical issue, regardless of comparisons with rates in the white population (Farley, 1984; Farley & Allen, 1988). Often race-comparative research has tended to either confuse or trivialize the important differences among families "within" the black population. Within a context that gives priority to whites as "the" normative standard, the often large average differences between blacks and whites tend to dominate the focus of study. In order to study the black family adequately, we need intraracial studies that assess variation within black families (Hatchett & Jackson, 1993). This does not necessarily imply that race-comparative research is always inappropriate. But, because of the reasons previously cited, race-comparative studies often result in a lack of attention to the possible cultural differences between blacks and whites, producing inappropriate types of research on black individuals and families (Allen, 1978; McAdoo, 1987; Dodson, 1981; Jackson et al., 1982).

ADEQUATE SAMPLES

Even if appropriately defined and conducted with sensitivity to race and cultural differences, much of the existing research on black families has not employed adequate samples (Jackson et al., 1982; Hatchett & Jackson, 1993; Staples & Mirande, 1980; Taylor, 1986). The majority of empirical studies have been based on nonprobability- selected samples of blacks and their families. Some attention has focused on the weaknesses of these samples, particularly on the generalizability of findings to larger populations (McAdoo, 1978; Taylor, 1986). Inadequately drawn samples of any population group do not permit justifiable generalization. For example, convenience samples of female-headed AFDC families reveal little about the functioning of black middle-class families. In fact, research on inadequate samples of female-headed AFDC families provides little information about possible differences by such factors as region or industrial sector in even these families. The bias introduced in nonprobability-selected samples has implications not only for the generalizability of findings, but also for the observed relationships among variables within a particular study (Jackson & Hatchett, 1986). The black family literature is replete with quantitative studies conducted on nonprobability or geographically restricted samples (Taylor, 1986). This lack of attention to appropriately defined samples of a sufficient size to meet both internal and external validity considerations undoubtedly contributes to the fragmented and conflicting findings in the contemporary literature on the black family (Staples & Mirande, 1980; Taylor et al., 1990).

NORMATIVE ROLE OF THE BLACK FAMILY

Related to the concern with race-comparative research is the lack of adequate attention to what the normative, functional role of the black family should be (McAdoo, 1978, 1988; Dodson, 1981; Stevens, 1984). While its role in socializing the young is generally assumed (Bowman & Howard, 1985; Dodson, 1981; Stevens, 1984), the black family may have other major roles as well.

These roles change in relation to contemporaneous events and with technological innovations. Elder (1985a) noted the need for a change in research orientation to one that places greater emphasis on context, process, and time, and the role of the black family as a buffer against systemically-caused disorganization. It is likely that historically in the United States, the normative role of the black family has been different from that of the white family (Nobles, 1978). The relationship of the black community to the family, particularly its extensions to other institutions such as the church (Taylor & Chatters, 1991), may mean that the black family assumes greater responsibilities than the white family in community integration processes. This may be simply a function of ethnicity, however, and not particularly unique to black families (Woehrer, 1978). Prior to conducting research, some attention should be given to defining the nature of normative roles (Burton & Dilworth-Anderson, 1991; Wilson, 1986). Failure to develop theoretical perspectives that include normative features of family functioning increases the difficulty in assessing the observed structures and functional forms of black families in research (Billingsley, 1968; Elder, 1985a; Staples & Mirande, 1980; Wilson, 1986).

SYSTEMIC AND CONTEXTUAL FACTORS IN BLACK FAMILY LIFE: CONCEPTUALIZATION AND MEASUREMENT

In a systems approach (Billingsley, 1968), adequate conceptualization and measurement of system-level variables and environmental factors that impinge upon the black family are imperative. Appropriate attention to this issue begins with theory, conceptualization, and measurement. A systems approach to the study of the family implies that there are factors that are external to the family but have extensive influence on family organization and functioning. Among these factors are changing economic, social, and political circumstances. Difficulties arise, however, in defining and operationalizing these factors. While the need for a systems approach in theories of the black family is well accepted (Billingsley, 1968; Farley & Allen, 1988), it has been difficult to operationalize these system factors into models of the black family.

Insufficient attention has been paid to the issues of operationalization, measurement, and analysis in research on black families. The very meaning of political, social, and economic context is often unclear. For example, Hill (1981b) noted the understated nature and deleterious affects of periodic recessions on the economic viability of the black community. He suggested that the timing of these cycles makes it impossible for economic recovery to occur within black communities. The continued comparatively low employment rates of blacks, compared to whites, even in periods of economic recovery, stand as a stark example of Hill's (1981a) major point. Yet the effects of such recessionary cycles have not been adequately modeled in research on the black family.

The Panel Study of Income Dynamics (PSID) is a 25-year ongoing study of American families (Duncan, 1984; Hill, 1983). Because the original focus of the PSID was the dynamics of poverty, the 1968 sample included a disproportionately large number of low-income households. This oversampling of poor families resulted in a sizable subsample of African Americans (Hill, 1992). Thus, the PSID provides an important data source for changing family norms among blacks over the last two and a half decades. This data set could be even more useful if both national and regional changes of a systemic, political, or social nature were assessed and included in the data set (Elder, 1985b).

APPROPRIATE UNIT OF ANALYSIS

Related to the issue of family definition and contextual variables is the appropriate unit of analysis in research on black families. The nature of family-level variables presents a variety of conceptual and methodological problems. For example, are simple aggregations of individual responses sufficient, or are there aspects of the family that transcend individual-level variables? How these units are defined, empirically assessed, and analyzed remains the subject of much conjecture (e.g., Mangen, Bengtson, & Landry, 1988). Thompson and Walker (1982) made a strong argument for the need for group-level data. They suggested that research be conceptualized at the group level, that measurement be relational, that analyses provide information about patterning, and that interpretations of the data refer to relational properties. On the other hand, Duncan and Hill (1985) suggested that measures of a longitudinal household unit are not feasible, and that assessment needs to focus on the individual. Other researchers, particularly in intergenerational research, have been very involved in this debate (e.g., Hagestad, 1982; Troll & Bengtson, 1979). Because of the reputed interdependence of the extended black family (Hatchett & Jackson, 1993; Mitchell & Register, 1984; Staples & Mirande, 1980), it may be that system- or group-level variables are more predictive of family and individual functioning. However, the issues of conceptualization, definition, measurement, analysis, and interpretation of such variables are far from having satisfactory answers. If Billingsley's (1968) assessment that the black family should be studied from a functional, systemic perspective is correct, then black family processes need to be understood within a temporal, adaptive, conceptual framework that considers changes in social, economic, and political circumstances (Elder, 1985a). Thus, research and research methodologies have to be adaptive and flexible as well.

We have conceptualized one systems-level approach to the study of family processes, operationalizing the notion of family environment (Brofenbrenner, 1979, 1986; Cauce, 1991; Garbarino, 1982; Zajonc, 1976, 1983; Zajonc & Markus, 1975). We hypothesize that three-generation lineages form family contexts that influence individual development in each lineage position, and that these different family environments are related to each other in systematic and predictable manners.

CONTRIBUTIONS OF MULTIGENERATION RESEARCH TO THE STUDY OF THE BLACK FAMILY

The study of the individual family must be considered within an analytic scheme that is responsive to time, process, and context (Elder, 1985a). These goals can best be achieved within a multigenerational family context (Hagestad, 1982; Hill & Konig, 1970; Jackson & Antonucci, 1994). It is within the multigenerational lineage framework that a sense of the individual family can be observed. We speculate that this is particularly true within black families which have historically included a broad array of tangible and intangible cross-generational transfers (Hatchett & Jackson, 1993; Mitchell & Register, 1984; Taylor, 1986; McAdoo, 1978; Stevens, 1984).

Substantively, for example, Burton's work (Burton & Bengtson, 1985; Hagestad & Burton, 1986) has revealed a great deal about on- and off-time grandparenthood and the accumulation of crises, as they affect individuals within multigenerational families. The critical nature of the early assumption of the grandparent role for black women would not have been revealed outside of the multigenerational family design. Second, issues of values and attitudinal transmission lie at the heart of much of today's public controversy regarding blacks, welfare, and welfare policy (Murray, 1985; Loury, 1985). Again, much can be learned about value and attitudinal transmission by examining family lineages within multigenerational families over time. The lack of good research designs has impeded an appropriate exploration of the nature and meaning of intergenerational value transmission.

Harriet McAdoo's work (1978) on single-parent families and support exchanges provided another example of the advantages of the multigenerational family design. A sense of the exchanges within multigenerational families, horizontally as well as vertically, was gained by studying these family lineages. McAdoo (1978, 1987) pointed out the importance of such exchanges across generations and for all socioeconomic levels among black families. This would not have been revealed in conventional cross-sectional or longitudinal research designs (Jackson & Antonucci, 1994).

STUDY DATA

Data from the 1981 national University of Michigan Three-Generation Family Study (Jackson et al., 1982; Jackson & Hatchett, 1986) of 510 three-generation lineage families are used in these analyses. The study consists of two linked samples collected from 1979 through 1981. The National Survey of Black Americans (NSBA) is the first cross-sectional nationally epresentative sample of 2,107 black Americans; the second study expands the sample by 2,443 respondents into a total of 510 complete three-generational lineages, and substantially more intergenerational dyads (Jackson, 1991). The two studies explored the role of family and intergenerational relations, the role of the church, physical and mental health, marriage and children, life satisfaction, racial ideology and identity, racial attitudes, education, employment, geographic proximity to children and parents, frequency and types of intergenerational contact, intergenerational transmission of information, advice, and affection, and the degree of psychological closeness between parents and children. The findings thusfar have revealed a great deal about the distribution of three-generation families, about family exchange patterns, the nature of family functioning, and some preliminary information about value and status transmission (Jackson & Hatchett, 1986).

STUDY VARIABLES AND DISTRIBUTIONS

Table 4.1 shows the major demographic variables used in the analyses. Generally, the distributions by generational position are consistent with expectations regarding changes across lineage position and historical occurrences. Thus, those in the oldest generation position reveal larger average ages than do those in the two lower positions. However, as is shown in the first panel in Table 4.1, there is considerable overlap in age, particularly among the middle and older lineage positions. Even without controls for age, blacks in the youngest position demonstrate considerably advanced educational attainment compared to those in either of the other two-generational positions. The family income distributions reveal the poor financial resources of all black fami-

Table 4.1. Distributions of Select Demographic Family Environment Measures by Generation Position (%)

Lineage Position by Age Categories								
Age	*13–24*	*25–34*	*35–45*	*46–54*	*55–64*	*65–74*	*75–84*	*85+*
Oldest	—	—	—	12.2	19.6	43.9	22.7	6.67
Middle	—	6.5	42.0	37.6	12.2	12.2	1.6	0.2
Youngest	64.7	32.1	2.4	0.6	—	—	—	—

Lineage Position by Years of Education					
Education	*Grade School*	*Some H.S.*	*H.S. Grad.*	*Some College*	*College Grad.+*
Oldest	47.2	40.2	8.5	2.4	1.8
Middle	9.3	43.1	29.4	10.8	7.4
Youngest	3.0	36.9	31.6	20.3	8.2

Lineage Position by Family Income Categories[1]							
Income	*$999*	*$4,999*	*$9,999*	*$14,999*	*$19,999*	*$24,999*	*$29,999*	*$30,000 +*
Oldest	5.2	41.3	31.6	10.6	4.3	3.1	2.2	1.8
Middle	2.0	14.5	24.3	19.3	12.2	11.2	8.1	8.6
Youngest	1.4	15.3	28.5	16.9	13.2	9.0	7.5	7.3

Lineage Position by Gender		
Gender	*Females*	*Males*
Oldest	72.4	27.6
Middle	70.4	29.6
Youngest	55.9	44.1

Lineage Position by Region		
Region	*South*	*Non-South*
Oldest	70.4	29.6
Middle	57.6	42.4
Youngest	58.4	41.6

[1] Figures represent upper limit of income category.

lies. As expected, those in the oldest lineage positions are the most skewed toward the lower end of the distribution. The middle and younger lineage members show a greater spread in income, but still remain relatively low in comparison to the general population.

The gender distributions, skewed toward females in the older two lineage positions, derive from sampling-selection factors in the study (Jackson & Hatchett, 1986), but more importantly from gender differences in all-cause mortality. Thus, females are heavily overrepresented in both the older and middle generations.

Chart 4.1 shows the distributions of the triads by generation position and gender. As shown, all-female triods are the predominant type (29.4%), contrasted with the all-male triads, which form only 3.9% of the 510 triads. Triads in which females are the largest number constitute

Chart 4.1.   Triad Gender Type

Gen 1	Gen 2	Gen 3	Frequency	Percentage
F	F	F	150	29.4
F	F	M	115	22.6
M	M	M	20	3.9
M	F	M	45	8.8
M	M	F	27	5.3
M	F	F	49	9.6
F	M	M	45	8.8
F	M	F	59	11.6
			510	100.0

43.8% of the total, and those in which males outnumber females contribute 22.9%.

In analyzing the gender environment variable, as shown in Table 4.1, the all-female triads are contrasted to all other triads. Table 4.1 also reveals a region pattern consistent with patterns of migration of the black population. In the oldest generation, approximately 70% of the respondents reside in the South, compared with the middle and the youngest generations, where approximately 58% of the sample reside in the South.

Chart 4.2 shows the heavy predominance of lineages in which all generation members reside in the same region, largely in the South. Because of the particular pattern shown in Chart 4.2, a set of two dummy variables representing all-lineage members residing in the South versus all-others and all-North versus all-others were used in the analyses summarized in Tables 4.4 through 4.8. In addition to the dummy variables described for gender and region types, education, age, and income were all averaged within lineages ($N = 3$) and scores assigned to each of the 510 triads.

Table 4.2 shows the items and distributions for the family proximity,

Chart 4.2.   Triad Region Type

Gen 1	Gen 2	Gen 3	Frequency	Percentage
S	S	S	269	52.7
S	S	N	13	2.5
N	N	N	130	25.5
N	S	N	2	0.4
N	N	S	9	1.8
N	S	S	10	2.0
S	N	N	67	13.1
S	N	S	10	2.0
			510	100.0

Table 4.2. Distributions of Family and Relative Proximity, Contact, Satisfaction Closeness and Exchange within Family Environments by Generation Position %

Lineage Position by Family Proximity

Where do most—that is, more than half—of your immediate family members live? (By immediate family, we mean your parents, children, brothers and sisters.)

Lineage Position	Household	Neighborhood	Same City	Same County	Same State	Other Place
Oldest	2.3	10.5	32.8	7.2	20.0	27.2
Middle	5.6	7.5	43.8	7.2	14.0	21.9
Youngest	29.5	7.5	33.2	4.9	13.9	11.4

Lineage Position by Relative Proximity (%)

A. How many of your relatives, not in your immediate family, live in this same house?

Lineage Position	Many	Some	A Few	None
Oldest	1.0	8.3	25.3	65.4
Middle	1.6	10.0	20.7	67.7
Youngest	5.7	11.2	18.5	64.7

B. How many of your relatives, not in your immediate family, live in this same neighborhood?

Oldest	10.5	11.8	34.3	43.5
Middle	7.8	11.2	24.0	57.0
Youngest	9.8	14.4	25.0	50.6

C. How many of your relatives, not in your immediate family, live in this same city?

Oldest	24.6	19.0	36.0	20.3
Middle	31.7	23.5	29.6	15.2
Youngest	46.1	18.8	21.6	13.5

D. How many of your relatives, not in your immediate family, live in this same county?

Oldest	18.1	19.2	30.4	32.3
Middle	21.9	18.4	28.8	30.9
Youngest	28.7	18.7	23.8	28.7

E. How many of your relatives, not in your immediate family, live in this same state?

Oldest	21.0	17.2	34.1	27.7
Middle	29.5	15.6	32.1	22.9
Youngest	35.7	20.0	24.9	19.5

(continued)

Table 4.2 Continued

Lineage Position	Household	Neighborhood	Same City	Same County	Same State	Other Place
F. How many of your relatives, not in your immediate family, live in another state?						
Oldest	25.2	25.2	39.0	10.6		
Middle	36.7	23.4	34.9	5.0		
Youngest	37.4	24.1	30.8	7.7		
G. How many of your relatives, not in your immediate family, live in another country?						
Oldest	1.3	1.3	12.2	85.2		
Middle	0.2	0.9	10.8	88.1		
Youngest	1.4	3.0	16.1	79.5		

Family Contact

How often do you see, write or talk on the telephone with family or relatives who do not live with you?

	Every Day	Once/ Week	Few Times/ Month	Once/ Month	Few Times/ Year	Never
Oldest	41.3	24.1	15.5	9.5	3.8	6.0
Middle	42.1	29.8	12.3	8.0	4.3	3.5
Youngest	34.6	30.7	15.8	5.9	7.1	6.0

Family Exchange

How often do people in your family—including children, grandchildren, grandparents, aunts, uncles, in-laws and so on—help out?

	Very Often	Fairly Often	Not Too Often	Never	You Never Need Help
Oldest	28.6	15.4	27.8	19.5	8.7
Middle	25.7	21.8	30.1	14.5	7.9
Youngest	42.8	30.4	19.1	4.9	2.8

Family Closeness

Would you say that family members are very close in their feelings to each other, fairly close, not too close or not close at all?

	Very Close	Fairly Close	Not Too Close	Not Close at All
Oldest	75.6	17.3	3.9	1.2
Middle	65.2	29.4	4.3	1.0
Youngest	59.8	33.7	5.1	1.4

(continued)

Table 4.2   Continued

Family Satisfaction

How satisfied are you with your family life—that is, the time you spend and the things you do with members of your family?

	Degree of Satisfaction			
Lineage Position	*Very Satisfied*	*Somewhat Satisfied*	*Somewhat Dissatisfied*	*Very Dissatisfied*
Oldest	79.2	18.0	1.8	0.6
Middle	55.0	35.8	8.4	0.6
Youngest	46.4	42.1	9.7	1.8

contact, satisfaction, closeness, and exchange variables by generational position. As shown, only a few significant differences in distributions by generational position are found. Since members of the third generation could be as young as 14, it is not surprising that nearly 30% report that most of their relatives live in the same household, as compared to 2.3 and 5.6% in the oldest and middle generations, respectively. For the most part, these distributions reveal strong similarities across generations; the bulk of the members in each generation report (52.6, 64.1, and 69.9% in the oldest, middle, and youngest, respectively) that their immediate family lives in the same county or closer. Although when asked about relatives, members of the oldest generation are slightly more likely that the others to report that their relatives live in their neighborhoods. For the most part, all generation members report relatively frequent contact with family and relatives.

Interestingly, both the oldest and youngest generations are equally likely (6.0%) to report never having contact with relatives. When asked about the frequency of exchanges, the youngest-generation members are most likely to indicate receiving assistance from relatives, followed by those in the oldest generation. On the other hand, the oldest-generation members are also the most likely to indicate that they never receive help and that they never need help. Overall, though, this item reveals that all generation members report receiving a great deal of family support.

While these differences in generation distributions are interesting, they reveal little about the nature of interactions within the lineages themselves. Just as with the sociodemographic factors, we hypothesize that lineages can be characterized as representing environments of contact, proximity, satisfaction, closeness, and intergenerational exchanges. Furthermore, these environments can be assessed through the measurement of perceptions and reports of each generation lineage member, and can then be averaged to represent the environmental context in which each lineage member resides (Zajonc, 1976). We propose that these environmental contexts are systematically related, ultimately influencing the nature of the exchange environments within lineages. Specifically, since the gender differences in help have been widely noted, we predicted that all-female lineages, controlling on resource environments, will be positively related to exchange environments. Similarly, we predicted that lineage environments having more all-South members will have higher exchange environments, again controlling on the resource environments.

We also hypothesized that the resource environmental factors of age, education, income, gender, and region will have little, if any, direct effects on the exchange environments, but instead will directly affect proximity, contact, satisfaction, and closeness environments, which, in turn, directly affect the exchange environments.

In the multivariate analyses described in the next section, the largest possible N is 510. Note that various lineage scores were developed based upon the standard deviation, variance, and position rank order of the size of the variables within the lineages. While these scores also show sufficient promise, the average-score approach to a family-level variable seems to demonstrate meaningful empirical relationships, is the easiest to understand conceptually, and is consistent with the approaches of prior studies that provide the theoretical rationale for developing our family environment framework (e.g., Jackson, Chatters, Taylor, & Chadiha, 1985; Zajonc & Markus, 1975).

In each of the variables, the average score was computed by taking the value on the variable within lineages and dividing by three. Each lineage was then assigned a score based upon this average. Table 4.3 provides a brief description of the averages for each variable. The nominal variables, gender and region, were described earlier in Charts 4.1 and 4.2. For age, the scores ranged from 31 to 69 with a mean of 46.3 average years for the lineages. Education environments ranged in average education from 3 to 17 years, with a grand mean of 9.8 years and a two-year standard deviation. Relative proximity environment, a summation and average of nonimmediate family living in each respondent's household, neighborhood, city, county, state, another state, and outside the United States, reveals a broad range of average scores. Approximately 2.2% of the sample indicate having environments in which no relatives live in close proximity, while a relatively small percentage (.2%) indicate having relatives in very close proximity.

The family proximity averages reveal a wide range of environment types with a high average proximal immediate family. Similarly, the

Table 4.3. Description of the Family Environment Averages[a]

Variable	Range	Mean	Standard Deviation	N
Age (years)	31–69	46.26	6.72	509
Education (years)	3–17	9.80	2.11	507
Income (categories)[b]	2–8	3.83	1.25	507
Relative Proximity (scale)	0–40	11.87	6.43	510
Family Proximity (scale)	2–6	3.55	1.12	309
Family Contact (scale)	1–5	2.26	1.02	320
Family Satisfaction (scale)	1–3	1.47	0.54	500
Family Closeness	1–3	1.34	0.52	502
Family Help	1–5	2.46	0.90	503

[a] Gender and Region are categorical and are not included in this table.
[b] Income ranged from categories of $000–999 to $30,000 plus. The average income of the lineages was in the range of $5,000 - $9,999.

average family contact is also relatively high. The original satisfaction scale (Table 4.2) was collapsed into three categories (Very, Some, and None) and as shown, the averages were high. Family closeness, collapsed in a similar manner, showed a similar pattern as satisfaction. Finally, the family help environments showed a reasonable spread across the index (Table 4.2).

MULTIVARIATE ANALYSES

Tables 4.4 through 4.8 present the results of the multivariate analyses, and explore possible indirect effects of these resource environments on the family help environment through their effects on proximity, contact, satisfaction, and closeness environments. We predicted that while the resource variables may have little or no independent effect on the help environment, they would influence family proximity, contact, closeness, and satisfaction environments.

Table 4.4 presents the results of the analyses that examine the effects of the resource environment variables on family and relative proximity. We expected age, income, and education to bear some relationship to reported proximity. As shown, all three are significantly related to proximity of relatives. Older average lineages, higher income, and highly educated environments are all related to lowered proximity of relatives. As has been reported, increased resources may be related to a thinning out of the support network. Somewhat surprisingly, the all-female triad, in contrast to all other compositions, is not a significant predictor of

Table 4.4. Ordinary Least Squares Hierarchical Regression Summary Tables—Relative and Family Proximity Environments

Family Environment Variables	Regression Coefficients	
	Relative Proximity b	*Family Proximity* b
Age	−0.11**	−.05**
Education	−0.20*	−.04
Income	−0.06**	−.09
Gender	−0.17	.03
(FFF = 1)		
Region	2.71**	.84**
(SSS = 1)	3.12**	.96**
(NNN = 1)		
R² (Adj.)	0.06**	.12**

FFF = All triad members Female
SSS = All triad members in South
NNN = All triad members in North
* $p < .05$
** $p < .01$

relative proximity environments. Region is also related to the proximity of relatives environment, such that both all-South and all-North lineages are significantly higher on the proximity measure than other regional groupings of the triads. For the proximity of family environment, average age of the lineage is again positively related. Increased age of the lineages is related to decreased proximity of family members within lineages. Education and income environments, unlike the case in the relative Proximity Model, are not related to proximity of immediate family environments. We found similar lack of effect for gender and a significant increase in proximal family environments for region homogeneity.

Table 4.5 shows the results of the regression of family contact environment on the base resource variables and proximity environments. The Base Model reveals a modest significant positive effect of increased income environments on the family contact environment. In addition, greater contact environments in all-female lineages and both all-South and all-North lineages, compared to all other patterns, report greater contact. The results of the Proximity Model analysis suggest that the region effects may be carried largely through reported relative contact, though some independent influence still remains. Notably, increased income, regardless of proximity, is significantly related to an increase in average contact environments. Similarly, female triads show greater contact regardless of other resources or relative proximity. Similarly, the

Table 4.5. Ordinary Least Squares Hierarchical Regression Summary Tables—Family Contact Environment

Family Environment Variables	Regression Coefficients	
	Base Model b	Proximity Model b
Age	.01	.01
Education	.04	.05
Income	.09+	.11*
Gender (FFF = 1)	.46**	.44**
Region		
(SSS = 1)	.36*	.29+
(NNN = 1)	.41*	.36+
Proximity		
family	NA	−.00
relatives	NA	.03**
R^2 (Adj.)	.06**	.09**
F (Increment)	NA	4.45*

FFF = All triad members Female
SSS = All triad members in South
NNN = All triad members in North
+ $p < .10$
* $p < .05$
** $p < .01$

region environments are not merely proxies for proximity; they do have an independent influence on contact, though a diminished one.

In Table 4.6 the results of the Base Model reveal that the positive family closeness environment can be predicted best by increased income environment and region of the country, with all-North triads showing significantly less family closeness in their environments than all other combinations of regionally distributed lineages. The Proximity Model, with a significant increase in explained variance ($F = 4.68$, $p < .01$), shows that these effects are independent of proximity, though increased relative proximity again shows a significant independent positive effect on family closeness. Region and income continue to exert independent influences. In fact, controlling on relative proximity results in a greater positive contribution of the income environment to the variation in the Family Closeness environment.

The Contact Model shows an even stronger effect of region (reduced closeness in northern triads) and the continued significant positive contribution of relative proximity. The family contact environment is highly significant, as indicated by the regression coefficient and the significant increment in the explained variance over Models 1 and 2. Income is no longer significant, suggesting that its effects on closeness of family envi-

Table 4.6. Ordinary Least Squares Hierarchical Regression Summary Tables—
Family Closeness Environment

	Regression Coefficients		
Family Environment Variables	Base Model b	Proximity Model b	Contact Model b
Age	.00	.00	.00
Education	.02	.02	.01
Income	.04+	.05*	.04+
Gender (Male = 0)	.10	.09	.05
Region	−.09	−.10	−.12
(South = 0)	−.29**	−.32**	−.34**
(North = 0)			
Proximity	NA	−.02	−.02
family	NA	.02**	.01*
relatives			
Family Contact	NA	NA	.08**
R² (Adj.)	.03**	.06**	.08**
F (Increment)	NA	4.68*	8.90**

FFF = All triad members Female
SSS = All triad members in South
NNN = All triad members in North
+ $p < .10$
* $p < .05$
** $p < .01$

ronment may be operating through its facilitative role in the positive family contact environment (See Table 4.6, Model 2).

Table 4.7 presents the models used to examine the relative influence of resource environments on the family satisfaction environment. First, no significant increment in explained variation is gained by adding the family proximity environment to the Base Model. Only a modest increase in explained variation is obtained by adding the family contact environment ($F = 2.20$, $p < .10$). As shown in all three models, family satisfaction is lowest in all-North lineages, perhaps indicating an impact of disorganized neighborhoods and living arrangements. This effect is independent of all other resources, and of proximity and contact.

Table 4.8 shows the nested hierarchial analysis on the family help environment. The Base Model reveals only one significant effect of the resource-related environments on the nature of the help environment in these lineages—the effect for income environment. Those families with higher average incomes report receiving higher average amounts of help. The Proximity Model that adds the two-family proximity variables reveals no significant effects. The income resource variable remains significant, although the overall regression accounts for only a modest proportion of the variance, which is not a significant increment over the

Table 4.7. Ordinary Least Squares Hierarchical Regression Summary Tables—Family Satisfaction Environment

Family Environment Variables	Regression Coefficients		
	Base Model b	*Proximity Model* b	*Contact Model* b
Age	.00	.00	.00
Education	−.02	−.02	−.02
Income	.02	.02	.02
Gender (Male = 0)	.06	.05	.05
Region			
(SSS = 1)	.04	.02	.01
(NNN = 1)	−.19*	−.22**	−.22*
Proximity			
family	NA	.01	.01
relatives	NA	.01	.01
Family Contact	NA	NA	.01
R² (Adj.)	.03*	.03*	.03*
F (Increment)	NA	.96(ns)	2.20+

FFF = All triad members Female
SSS = All triad members in South
NNN = All triad members in North
+ $p < .10$
* $p < .05$
** $p < .01$

Base Resource Model. Interestingly, the family proximity environment bears no relationship to the family help environment.

The third model adds the family contact environment variable to the previous equation. As shown, the regression is significant and the proportion of variation accounted for is a modest increment, though significant, over the Proximity Model alone. Income remains the only significant predictor, although those families with high average contact also tend to report higher average family help ($p < .11$). The Closeness Model is significant, and adds a significant increment to the variation explained over that provided by the Contact Model ($F = 7.09$, $p < .01$). While income remains a significant positive predictor of family help environment, positive family closeness environments account for a significant proportion of the variation in average family help over that of the Base and Proximity Models. The final regression, the Satisfaction Model, examines the incremental contribution of satisfaction to the average family help environments. This regression is significant, and adds a modest increment over the variation accounted for by the Closeness Model. High income and family closeness average family environments remain significantly related to high average help environments. In addition, reflecting the marginal increment in the variation explained by the

Table 4.8. Ordinary Least Squares Hierarchical Regression Summary Tables—
Family Help Environment

Family Environment Variables	*Regression Coefficients*				
	Base Model b	Proximity Model b	Contact Model b	Closeness Model b	Satisfaction Model b
Age	−.01	−.01	−.01	−.01	−.01
Education	−.00	−.00	−.01	−.01	−.00
Income	.13**	.13**	.12**	.11**	.11**
Gender (FFF = 1)	−.03	−.03	−.06	−.04	−.08
Region					
(SSS = 1)	.11	.07	.05	.08	.08
(NNN = 1)	−.03	−.07	−.10	−.00	.03
Proximity					
family	NA	.03	.03	.03	.03
relatives	NA	.01	.01	.00	.00
Family Contact	NA	NA	.07	.05	.05
Family Closeness	NA	NA	NA	.25**	.23**
Family Satisfaction	NA	NA	NA	NA	.17+
R^2 (Adj.)	.02*	.02+	.03*	.05**	.06**
F (Increment)	NA	.39(ns)	2.48+	7.09**	3.67+

FFF = All Triad Members Female
SSS = All Triad Members in South
NNN = All Triad Members in North
$^+ p < .10$
$^* p < .05$
$^{**} p < .01$

Satisfaction Model ($F = 3.67$, $p < .10$), family satisfaction environment is positively related to the average Help environment.

Thus, Table 4.8 reveals that a significant model of the interrelations among family environments does exist and that a model that includes closeness and satisfaction can account for a respectable proportion of the variation ($R^2 = 06$, $p < .01$). As predicted, most of the family resource environment variables bear no independent or joint relationships to the variance in the average amount of help found in black American three-generation families. Income is the only exception and, as might be expected, high average income environments are significantly related to higher average help environments, independent of any other variables. Contact, satisfaction, and closeness, all have independent relationships. High levels of perceived family closeness clearly constitutes the most important variable, while both proximity of relatives and family contact do not independently contribute to the overall explained variation in family help. These findings are consistent with some prior research on individual nonlineage, cross-sectional relationships that have found other network characteristics, in addition to family resources such as satisfaction, closeness, and proximity, to be important predictors of family assistance (e.g., Hatchett & Jackson, 1993; Jayakody, Chatters, & Taylor, 1993; Taylor, Chatters, & Jackson, 1993, 1993; Taylor & Chatters, 1991).

Though predicted, the lack of an effect on the environment of help received by age, gender, and educational resource environments is somewhat disconcerting. The income effect is reasonable and predictable. McAdoo (1987) has suggested that because of greater resources, black middle-class families might provide greater assistance to their members. Conversely, the seminal work by Stack (1974) suggested that a lack of tangible resources may contribute a great deal to the amount of help exchanged among multigeneration families. In either case, resources, in addition to the observed income effect, should bear some relationship to help environments.

Overall, these analyses reveal significant effects of age and education environments as resources for family proximity, but not family contact, family satisfaction, nor family closeness environments. Income appears to act as a facilitative factor in relative proximity and family contact environments which, in turn, are important predictors of perceived closeness environments. Region appears important as a proxy for proximity, facilitating contact, but also seems to have an independent role, perhaps indicating poor quality of life and thus low family satisfaction and closeness among lineages not in the South.

SUMMARY AND CONCLUSIONS

The Family Environment Context Model and approach address many of the issues raised earlier in the Introduction. We believe that it is the appropriate unit of analysis needed to understand the systemic, ecological nature of black family life. It may provide a useful approach to what has been a thorny set of issues in the family and multigenerational literature. The preliminary analyses reported in this chapter are a positive first step in ascertaining the theoretical and empirical advantages of conceptualizing and operationalizing measures of family environments as within-lineage averages of reports of a probability sample of multigenerational family members, and demonstrating that these measures would reveal predicted systematic and theoretically meaningful sets of relationships.

We have focused on the aggregate family level, attempting to understand how environmental contexts may be influenced by the relative presence or absence of other environmental features (Hoffman, 1991).

Zajonc (1976) has argued that intellectual environments exist and that they influence the intellectual development of their members. He conceded, however, that the intellectual properties of the social and physical environments were not the only features important for intellectual development. Others (e.g., Alwin, 1990; Blake, 1989) have argued that the appropriateness of the Confluence Model in accounting for intellectual functioning may be questioned.

To our knowledge, the fundamental issue of the existence, nature, and influence of aggregate family environments has not been seriously confronted (Alwin, 1990; Hermalin, 1983). We extend the thinking of Zajonc (1983) and others (e.g., Alwin, 1990; Blake, 1989; Hermalin, 1983) to argue that intellectual development is not the only feature; in fact, it may not even be the most important one (Alwin, 1990). Environmental factors other than the intellectual environment may be related in predictable and systematic ways to each other and to individual outcomes.

Our preliminary results are provocative, and they indicate significant interrelationships among lineage environments. The next steps will be to refine our measures and to examine more complicated and sophisticated multivariate models. Finally, we believe that structural equation modeling is the appropriate final outcome of this work (Godwin, 1985). In this approach, family environment is conceived as a latent variable with observed indicators represented by each lineage member's score on a particular construct measure. These latent variables should show the same types of relationship demonstrated in this chapter, which used a relatively crude analysis approach.

Finally, just as in the Confluence Model (Zajonc, 1983), we believe that each member of the lineage contributes to the environment and is also influenced by the environment that he or she helps to create. In fact, as we would also predict, the Confluence Model does not work without including the target of the influence environment as part of that environment (Zajonc, 1983). Thus, individual actors stand in reciprocal relationships, contributing to family environment features as well as being influenced by them. The Family Environment Context Model may provide a more ecologically valid and heuristically useful framework for studying and understanding the nature of reciprocal interactions and individual functioning within multigenerational families (Hagestad, 1981).

ACKNOWLEDGMENTS

This chapter is based on a paper presented at Conference on Aging and Generational Relations: A Historical and Cross-Cultural Perspective, Center for Family

Research, University of Delaware, October 10–13, 1991. Our appreciation goes to Donna Cochran, Keith Hersh, Linda Shepard, and Estina Thompson for assistance in the preparation and analysis of the data. We would like to thank our colleague Elizabeth Douvan, whose thinking and work on family issues contributed to the literature review in this chapter. We appreciate the Milbank Memorial Fund's support of the work by the third author.

REFERENCES

Allen, W. R. (1978). The search for applicable theories of black family life. *Journal of Marriage and the Family, 40,* 117–129.

———. (1979). Class, culture, and family organizations: The effects of class and race on family structure in urban America. *Journal of Comparative Family Studies, 10,* 301–313.

Alwin, D. F. (1990). *Family of origin and cohort differences in verbal intelligence.* Unpublished paper. Ann Arbor, MI: Institute for Social Research.

Antonucci, T. C. (1990). Social supports and social relations. In R. H. Binstock, & L. George (Eds.), *Handbook of aging and the social sciences,* 3rd ed. (pp. 105–117) New York: Academic Press, 205–227.

Antonucci, T. C., & Akiyama, H. (1987). An examination of sex differences in social support among older men and women. *Sex Roles, 17,* 737–749.

Antonucci, T. C., & Jackson, J. S. (1990). The role of reciprocity in social support. In I. G. Sarason, B. R. Sarason, & G. R. Pierce (Eds.), *Social support: An interactional view* (pp. 173–198). New York: John Wiley & Sons.

Belle, D. (1982). The stress of caring: Women as providers of social support. In L. Goldberg & S. Breznitz (Eds.), *Handbook of stress: Theoretical and clinical aspects* (pp. 496–505). New York: Free Press, 496–505.

Bengtson, V., Cutler, N., Mengen, D., & Marshall, V. (1985). Generations, cohorts, and relations between age groups. *Handbook of aging and the social sciences.* New York: Van Nostrand Reinhold.

Bengtson, V., Rosenthal, C., & Burton, L. (1990). Families and aging: Diversity and heterogeneity. In R. H. Binstock & L. George (Eds.), *Handbook of aging and the social sciences* (pp. 263–287). New York: Academic Press.

Berkman, L. S., & Syme, S. L. (1979). Social networks, host resistance, and morality: A nine-year follow-up study of Alameda County residents. *American Journal of Epidemiology, 109,* 186–204.

Billingsley, A. (1968). *Black families in white America.* Englewood Cliffs, NJ: Prentice Hall.

Blake, J. (1989). *Family size and achievement.* Berkeley: University of California Press.

Blazer, D. G. (1982). Social support and mortality in an elderly population. *American Journal of Epidemiology, 115,* 684–694.

Bowman, P. J. & Howard, C. (1985). Race-related socialization, motivation and academic achievement: A study of black youth in three-generation families. *Journal of the American Academy of Child Psychiatry, 24,* 134–141.

Bronfenbrenner, U. (1979). *The ecology of human development: Experiments by nature and design.* Cambridge, MA: Harvard University Press.

———. (1986). Ecology of the family as a context for human development: Research perspectives. *Developmental Psychology, 22,* 723–742.

Burton, L., & Bengtson, V. (1985). Black grandmothers: Issues of timing and continuity of roles. In V. L. Bengtson & J. F. Robertson (Eds.) *Grandparenthood.* Beverly Hills, CA: Sage.

Burton, L., & Dilworth-Anderson, P. (1991). The intergenerational family roles of aged black Americans. In S. K. Pifer, & M. B. Sussman (Eds.), *Families: Intergenerational and generational connections* (pp. 311–330). New York: Hayworth Press.

Cauce, A. M. (1991). *Ecological correlates of development in African American early adolescents.* Paper presented at the University of Denver, January.

Cheal, D. (1983). Intergenerational family transfers. *Journal of Marriage and the Family, 45,* 805–813.

Clark, M. S. (1984). Record keeping in two types of relationships. *Journal of Personality and Social Psychology, 47,* 549–557.

Cohen, S., & Syme, L. (Eds.) (1985). *Social support and health.* New York: Academic Press.

Demos, J. (1970). *A little commonwealth: Family life in Plymouth colony.* New York: Oxford University Press.

Dodson, J. (1981). Conceptualizations of black families. In H. P. McAdoo (Ed.), *Black families* (pp. 77–90). Beverly Hills, CA: Sage.

Dowd, J. J. (1984). Beneficence and aged. *Journal of Gerontology, 39,* 102–108.

Dowd, J. J., & Bengston, V.L. (1978). Aging in minority populations: An examination of the double jeopardy hypothesis. *Journal of Gerontology, 33,* 427–436.

Duncan, G. J. (1984). *Years of poverty—Years of plenty.* Ann Arbor: Institute for Social Research, University of Michigan.

Duncan, G. J., & Hill, M. S. (1985). Conceptions of longitudinal households: Fertile or futile? *Journal of Economic and Social Measurement, 13,* 361–375.

Elder, G. H., Jr. (1985a). Household, kinship and the life course: Perspectives on black families and children. In M. Spencer, G. Brookins, & W. Allen (Eds.), *Beginnings: The Social and Affective Development of Black Children* (pp. 29–43). Hillside, NJ: Lawrence Erlbaum Associates.

———. (Ed.) (1985b). *Life course dynamics: Trajectories and transitions, 1968–1980.* Ithaca: Cornell University Press.

Farley, R. (1984). *Blacks and whites: Narrowing the gap?* Cambridge, MA: Harvard University Press.

Farley, R., & Allen, W. (1988). *Across the color line: Race differences in the quality of U. S. life.* New York: Russell Sage Foundation.

Foa, U., & Foa, E. (1974). *Societal structures of the mind.* Springfield, IL: Charles C. Thomas.

Garbarino, J. (1982). *Children and families in the social environment.* Hawthorne, NY: Aldine de Gruyter.

Glass, J., Bengtson, V. L., & Dunham, C. C. (1986). Attitude similarity in three-generation families: Socialization, status, inheritance, or reciprocal influence. *American Sociological Review, 51*, 685–698.

Godwin, D. D. (1985). Simultaneous equations methods in family research. *Journal of Marriage and the Family, 47*, 9–22.

Goldman, N. (1986). Effects of mortality and fertility levels on kinship. In *Consequences of mortality trends and differentials* (pp. 79–87). New York: The United Nations.

Hagestad, G. O. (198l). Problems and promises in the social psychology of intergenerational relations. In J. March (Ed.), *Aging: Stability and change in the family.* New York: Academic Press.

———. (1982). The continuous bond: A Dynamic, Multigenerational Perspective on Parent-Child Relations Between Adults. In M. Perlmutter (Ed.), *Parent-child interaction and parent-child relations in child development.* The Minnesota Symposium on Child Psychology, Volume 17.

———. (1990). Social perspectives on the life course. In R. H. Binstock, & L. Goerge (Eds.), *Handbook of Aging and the Social Sciences* (pp. 151–168). New York: Academic Press.

Hagestad, G. O., & Burton, L. (1986). Grandparenthood, life context and family development. *American Behavioral Scientist, 29*, 471–484.

Hatchett, S. J., & Jackson, J. S. (1993). African American extended kin systems: An assessment. In H. P. McAdoo (Ed.), *Family ethnicity: Strengths in diversity.* Newbury Park, CA: Sage.

Hermalin, A. I. (1983). *Individuals, siblings and the family: Perspectives on the sociology of the family.* Paper presented at a Workshop on Family Research in Asia, East-West Population Center, Honolulu, Hawaii.

Hill, M. S. (1983). Trends in the economic situation of U.S. families and children: 1970–1980. In R. R. Nelson & F. Skidmore (Eds.), *American families and the economy* (pp. 9–58). Washington, DC: National Academy Press.

———. (1992). *The panel study of income dynamics: A user's guide.* Newbury Park, CA: Sage Publications.

Hill, R. (1970a). *Family development in three generations: A longitudinal study of changing family patterns of planning and achievement.* Cambridge, MA: Schenkman.

———. (1970b). The three-generation research design: Method for studying family and social change. In R. Hill & R. Konig (Eds.), *Families in east and west* (pp. 536–551). Paris: Mouton.

Hill, R., & Konig R. (1970). *Families in east and west.* Paris: Mouton.

Hill, R. B. (1981a). *Economic policies and black progress: Myths and realities.* Washington, DC: National Urban League.

———. (1981b). Multiple public benefits and poor black families. In H. P. McAdoo (Ed.), *Black families* (pp. 306–318). Beverly Hills, CA: Sage.

Hoffman, L. W. (1991). The influence of family environment on personality: Accounting for sibling differences. *Psychological Bulletin, 110*, 187–203.

House, J. S., Landis, K. R., & Umberson, D. (1988). Social relationships and health. *Science, 241*, 540–544.

House, J. S., Robbins, C., & Metzner, H. C. (1982). The association of social relationships and activities with mortality: Perspective evidence from the Tecumseh health study. *American Journal of Epidemiology. 116*, 123–140.

Huston, T. L., & Robins, E. (1982). Conceptual and methodological issues in studying close relationships. *Journal of Marriage and the Family, 44*, 901–925.

Ingersoll-Dayton, B., & Antonucci, T. C. (1988). Non-reciprocal social support: Another side of intimate relationships. *Journal of Gerontology: Social Sciences, 43*, 65–73.

Jackson, J. S. (Ed.) (1991). *Life in black America.* Newbury Park, CA: Sage.

Jackson, J. S., & Antonucci, T. C. (1994). Survey methodology in life-span human development research. In S. H. Cohen & H. W. Reese (Eds.), *Life-span developmental psychology: Methodological interventions.* Hillsdale, NJ: Lawrence Erlbaum Associates.

Jackson, J. S., Antonucci, T. C. & Gibson, R. C. (1990). Cultural, racial and ethnic influences on aging. In J. E. Birren & K. W. Schaie (Eds.), *Handbook of the psychology of aging,* 3rd ed. (pp. 103–123). New York: Academic Press.

Jackson, J. S., Chatters, L. M., Taylor, R. J. & Chadiha, L. (1985). *Well-being in three generation family lineage environments.* Paper presented at the International Association of Gerontology XIII Meeting, New York.

Jackson, J. S., & Hatchett, S. J. (1986) Intergenerational research: Methodological considerations. In N. Datan, A. L.Greene, & H. W. Reese (Eds.), *Intergenerational relations.* Hillsdale, NJ: Lawrence Erlbaum Associates.

Jackson, J. S., Tucker, M. B., & Bowman, P. J. (1982). Conceptual and methodological problems in survey research on black Americans. In W. T. Liu (Ed.), *Methodological problems in minority research* (pp. 11–40). Pacific/Asian American Mental Health Research Center.

Jayakody, R., Chatters, L. M., & Taylor, R. J. (1993). Family support to single and married African American mothers: The provision of financial, emotional, and child-care assistance. *Journal of Marriage and the Family, 55*(2).

Kitson, G. C., Sussman, M. B., Williams, G. K., et al. (1982). Sampling issues in family research. *Journal of Marriage and the Family, 44*, 965–981.

LaRossa, R., & Wolf, J. H. (1985). On qualitative family research. *Journal of Marriage and the Family, 41*, 531–541.

Lasch, C. (1977). *Haven in a heartless world: The family besieged.* New York: Basic Books.

Lee, G. R. (1988). Aging and intergenerational relations. *Journal of Family Issues, 8*, 448–450.

Loury, G. (1985). Beyond civil rights. *The New Republic,* October 7.

Mangen, D. J., Bengtson, V. L., Landry, P. H., Jr. (Eds.) (1988). *Measurement of intergenerational relations.* Beverly Hills, CA: Sage.

Markides, K. S., Boldt, J. S., & Ray, L. A. (1986). Sources of helping and intergenerational solidarity: A three generational study of Mexican Americans. *Journal of Gerontology, 41*, 506–511.

Markides, K. S., & Cole, T. (1984). Change and continuity in Mexican American religious behavior: A three-generation study. *Social Science Quarterly, 65*, 618–625.

Markides, K. S., & Krause, N. (1985). Intergenerational solidarity and psychological wellbeing among older Mexican Americans: A three-generation study. *Journal of Gerontology, 40*, 390–392.

McAdoo, H. P. (1978). Factors related to stability in upwardly mobile black families. *Journal of Marriage and the Family, 40*, 762–778.

———. (1987). *Black families.* 2nd Ed. Beverly Hills, CA: Sage.

Medalie, J. H., & Goldbourt, U. (1976). Angina pectoris among 10,000 men: Psychological and other factors evidenced by a multivariate analysis of a 5-year incidence study. *American Journal of Medicine, 60*, 910–921.

Mitchell, J., & Register, J. C. (1984). An exploration of family interaction with the elderly by race, socioeconomic status and residence. *The Gerontologist, 24*, 48–54.

Moynihan, D. (1965). *The negro family: The case for national action.* U.S. Department of Labor: Office of Planning and Research.

Murray, C. (1985). *Losing ground: American social policy 1950–1980.* New York: Basic Books.

Mutran, E. (1985). Intergenerational family support among blacks and whites: Response to culture or to socioeconomic differences. *Journal of Gerontology, 40*, 382–89.

Nobles, W. (1978). Toward an empirical and theoretical framework for defining black families. *Journal of Marriage and the Family, 40*, 679–698.

Orth-Gomer, D., & Johnson, J. V. (1987). Social network interaction and mortality: A six year follow-up study of a random sample of the Swedish population. *Journal of Chronic Disease, 40*(10), 949–57.

Roberts, R. E. L., & Bengtson, V.L. (1990). Is intergenerational solidarity a unidimensional construct? A second test of a formal model. *Journal of Gerontology, 45*, S12–20.

Ryder, N. B. (1974). *Reproductive behavior and the family life cycle. In The Population Debate: Dimensions and Perspectives.* Papers presented at the World Population Conference, Bucharest, Vol 2 (pp. 278–288). New York: The United Nations.

Schoenbach, V. J., Kaplan, B. H., Fredman, L., & Kleinbaum, D. H. (1986). Social ties and mortality in Evans County, Georgia. *American Journal of Epidemiology, 123*, 577–591.

Stack, C. B. (1974). All our kin: Strategies for survival in a black urban community. New York: Harper and Row.

Staples, R., & Mirande, A. (1980). Racial and cultural variations among American families: A decennial review of the literature on minority families. *Journal of Marriage and the Family, 42*, 157–173.

Stevens, J. H. (1984). Black grandmothers' and black adolescent mothers' knowledge about parenting. *Developmental Psychology, 20*, 1017–1025.

Taylor, R. J. (1986). Receipt of support from family among black Americans: Demographic and familial differences. *Journal of Marriage and the Family, 48*, 67–77.

———. (1988). Aging and supportive relationships among black Americans. In J. S. Jackson (Ed.), *The black American elderly: Research on physical and psychosocial health.* Springer: New York.

Taylor, R. J., Chatters, L. M., & Jackson, J. S. (1993). A profile of familial relations among three generation black American families. *Family Relations, 42*, July, 332–341.

Taylor, R. J., & Chatters, L. M. (1991). Extended family networks of older black adults. *Journal of Gerontology: Social Sciences, 46*, S210–217.

Taylor, R. J., Chatters, L. M., Tucker, M. B., & Lewis, E. (1990). Developments in research on black families: A decade review. *Journal of Marriage and the Family, 52*, 993–1014.

Thompson, L., & Walker, A. J. (1982). The dyad as the unit of analysis: Conceptual and methodological issues. *Journal of Marriage and the Family, 44*, 889–900.

Thornton, A., & Rodgers, W. (1987). The influence of individual and historical time on marital dissolution. *Demography, 24*, 1–22.

Troll, L. E., & Bengtson, V. L. (1979). Generations and the family. In W.R. Burr, R. Hill, F. I. Nye, & I. L. Reiss (Eds.), *Contemporary theories about the family.* Vol 1 (pp. 127–160). New York: Free Press.

Veroff, J., Kulka, R. A., & Douvan, E. (1981). *Mental health in America: Patterns of help-seeking from 1957 to 1976.* New York: Basic Books.

Wilson, M. N. (1986). The black extended family: An analytical consideration. *Developmental Psychology, 22*, 246–256.

Woehrer, C. E. (1978). Cultural pluralism in American families: The influence of ethnicity on social aspects of aging. *The Family Coordinator*, October, 329–339.

Zajonc, R. B. (1976). Family configuration and intelligence. *Science, 192*, 227–236.

———. (1983). Validating the confluence model. *Psychological Bulletin, 93*, 457–480.

Zajonc, R. B., & Markus, G. B. (1975). Birth order and intellectual development. *Psychological Review, 82*, 74–88.

5

The Demography of Family Care
for the Elderly

Douglas A. Wolf, Beth J. Soldo, and Vicki Freedman

INTRODUCTION

In theory, older Americans can draw upon three types of resources: their own economic resources resulting from savings and investments made over the life cycle; informal transfers of resources from family, friends, and other nonmarket sources, such as charitable programs; and public transfers provided through programs operated by governments. Over time, a pattern has emerged in which the public sector has assumed primary responsibility for acute health care and income maintenance programs for the elderly (Moroney, 1986). The responsibility for chronic health care, however, has come to be shared by the private and public sectors.

The alliance of state, market, and family in providing and financing long-term care is neither systematic nor comprehensive (Soldo, Agree, & Wolf, 1989). The public sector has committed vast resources to financing institutional care for impoverished elderly, assigning almost exclusive responsibility for community care to the private sector. Medicaid covers about half the cost of nursing home episodes for older Americans; nursing home residents and their families finance the other half, primarily with out-of-pocket expenditures (Levit, Freeland, & Waldo, 1990). For the noninstitutionalized elderly with chronic care needs, however, Medicare and Medicaid offer only restricted benefits for paid care and for limited periods of time. The vast majority of noninstitutionalized frail elderly, therefore, depend on informal helpers, primarily their kin. Even at extreme levels of disability, nearly 60% of the disabled elderly rely

primarily on family caregivers (Soldo, Agree, & Wolf, 1989; Stone, Cafferata, & Sangl, 1987).

The demand for informal care in response to chronic disability is
substantial, and is likely to increase as the U.S. population continues to
age (Soldo & Agree, 1988). Estimates from the 1982 National Long Term
Care Survey (NLTCS) indicate that nearly 20% of noninstitutionalized
elderly have at least some limitation in their ability to care for themselves. Of these 4.6 million elderly, 850,000 had severe limitations in
daily activities. The prevalence of disability increases with age, such that
49% of those 85 and over and living in the community have difficulty
with at least some self-care activities. Recent research in the United
States has addressed the ways in which the family organizes itself in
response to the personal care needs of its elderly members (e.g., Cantor,
1980; Doty, 1986; Horowitz, 1985; Wolf & Soldo, 1990).

This chapter addresses issues in the demography of family care of the
elderly. We raise several questions from the perspective of potential
caregivers: What proportion of the population is liable to be called upon
to care for an elderly parent? And how is this potential care burden
distributed among siblings? We also consider these issues from the perspective of the elderly: What is the availability of children to serve as
potential caregivers: What are the chances of being without spouse or
children in old age?

At the *family* level, these questions are related to patterns of fertility,
mortality, and marriage. At the *population* level, changes in fundamental
demographic processes alter the relative size of the elderly and nonelderly populations, and raise questions about the allocation of public
resources to competing ends. In this chapter we focus on the family level.

Our goal is to identify issues that should be addressed in quantitative
models whose scope is defined by the intersection of three key areas of
demographic research: family patterns, health, and care of the elderly.
Many of the questions raised are somewhat technical, and in some cases
there is a clear need for better theoretical groundwork. Our intention,
however, is not to suggest answers, but to pose questions that should
guide later model-building efforts.

First, we consider the structure of kin networks, from the perspective
of both the older and younger generations. We then examine health and
disability—the factors that create demands for personal care, whether
provided by family members or by others. Finally, we discuss the consequences of kin patterns and care needs jointly: Given a particular
pattern of health or functional problems, and given a particular configuration of available kin, what family-care patterns are likely to be
observed?

KIN NETWORKS OF THE ELDERLY: DESCRIPTIVE DATA
ON THE COMPOSITION OF KIN NETWORKS

Data that allow us to describe an individual's position in his or her kin network is rare. In recent decades only a few sample surveys have included information on the number of—and, less often, the characteristics of—relatives living outside the sample households. Two new data bases containing unusually rich data on the composition of the extended family and transfer behaviors are the Health and Retirement Survey (HRS) and the Survey of Asset and Health Dynamics (AHEAD). The HRS targets persons age 51 to 61 in 1992; the AHEAD draws on the HRS screening activity to identify persons age 70 and over in 1993. Both surveys provide extensive data on children, parents, and siblings of respondents, and their spouses. Transfers of time and money between specified family members can also be identified. Data from both the HRS and the AHEAD are publicly available. Data from a second round of HRS interviewing, collected in 1994, was released in 1995.

Another relatively recent survey that has collected detailed information on the kin networks of respondents is the 1987–88 National Survey of Families and Households (NSFH). The NSFH is a nationally representative survey of noninstitutionalized adults living the United States designed to provide comprehensive information on a variety of family issues (Sweet, Bumpass, & Call, 1988). Each respondent was asked to provide information on children, siblings, and parents (both in and outside of the household). Similar information was collected from spouses.

Data from the NSFH allow us to identify the proportion of the adult population potentially at risk of providing care for an elderly parent. Table 5.1 shows the distribution of the adult population by age, number of siblings, and the existence of an elderly mother. The columns display for several age groups the percentage of respondents with a living mother age 65–84, followed by the corresponding percentage of adults with a mother age 85 or older, and finally by those whose mother is either nonelderly or deceased. Adults with a living mother are further classified by the number of living siblings.

Although adults with either a nonelderly or a deceased mother constitute the majority of all three age groups shown in the table, nearly half of persons age 40–64 have a living elderly mother (44.6%). Over one-quarter of the adults in this age group with a living mother have no siblings of their own; such children have a higher risk than their counterparts with siblings of providing parental care.[1]

Table 5.1. Distribution of Adult Population by Age, Existence and Age of Mother and Number of Siblings (%)

	Age Group			
	Age 19–39	Age 40–64	Age 65+	Total
Mother age 65–84				
0 siblings	2.7%	10.5	0.1	5.0
1 sibling	1.9	7.1	0.3	3.5
2 siblings	2.5	7.5	0.1	3.9
3 siblings	1.5	4.8	0.1	2.4
4+ siblings	3.4	10.0	0.2	5.3
Mother age 85+				
0 siblings	0.0	1.2	1.4	0.7
1 sibling	0.0	0.9	0.6	0.4
2 siblings	0.0	0.8	0.6	0.4
3 siblings	0.0	0.4	0.3	0.2
4+ siblings	0.0	1.3	1.3	0.7
Other				
(mother <65 or deceased)	87.9	55.4	95.0	77.7
Total	100.0	100.0	100.0	100.0

Source: 1987–1988 National Survey of Families and Households.

Kin availability from the perspective of an older woman is reflected in Table 5.2, in which we present the distribution of older women in the NSFH by age and number of living children. In 1988, one in five elderly women had no living children; among the oldest elderly (those age 85 and older), 37% were without a living child. Assuming continued improvements in life expectancy at age 65, the proportion of adults with a living elderly mother is likely to increase. Projections of family caregivers indicate that the proportion of childless elderly women will decline modestly over the next 20 years (Himes, 1992); however, as the baby boom generation reaches old age, this trend is expected to reverse. Thus, in the short run, more adult children will be at risk for providing parent care, and a greater proportion of the elderly will have children potentially available to provide such care.

Whether or not adult children actually deliver personal care services to parents is related to a host of demographic, economic, and health-related factors. Despite increased numbers of adult children at risk for parent care, the prevalence of family caregiving may decline in the future if more adult children are faced with competing demands from child or grandchild care and from market activity (Doty, 1986; Stone & Short, 1990). Such trends do not necessarily translate into a reduction in care received by disabled parents, since children may use their earnings to finance private care of parents or to purchase assistive equipment not covered by public insurance programs.

Table 5.2.   Distribution of Older Women by Age and Number of Living Children (%)

Number of Living Children:	Age Group		
	65–84	*85+*	*Total*
0	19.8	37.0	21.0
1	15.7	15.7	15.7
2	22.2	22.5	22.3
3	17.9	08.7	17.3
4	09.9	04.7	09.5
5+	14.5	11.4	14.3
Total	100.0	100.0	100.0
Percent of Older Women	92.8	07.2	100.0

Source: 1987–1988 National Survey of Families and Households

MODELING KIN NETWORKS

In order to understand better why kin networks look the way they do and to investigate their dynamics, we must go beyond descriptive data and develop models of kin networks. This has been an area of considerable activity among demographers in recent years. Some effort has gone into analytic models—the best-known being that of Goodman, Keyfitz, and Pullum (1974, 1975), who derived expressions for the expected number of female kin for several ascending and descending generations and degrees of remove from the reference person (ego), by age of ego. This model is limited in that the kin are not themselves classified by age; nor does the model yield the frequency distributions underlying the expectations. Another class of analytic kin models are those based upon branching processes (Pullum, 1982). These models can be used to produce full frequency distributions of kin numbers, but generally dispense with the age dimension altogether, greatly limiting their usefulness.

Microsimulation techniques have been used to develop still more detailed kin models. The microsimulation models are operationalized as computer programs, often bearing descriptive names such as MOMSIM (Ruggles, 1987), SOCSIM (Hammel et al., 1989), or KINSIM (Wolf, 1988); for a survey of these and related efforts see De Vos and Palloni (1989). The common feature of such models is their use of probabilistic techniques (the Monte Carlo method) to assign attributes to individuals in a population, such as dates of birth, death, marriage, and birth of own children. Data fields that record linkages between individuals in the simulated population can be manipulated to provide details of kin networks at a point in time or, in some approaches, over the life cycle.

An assumption made in virtually all kin models is that the various demographic events underlying kin patterns are independent—that is, that the fertility of mothers and daughters is uncorrelated, that mortality is independent within and across generations, and that mating is random with respect to kin patterns across potential mates. Ruggles (1987), speaking specifically of fertility, called this the "whopper assumption," highlighting its highly questionable nature. In the remainder of this section, we focus on the issue of independence, or lack thereof, of these demographic outcomes.

Correlations between Counts of Living Kin

If demographic events are correlated along family lines, then we would expect to see correlations of various counts of kin by type: For example, if women whose mothers had many children also have many children of their own, then there should be a positive correlation between numbers of siblings and numbers of aunts and uncles, and between numbers of siblings and numbers of children. Similar associations could be anticipated if longevity were passed from generation to generation. The converse, however, is not necessarily true: Pullum and Wolf (1991) demonstrated that there are "built-in" correlations among certain kin counts, such as number of children and number of grandchildren, even when all demographic events are independent.

In Table 5.3, we again use the NSFH data to illustrate the magnitude of correlations between selected indicators of kin network composition. With the NSFH data, our analysis is limited to counts of parents, siblings, and children. The correlations shown in the table pertain to *living* kin, and therefore reflect the combined effects of fertility and mortality. Table 5.3 shows a fairly consistent pattern of significant positive correlation between numbers of siblings and numbers of children. Particularly for the younger age groups (ages 19–59), the most likely explanation for the correlations is positively correlated fertility between mothers and daughters. A number of scholars have provided evidence of such a correlation, including Anderton, Tsuya, Bean and Mineau (1987), Hodge and Ogawa (1986), and Danziger and Newman (1989).

One initially puzzling aspect of Table 5.3 is the negative correlation between the number of living parents (which can only equal 0, 1, or 2) and the number of children, for those under age 50. However, this may reflect intergenerational transmission of fertility patterns as well: That is, if having fewer living parents is associated with being born late in one's parents' lives (as is likely), then it may also be associated with having more siblings (most or all of whom are older). This would lead to a

Table 5.3. Correlations between Counts of Kin, by Age

Age Group	N	Correlation Coefficients Parents/Siblings	Correlation Coefficients Parents/Children	Correlation Coefficients Siblings/Children
19–29 Years	1795	−0.07**	−0.07**	0.18**
30–39 Years	1889	−0.07**	−0.08**	0.16**
40–49 Years	1025	−0.08**	−0.09**	0.07*
50–59 Years	759	−0.05	−0.00	0.14**
60–69 Years	738	0.04	0.02	0.01
70–84 Years	705	−0.02	0.03	0.12**
85+ Years	86	0.00	0.00	−0.01

* $.01 \leq p < .05$
** $p < .01$
Source: 1987–88 National Survey of Families and Households

negative association between number of living parents and number of children, operating through the hypothesized positive association between number of siblings and number of children. There is, in fact, direct evidence of the negative association between number of parents and number of siblings, shown in the first column of the table.

It must be acknowledged, however, that alternative explanations for some of the patterns shown in Table 5.3 can be imagined. For example, it may be that people who experience a parent's death while young tend to marry early, hastening their own likelihood to bear children. The negative correlation between numbers of parents and siblings may arise in part because the death of a parent removes the parent from risk of further childbearing, but it may also reflect intergenerational transmission of longevity.

There is more direct evidence of such intergenerational correlations of mortality in other research. A number of researchers have addressed the "heritability of longevity" (Abbot, Abbey, Bolling, & Murphy, 1978; Desjardins & Charbonneau, 1990; Pearl, 1931; Pearl & Pearl, 1934; Phillipe, 1978). These studies have indicated that any index of such heritability must be very small, although positive. Recent models of mortality that incorporate unobserved "frailty" parameters fixed over the lifetime suggest that the upper bound on correlations between observed ages at death is quite small, even with perfect inheritance of frailty (Vaupel, 1988). The newest empirical research directed at the heritability of longevity has employed data on twins (e.g., Hougaard, Harvald, & Holm, 1992), and has found evidence of within-pair dependence of lifetimes; however, the estimated dependence is so small that knowing one twin's survival status provides only slight improvement in the ability to predict the other twin's survival.

Assortive Mating and Kin Patterns

Another possible departure from independence among the behaviors underlying kin patterns concerns mate selection. In particular, if husbands' and wives' sibling counts are not randomly distributed, there may be consequences for the competition between husbands' and wives' elderly parents for care. A related issue concerns the possibility of non-random mating with respect to genetic determinants of longevity (or, more plausibly, with respect to health and environmental conditions that influence mortality). The latter sort of nonrandomness also would have consequences for the overall distribution of kin networks, and for possible correlations between the counts of own and in-law kin.

The distribution of married men and women according to the number of husband's and wife's siblings is shown in Table 5.4. There is some evidence of positive assortive mating—that is, of a tendency to marry those with similar sibling counts (the χ^2 statistic for the cross-tabulation is 164.38, which with 25 degrees of freedom easily exceeds the .001 level of statistical significance). The sum of the diagonal elements of the table is 21.03%, well above the 14.55% figure that would be expected under random mating. We do not mean to suggest that mate selection takes place on the basis of the number of siblings a potential spouse has. Undoubtedly, family size is correlated with other social and economic factors, such as race, religion, ethnicity, economic status, and educational attainment, which intervene more directly in shaping the pools from which spouses are selected. Nevertheless, the patterns we have observed, whatever their origin, have implications for family care for the elderly.

Table 5.4. Distribution of Married Couples by Husband's and Wife's Number of Siblings (%)

Husband's Number of Siblings	Wife's Number of Siblings						
	0	1	2	3	4	5+	Total
0	2.17	2.99	1.61	2.32	2.36	1.76	13.20
1	2.01	3.43	4.51	1.67	1.16	3.80	16.57
2	2.24	4.39	5.12	3.35	2.42	2.52	20.04
3	2.35	2.66	3.56	3.56	2.27	4.19	18.60
4	1.57	1.24	2.52	2.04	1.31	2.72	11.39
5+	2.72	3.03	2.46	3.78	2.76	5.44	20.19
Total	13.05	17.74	19.79	16.72	12.28	20.43	100.00

Source: 1987–1988 National Survey of Families and Households

DEMOGRAPHIC MODELS OF HEALTH

Unprecedented increases in life expectancy at age 65 and even at ages 85 and 95 have spurred interest in the extent to which improvements in survivorship translate into improved health of the elderly. Research addressing this issue has proceeded along two not entirely independent lines. At the population level, considerable work has been done over the last ten years on strategies for estimating what has become known as "active" or disability-free life expectancy (Manton & Stallard, 1991; Rogers, Rogers, & Belanger, 1989; Wilkins & Adams, 1983). While the methods used vary considerably, as do the assumptions employed about the nature of disease processes, there appears to be a consensus that a direct correspondence does not exist between additional years of *total* life expectancy and of *disability-free* life expectancy. Estimates of the ratio of increases in disability-free life expectancy to total life expectancy range from 60 to 78%.

Of more direct concern for this chapter are studies that attempt to model the disease process itself. In a series of papers, Manton and his colleagues have called attention to three aspects of disease processes which models of underlying disease-disability processes must take into account. First, because these processes are both multidimensional in nature and variable in intensity (Manton & Stallard, 1991), modeling disability with simple discrete indicators does not accurately represent the heterogeneity of the older population (Manton, Corder, & Clark, 1991). Second, contrary to popular assumptions, chronic disease and disability are not necessarily degenerative. Evidence from two U.S. data sources—the 1984–86 Longitudinal Survey of the Aged (LSOA) of elderly living in the community and the 1982–84 NLTCS data for frail elderly—indicates that the potential to recover function is far greater than once envisioned. Approximately one in five impaired elderly improve in functional capacity over a 24-month period (Kovar, 1988; Manton, 1988). Third, a true representation of disease and disability processes in the elderly must take into account the substantial co-morbidities—the presence of multiple, nonindependent, potentially interacting chronic diseases or conditions—found in this population. Failure to account for this phenomenon results in exaggerated claims of improvements in life expectancy and reductions in health care costs (Manton et al., 1991).

While complex models of disease states and transitions have been developed in which disease processes are represented by markers of specific pathologies and functional capacities (see, for example, Manton & Soldo, 1985), these models so far have treated measures of kin availability and family caregiving patterns as exogenous factors. From a life-

Table 5.5. Percentage Distribution of Women Age 70 and Older in 1984, by Health Outcome in 1986, Family Size and Health Outcome in 1984

Number of Children, 1984	Outcome State in 1986			
	Not Disabled[1]	Disabled[2]	Nursing Home	Dead
A. All women 70 and older				
none[3]	38.7	39.9	3.8	17.7
one or two	40.9	39.2	3.2	16.7
three or more	37.9	38.6	3.6	19.9
B. Not disabled in 1984[1]				
none	51.3	32.4	3.2	13.1
one or two	53.6	34.1	1.6	10.7
three or more	51.3	33.9	2.1	12.7
C. Disabled in 1984[2]				
none	3.5	60.7	5.3	30.5
one or two	11.3	51.1	7.1	30.6
three or more	9.1	48.6	6.9	35.4

[1] No reported problems with self care as measured by Katz's Activities of Daily Living (ADL) scale.
[2] One or more reported problems with self care as measured by Katz's ADL scale.
[3] Rows sum to 100%.
Source: Weighted tabulations from the *1984–86 Longitudinal Survey of the Aged.*

cycle perspective, however, it is likely that health during childhood and young adulthood influences both marital and fertility outcomes, and therefore influences subsequent kin patterns. Given that the dynamics of health and kin may be interdependent over an individual's lifetime, joint modeling of health trajectories and family status is warranted.

Tentative evidence from animal models that treat kin as an exogenous factor supports an inverse relationship between fertility and survivorship (Roderick & Storer, 1961). Evidence from the 1984–86 LSOA data also suggests a possible relationship, as shown in Table 5.5. This table presents the distribution of older women across survivorship/disability states in 1986, according to baseline functional status and number of living children in the baseline year, 1984. While no relationship can be discerned between functional status at follow-up and family size at baseline (in the upper panel of the table), estimates that condition on baseline functional status suggest the operation of a possible biosocial selection effect associated with family size. For women age 70 and older and not disabled at baseline, family status affects only the relative risk of being in a nursing home. This finding is consistent with earlier research on the effect of childlessness on nursing home transitions (Dolinsky & Rosenwaike, 1988; Garber & MaCurdy, 1989; Townsend, 1965).[2] Among women with any functional disability in 1984, however, those with three or more children have a higher probability of improved functioning.

The mechanism underlying the patterns shown in this table may be some form of biological selection of the sort suggested in animal studies, or an expression of the cumulative effects of the socioeconomic correlates of fertility. A contrasting possibility is that family size is an index of potential social support resources, which some have argued enhance recovery, subsequent survivorship, and health.[3] Both the selection argument and the social-support argument imply, however, that models in which both family patterns and health and/or functional status are determined should not treat the effects as unidirectional. Whether or not elderly with the greatest needs for care are also relatively richer in kin who could act as caregivers—or, indeed, whether generalizations this sweeping are even appropriate—are questions for which existing research does not provide a clear answer.

KIN NETWORKS, HEALTH, AND FAMILY CARE OF THE ELDERLY

Having considered possible complications in models of kinship and in models of disease and functional status—including the possibility that the two should be jointly modeled—we turn now to the question that originally motivated this chapter: the combined consequences of kin patterns and of health status for family care of the elderly.

Considerable research in recent years has attempted to relate family patterns and health status to various behavioral outcomes in the lives of the elderly—particularly coresidence of the elderly and their children—and the provision by children of personal care for their elderly parents. Nearly all of this literature is empirical and is based upon cross-sectional data. Thus, the modeling issues that arise in this literature tend to be statistical, in contrast to some of the more theoretical or formal modeling issues previously discussed. They also reflect the limitations of usual data-collection designs, many of which severely limit the inferences that can be drawn about the inevitably more complex processes being analyzed.

In a series of studies, we have developed a "microanalytic" approach to these questions using models in which a detailed representation of the kin network—one using data that records attributes of individual network members—is mapped into behavioral outcomes of interest. For example, Wolf and Soldo (1988) addressed the question, "What is the probability that an older mother will co-reside with one of her children, given the characteristics of the mother and each of the children?" The statistical approach used takes account of differences across observations in the numbers and attributes of living children. Wolf, Freedman, Soldo, and Stephen (1991) addressed parent-child coresidence from the perspective of married couples, in which the husband, the wife, or both may have an elderly unmarried (i.e., widowed or divorced) mother. Here, as well, differences can occur across observations in at-risk status, depending on which spouse's mother is elderly and unmarried.

While coresidence between the elderly and their children tends to be limited to no more than a single parent-child pair at any one time, more than one child may be simultaneously involved in providing care to a needy parent. To address this phenomenon, Wolf and Soldo (1990) developed a model of the entire "portfolio" of caregivers assembled to assist frail older women. This model, however, is based on the restrictive assumption that caregiving choices are made hierarchically; that is, that the primary caregiver is chosen first, followed by the secondary caregiver (if any)—the choice of whom is made conditional upon the choice of primary caregiver—followed in turn by the tertiary caregiver (if any), and so on. Here we present new results from an alternative model, one in which children's caregiving choices are treated as *simultaneously* determined.

A SIMULTANEOUS LOGIT MODEL OF CHILDREN'S CAREGIVING BEHAVIOR

Statistical Framework

Our starting point is a logit model of a binary variable representing whether a child is a caregiver. We then consider the joint probability distribution of all children's caregiving behavior. Let i, j, and k refer to children in a family containing n children. To each child there corresponds a binary dependent variable Y_i and a scalar θ_i that depends upon the attributes of the parent, represented by the array X; the attributes of the child, represented by the array S_i, and unknown parameters.

Adopting the logit functional form, the probability expressions for Y_i are:

$$pr(Y_i = 1) = e^{\theta_i}/(1 + e^{\theta_i}) \quad \text{and} \quad pr(Y_i = 0) = 1/(1 + e^{\theta_i}).$$

Analogous expressions are used for the other children. Suppose that there are just two children, i and j. Such a case produces four possible outcomes: $Y_i = 0$ and $Y_j = 0$; $Y_i = 0$ and $Y_j = 1$; $Y_i = 1$ and $Y_j = 0$; and $Y_i = 1$ and $Y_j = 1$. Each possibility can be treated as one cell of a four-category variable, the probability of which is given by a multinomial logit expression. For example:

$$pr(Y_i = 0; Y_j = 1) = \frac{e^{\theta_j}}{1 + e^{\theta_i} + e^{\theta_j} + e^{\theta_i + \theta_j + \theta_{ij}}} . \tag{1}$$

The denominator of (1) contains four terms, one for each of the possible joint outcomes of Y_i and Y_j. The scalar θ_{ij} is a function of both S_i and S_j, the variables describing the children, and may depend upon parental characteristics as well, through interactions with the children's variables. If $\theta_{ij} = 0$, then the probabilities for Y_i and Y_j are independent, and the expression for the joint probability of Y_i and Y_j is simply the product of the corresponding univariate probability expressions given before. So if we are willing to assume that $\theta_{ij} = 0$, then each child's caregiving activity can be treated as an independent observation in a binary-logit estimation. The latter approach has, in fact, been used by some researchers, including Dwyer and Coward (1991), Dwyer, Henretta, Coward, and Barton (1992), and Lee, Dwyer, and Coward (1993). The studies cited all implicitly maintained the assumption that each child's decision to provide help to his or her elderly parent is independent of the corresponding decisions of any siblings. In contrast, in equation (1) the term θ_{ij} provides the basis for a statistical test of whether the children's care activities are in fact independent.

More generally, in families with n children there will be an equation like (1), the denominator of which will contain one term for each possible combination of values $Y_1, \ldots, Y_n$. The first term in the denominator corresponds to the outcome $Y_1 = Y_2 = \ldots = Y_n = 0$. The number of terms in the denominator is equal to 1, plus the number of ways in which only one child can have $Y = 1$, plus the number of ways in which exactly two children can have $Y = 1$, and so on, ending with the number of ways in which m children can have $Y = 1$, where m is the maximum number of children observed providing care at once.[4]

Since (1) is a multinomial logit expression, the statistical theory and estimation algorithms necessary to implement the model are readily available. However, the practical problem of obtaining estimation software for multinomial logit problems with large numbers of dependent-variable categories must be overcome. Also, the analyst must choose a parsimonious parameterization of the terms $\theta_1, \theta_2, \ldots, \theta_{12}, \ldots$ in order to avoid overwhelming the data with unknown parameters to be estimated.[5]

Parameterization of the Caregiving Model

Below we present results for a simultaneous logit model of elder care in which individual families have as many as 84 distinct behavioral outcomes. We limit our attention to the provision of personal-care services by the children of older unmarried women. The question addressed is that of interdependencies among the children—that is, how is the probability that child i helps his or her mother influenced by the caregiving behavior of the other $n - 1$ children?

In the case of personal care, an additional complexity must be addressed: Older women make extensive use of informal and formal services provided by sources other than their children, and it is reasonable to suppose that such service use is also determined jointly with that of children. In order to incorporate this type of caregiving into our model, we create an additional "pseudo-child," the $n+1^{th}$ child, with no observed attributes, and let this $n+1^{th}$ possible caregiver stand for all "other" caregivers. This doubles the number of outcome categories in the model, since each type of care arrangement involving a child can appear with or without an "other" caregiver as well.

To facilitate the subsequent discussion, we adopt a terminology in which children who provide care singly are called "solos," pairs of children providing care are "duets," and triples of children providing care are "trios." In our empirical analysis, in no case do more than three children simultaneously provide care, thus reducing the number of terms to be evaluated in each multinomial-logit expression.

Besides the independent variable arrays X and $S_1, \ldots, S_n$ already defined (where S_i can be associated with child i acting as a "solo" provider), we can define additional arrays D_{ij}—variables measuring attributes of the duet containing i and j—and T_{ijk}—similarly, descriptors of the trio containing i, j, and k. The unknown parameters to be estimated are distinguished as follows: B_1 = coefficients on parental variables determining use of "other" caregivers; B_2 = coefficients on parental variables determining whether children are care providers; B_3 = coefficients on a child's variables determining that child's provision of care as a "solo"; B_4 = coefficients on "duet" variables; and B_5 = coefficients on "trio" variables. To illustrate the model actually estimated, the equation for the probability that $Y_i = Y_j = Y_k = 1$ while all other Ys equal 0, is:

$$\frac{e^{B_2(3X)+B_3(S_i+S_j+S_k)+B_5T_{ijk}}}{1 + e^{B_1X} + e^{B_2X+B_3S_1} + \ldots + e^{B_2(3X)+B_3(S_i+S_j+S_k)+B_5T_{ijk}+} \ldots},$$

where the denominator contains all the terms described above.

Data

We use data from the 1982 NLTCS. This was a nationally representative sample of noninstitutionalized elderly with a confirmed disability in either Instrumental Activities of Daily Living (IADL) or Activities of Daily Living (ADL). The analysis is limited to unmarried women 65 or older, with at least one ADL limitation, and with one to six living children. The six types of ADL conditions checked were eating, getting in and out of bed, walking around indoors, dressing, bathing, and toileting. Women with no children were eliminated because the study focuses on simultaneity of children's caregiving behavior. Women with seven or more children, about eight percent of the women with children, were eliminated in order to contain the size of the estimation problem in this first, exploratory analysis. And, finally, two observations were deleted in which four children provided care simultaneously; it would have been impossible to estimate parameters for only two "quartets." Thus we analyzed a sample of 1,183 mothers, with an average of 2.55 children, who receive care from one, two, or three of their children, possibly in combination with care from "others."

Independent variables used in the analysis include characteristics of the women and of their children. For women, the variables are the number of children; a dummy variable indicating black women; age; income; and dummy variables indicating women with three or four ADL limitations, and those with five or six ADL limitations (the omitted group is women with one or two ADL limitations). For children, the variables used are age; as well as dummy variables indicating daughters and married children. Average values for these variables, for the 1,183 mothers and 3,012 children included in the sample, are presented in Table 5.6. The mothers are on average 80 years old; a substantial portion of the sample consists of women in the "oldest old" group. These mothers' children are, on average, almost 53 years old; slightly more than half are daughters, and about three-quarters are married.

We included additional variables in the simultaneous logit model, as follows: for duets, a dummy variable indicating duets containing an only daughter ("Only daughter"); a dummy variable indicating duets containing one of a woman's two or more daughters ("1/2+ daughters"); and a dummy variable indicating duets containing two daughters ("2 daughters"). The omitted category is duets containing two sons. The sample averages of these variables for the 3547 possible duets found in the sample are shown in Table 5.6. Of these 3562 duets, 67 were observed to be the chosen care arrangement. Finally, we used a single dummy variable to indicate all outcomes containing a trio of child caregivers, whether or not there is also caregiving by "others." There are

Table 5.6.   Average Values of Variables used in Model: 1982 LTC Survey Sample

Mothers		Children		Duets	
Variable	Sample Mean	Variable	Sample Mean	Variable	Sample Mean
No. of Children	2.55	Daughter	0.52	Only daughter	0.14
Black	0.10	Age	52.60	1/2+ daughters	0.36
Age	80.02	Married	0.74	2 daughters	0.27
ADL3,4	0.21				
ADL5,6	0.24				
Income	$1,073				
N	1183	N	3012	N	3547

2,773 possible trios in the sample, but only 13 observations in which a trio actually provides ADL assistance.

Results.   Estimates of the model parameters are shown in Table 5.7. We estimated both a "naive" model—one that ignores the possible simultaneity of children's caregiving behavior—and the fully simultaneous model described above.

The estimated parameters pertaining to the propensity to receive care from "others" are almost identical in the two models. Only the parameters corresponding to the ADL indicators are significantly different from zero, and show the expected pattern: Women with more severe impairments are more likely to receive care. Of the parameters pertaining to the propensity for a child to be a caregiver, those corresponding to the mothers' and children's variables are generally larger in absolute value in the simultaneous model than in the naive model. Again, the ADL indicators have large effects, but the parameters for number of children, income, and the dummy variables for daughters and married children are also significantly different from zero.

The simultaneous model has nine more parameters than does the naive model, and a likelihood-ratio test for the two models produces a χ^2 statistic of 12.44, which with nine degrees of freedom fails to meet the .10 significance criterion. However, two of the estimated parameters of the simultaneous model are individually significant. The results indicate that duets containing one daughter, in families when one or more *other* daughters are available, are less likely to provide care than would be indicated by the naive model. The same is true for duets containing two daughters. In other words, we find evidence—albeit limited—of interdependencies in the caregiving behavior of an older woman's children.

Table 5.7. Results: Alternative Models of Caregiver Outcomes: 1982 LTC Survey Sample

Independent Variables	Naive Model		Simultaneous Model	
	Children	Others	Children	Others
Intercept	−1.987***	−1.261***	2.078***	−1.260***
Number of children	−0.276***	−0.015	−0.242***	−0.016
Black	−0.021	0.389	−0.008	0.388
Mother's age	0.018	−0.016	0.020*	−0.016
ADL 3,4	0.809***	0.867***	0.879***	0.868***
ADL 5,6	1.666***	2.235***	1.811***	2.238***
Income	−0.075*	−0.039	−0.081*	−0.038
Daughter	1.613***	—	1.690***	—
Child's age	0.009	—	0.001	—
Married	−0.888***	—	−0.897***	—
Duet without "other"	—	—	0.673	—
Duet: only daughter	—	—	−1.195	—
Duet: 1/2 daughter	—	—	−1.666*	—
Duet: 2 daughters	—	—	−1.302*	—
Duet plus "other"	—	—	−0.854	—
Duet + 0: only daughter	—	—	0.516	—
Duet + 0: 1/2 daughter	—	—	0.718	—
Duet + 0: 2 daughters	—	—	0.065	—
Trio	—	—	0.739	—

* $p < .1$
*** $p < .01$

Implications of Results.   What interpretations or implications can be extracted from the simultaneous-logit results, beyond those that would emerge from the more usual (and possibly mis-specified) independent-behavior model? We provide one example of the usefulness of the simultaneous approach, considering the implied probabilities of caregiving behavior of sons, according to the existence of various patterns of siblings.

Table 5.8 presents probabilities of providing ADL assistance for a married son in several situations distinguished by the number and types of siblings. In all cases, we hold constant the mother's characteristics as follows: age = 80, income = $1,073—the sample averages for these variables—black = 0, ADL34 = 0, and ADL56 = 1. All children are married, and all are assigned an age of 53 (the sample average) in order to avoid introducing age effects into the computations. The number and sexes of children are varied as indicated in the rows of the table. The computations are performed by substituting the indicated values for the mothers' and children's characteristics, plus all the relevant variables for duets and trios, as appropriate, along with the estimated parameters

Table 5.8. Computed Probability of Providing ADL Assistance for a Reference Child, given Existence of other Children.

Reference Child	Other Child(ren)	Result from Simultaneous Model				Result from Naive Model
		As Solo	In Duet	In Trio	Total	Total
Married son	none	0.238	—	—	0.238	0.222
Married son	1 married daughter	0.088	0.078	—	0.166	0.178
Married son	1 married son; 1 married daughter	0.070	0.062	0.007	0.139	0.141
Married son	2 married daughters	0.046	0.067	0.024	0.137	0.141
Married son	1 married son; 2 married daughters	0.040	0.052	0.018	0.110	0.111
Married son	2 married sons; 3 married daughters	0.025	0.031	0.013	0.070	0.067

shown in Table 5.7, into the multinomial logit expressions, which produce probabilities for every possible caregiving outcome. In some cases our reference child—a married son—appears in more than one caregiving duet, or in more than one caregiving trio. In such cases the corresponding probabilities are summed, producing the numbers shown in the columns of Table 5.8.

Our illustrative calculations pertain to an older woman in the most severe category of ADL impairments. The model implies that a married son who is an only child has a probability of 0.238 of providing ADL assistance to his mother. However, if he has any siblings, the probability that he will provide ADL assistance in any capacity, and especially the probability that he will be a solo provider of ADL assistance, falls considerably. This finding agrees with those of several previous studies; sons, and particularly married sons, are relatively infrequent providers of ADL assistance to their older mothers. Yet some rather interesting patterns emerge in Table 5.8: A son is, relatively, rather likely to appear as part of a caregiving duet. When a married son has a married sister (rows 2 and 3 of the table) he is almost as likely to be part of a caregiving duet as to be a solo caregiver; when he has two or more married sisters (rows 4–6 of the table) he is more likely to be part of a caregiving duet than to be a solo caregiver. The last two columns of the table compare the total probability of being a caregiver—as part of any sort of arrangement— calculated from the simultaneous model with the probability of caregiving implied by the naive model, all other factors held constant. The two columns contain strikingly similar numbers. The value of the simultaneous model clearly lies in its ability to reveal the interdependencies of the children's behavior.

SUMMARY

We have examined several issues concerning the way in which family composition—construed broadly to include not only the size of kin networks, but also a detailed rendering of each member's attributes—is related to elder care arrangements. Of particular concern has been the formulation of models that, on the one hand, help us to understand the nature and dynamics of kin networks themselves, and, on the other, help us to map kin networks into care arrangements, taking account of intervening relationships with health and functional status.

Our discussion of issues relevant to modeling kin networks suggests that interdependencies across dimensions of behavior, and along family lines, exist and influence the distribution of kin counts. It would be useful if more attention were paid to such issues in future demographic research.

With respect to associations between family composition and the dynamics of health and functional status, the picture is less clear. We present evidence that there may be such an association. However, this issue requires further conceptual and theoretical developments.

We also have summarized several "microanalytic" studies of parent-child coresidence and helping activities, including new results based on a simultaneous-logit approach to caring for a frail parent. A finding common to these studies is that from the perspective of the elderly, living children constitute a *heterogeneous* resource: The extent to which a particular child is a potential provider of care or of a shared residence varies according to the child's characteristics, particularly sex and marital status. A further source of heterogeneity, in the case of married children, is found in the kin networks of the children's *spouses*, since members of these networks may compete for the child's resources.

The issues identified in this chapter relate to model building in more general ways as well. First, they have implications for the state space of the model—for example, a marriage model might be improved by adding variables for potential mates' number of siblings. Second, they have implications for data collection. The HRS and AHEAD surveys mentioned earlier ultimately will provide longitudinal observations on the composition and functioning of family groups containing elderly parents. These data will support the estimation of models richer in structure than any surveyed in this chapter. Beyond this, our understanding of intrafamilial behavior could be further enhanced by using *linked* longitudinal data files that allow us to analyze of behaviors in the lives of individuals related through blood or marriage.

On a more substantive note, our findings suggest that the family, rather than its individual members, is the proper unit of analysis with which to study the mobilization of informal-care resources. Interdependencies among the caregiving activities of siblings is indicative of coordinated decision making, and of conscious sharing of the "burden" of elder care. In the current policy environment community-based long-term care is receiving particular emphasis. Any new public initiatives to promote this type of care will inevitably interact with family decision making. A full understanding of the net benefits of these initiatives, whether from the perspective of those receiving care, or of family members who might potentially provide it, or indeed of society as a whole, must rest on knowledge of the coordinated, interdependent actions of family members on behalf of their elderly members.

ACKNOWLEDGMENTS

This paper was prepared for presentation at the U.S.-USSR Population Symposium, held at The Urban Institute, March 18–20, 1991. Support for this research was provided by the National Institute on Aging, through grant number R01 AG08651.

NOTES

1.   Because the NSFH is cross-sectional, the effect of age on kin structure cannot be identified mathematically; instead, age effects represent the *combined* influences of age and cohort on kin availability. Dynamic interpretations of such estimates as trends over the life course are reasonable only in the absence of cohort effects.

2.   These data may also reflect the operation of unobserved selection mechanisms, since 98% of women with *no* children were not disabled at baseline, while 92% of those with *any* children were without disabilities in 1984. The sample excludes women living in institutions at baseline. Childless women with disabilities may have previously selected out of the community and into nursing homes at higher rates than did women with children.

3.   See Berkman (1985) for a review of the clinical epidemiological evidence on the relationship between family size and survivorship, and Antonucci (1990) for a review of the literature on social support and aging.

4.   The number of terms in the denominator is, in fact, the sum of binomial coefficients; that is, it equals

$$1 + \frac{n!}{(n-1)!} + \frac{n!}{(2!)(n-2)!} + \cdots + \frac{n!}{(n!)(n-m)!} \; .$$

5.   The method described here has also been used by Ofstedal and Chi (1992), in an analysis of parent-child coresidence in Taiwan. In their data, Ofstedal and Chi found a substantial proportion of elderly parents co-residing with two or more of their adult children simultaneously.

REFERENCES

Abbot, M., Abbey, H., Bolling, D., & Murphy, E. (1978). The familial component in longevity: A study of offspring of nonagenarians. III. Intrafamilial studies. *American Journal of Medical Genetics, 2,* 105–120.

Anderton, D. L., Tsuya, N. O., Bean, L. L., & Mineau, G. P. (1987). Intergenerational transmission of relative fertility and life course patterns. *Demography,* *24,* 467–480.

Antonucci, T. C. (1990). Social supports and social relationships. In R. H. Binstock & L.K. George (Eds.), *Handbook of aging and the social sciences.* New York: Academic Press.

Berkman, L. F. (1985). The relationship of social networks and social support to morbidity and mortality. In S. Cohen & S. L. Syme (Eds.), *Social support and health.* New York: Academic Press.

Cantor, M. (1980). The informal support system: Its relevance to the lives of the elderly. In E. Borgatta & N. McClusky (Eds.), *Aging and society.* Beverly Hills, CA: Sage.

Danziger, L., & Newman, S. (1989). Intergenerational effects on fertility: Theory and evidence from Israel. *Journal of Population Economics, 2,* 25–38.

De Vos, S., & Palloni, A. (1989). Formal models, and methods for the analysis of kinship and household organization. *Population Index, 55,* 174–198.

Desjardins, B., & Charbonneau, H. (1990). L'héritabilité de la longévité. *Population, 3,* 603–616.

Dolinsky, A., & Rosenwaike, I. (1988). The role of demographic factors in the institutionalization of the elderly. *Research on Aging, 10,* 235–257.

Doty, P. (1986). Family care of the elderly: The role of public policy. *Milbank Memorial Fund Quarterly, 64,* 34–75.

Dwyer, J. W., & Coward, R. T. (1991). A multivariate comparison of the involvement of adult sons versus daughters in the care of impaired adults. Journals of Gerontology: *Social Sciences, 46,* S259–269.

Dwyer, J. W., Henretta, J. C., Coward, R. T., & Barton, A. J. (1992). Changes in the helping behaviors of adult children as caregivers. *Research on Aging, 14,* 351–375.

Garber, A., & MaCurdy, T. (1989). *Predicting nursing home utilization among the high-risk elderly.* National Bureau of Economic Research Working Paper No. 2843.

Goodman, L. A., Keyfitz, N., & Pullum, T. W. (1974). Family formation and the frequency of various kinship relationships. *Theoretical Population Biology, 5,* 1–27.

———. (1975). Addendum. *Theoretical Population Biology, 8,* 376–381.

Hammel, E. A., Mason, C., Wachter, K., Wang, F., & Yang, H. (1989). *Microsimulation as a tool in exploring social and demographic interrelationships, with an example from China, 1750–2250, or, how tradition is achieved by modernity.* Graduate Group in Demography Working Paper #27, Berkeley: University of California.

Himes, C. L. (1992). Future caregivers: Projected family structures of older persons. Journal of Gerontology: *Social Sciences, 47,* S17–26.

Hodge, R. W., & Ogawa, N. (1986). *Siblings and family size from generation to generation.* NUPRI Research Paper Series No. 29. Population Research Institute, Nihon University, Tokyo, Japan.

Horowitz, A. (1985). Family caregiving to the frail elderly. In C. Eisendorfer (ed.), *Annual review of gerontology and geriatrics,* vol. 5 (pp. 194–246). New York: Springer.

Hougaard, P., Harvald, B., & Holm, N. V. (1992). Measuring the similarities between the lifetimes of adult Danish twins born between 1881–1930. *Journal of the American Statistical Association, 87,* 17–24.

Kovar, M. G. (1988). *Some estimates of change: Preliminary data from the longitudinal survey of aging.* Proceedings of the 1987 Public Health Conference on Records and Statistics, Data for an Aging Population. Washington, DC: Government Printing Office.

Lee, G. R., Dwyer, J. W., & Coward, R. T. (1993). Gender differences in parent care: Demographic factors and same-gender preferences. *Journal of Gerontology: Social Sciences, 48,* S9–S16.

Levit, K. R., Freeland, M. S., & Waldo, D. R. (1990). National health care spending trends: 1988. *Health Affairs, 9,* 171–184.

Manton, K. G. (1988). A longitudinal study of functional change and mortality in the United States. *Journal of Gerontology, 41,* 486–99.

Manton, K. G., & Soldo, B. J. (1985). Dynamics of health changes in the oldest old: New perspectives and evidence. *Milbank Memorial Fund Quarterly, 63,* 206–285.

Manton, K. G., & Stallard, E. (1991) Cross-sectional estimates of active life expectancy for the U.S. elderly and oldest-old populations. *Journal of Gerontology, 46,* 170–182.

Manton, K. G., Corder, L. S., & Clark. R. (1991). *Estimates and projections of dementia-related service expenditures.* Center for Population Studies Working Paper, Duke University.

Moroney, R. M. (1986). *Shared responsibility: Families and social policy.* Hawthorne, NY: Aldine deGruyter.

Ofstedal, M. B. & Chi, L. (1992). *Coresidence choices of elderly parents and adult children in Taiwan.* Paper presented at the annual meeting of the Gerontological Society of America, November.

Pearl, R. (1931). Studies on human longevity. IV. The inheritance of longevity. Preliminary report. *Human Biology, 3,* 245–269.

Pearl, R., & Pearl, R. D. (1934). Studies on human longevity. VI. The distribution and correlation of variation in the total immediate ancestral longevity of nonagenarians and centenarians in relation to the inheritance factor in duration of life. *Human Biology, 6,* 98–222.

Phillipe, P. (1978). Familial correlations of longevity: An isolate-based study. American Journal of Medical *Genetics, 2,* 121–129.

Pullum, T. W. (1982). The eventual frequencies of kin in a stable population. *Demography, 19,* 549–565.

Pullum, T. W., & Wolf, D. A. (1991). Correlations between frequencies of kin. *Demography, 28,* 391–410.

Roderick, J. H., & Storer, J. B. (1961). Correlation between mean litter size and mean life span among 12 inbred strains of mice. *Science, 134,* 48–49.

Rogers, A., Rogers, R. G., & Belanger, A. (1989). Longer life but worse health? Measurement and dynamics. *The Gerontologist, 30,* 640–649.

Ruggles, S. (1987). *Prolonged connections: The rise of the extended family in nineteenth century England and America.* Madison: University of Wisconsin Press.

Soldo, B. J., & Agree, E. (1988). America's elderly. *Population Bulletin, 43*(3).

Soldo, B. J., Agree, E., & Wolf, D. A. (1989). The balance between formal and informal care. In M. Ory and K. Bond (Eds.), *Aging and health care: Social science and policy perspectives.* London: Routledge.

Stone, R., Cafferata, G. L., & Sangl, J. (1987). Caregivers of the frail elderly: A national profile. *The Gerontologist, 27,* 616–626.

Stone, R., & Short, P. F. (1990). The competing demands of employment and informal caregiving to disabled elders. *Medical Care, 28,* 513–526.

Sweet, J., Bumpass, L., & Call, V. (1988). *The design and content of the national survey of families and households.* NSFH. Working Paper No. 1. Madison: Center for Demography and Ecology, University of Wisconsin.

Townsend, P. (1965). The effects of family structure on the likelihood of admission to an institution in old age: The application of a general theory. In E. Shanas & F. Streib (Eds.), *Social structure and the family.* Englewood Cliffs, NJ: Prentice-Hall.

Vaupel, J. (1988). Inherited frailty and longevity. *Demography, 25,* 277–287.

Wilkins, R., & Adams, O. B. (1983). Health expectancy in Canada, late 1970s, Demographic, regional, and social dimensions. *American Journal of Public Health, 73,* 1073–1080.

Wolf, D. A. (1988). Kinship and family support in aging societies. In *Economic and social implications of population aging.* Population Division, Department of International Economic and Social Affairs. New York: United Nations.

Wolf, D. A., & Soldo, B. J. (1988). Household composition choices of older unmarried women. *Demography, 25,* 387–403.

———. (1990). *Family structure and caregiving portfolios.* Paper presented at the Annual Scientific Meeting of the Gerontological Society of America, November, 1990.

Wolf, D. A., Freedman, V. A., Soldo, B. J., & Stephen, E. H. (1991). *Making room for mom: Coresidence of married couples and their elderly mothers.* Paper presented at the Annual Meeting of the Population Association of America, March, 1991.

6

Asymmetry in Intergenerational Family Relationships in Italy

Marzio Barbagli

This chapter concerns the relationship between parents and adult children in some of the regions of contemporary Italy. I will attempt to answer three basic questions: First, how strong are intergenerational ties in Italy, and are they stronger or weaker than those in other Western nations for which there are comparable data? Second, are relationships between parents and adult children influenced by the particular phase of life in which the former and latter live, and to what extent? Finally, and most important, is the dominant kinship pattern in the various regions of Italy bilateral, patrilateral, or matrilateral—that is, is there a tendency toward one of the two lines of kinship and, if so, is this the male or female line?

The chapter is based on an inquiry carried out with two colleagues on a large sample of families in one of the most economically developed regions of Italy, Emilia-Romagna.[1] However, data from recently conducted inquiries on the relationship between parents and adult children in other Italian regions (Veneto and Sardinia) as well as information obtained from historical research is included.

THE STRENGTH OF INTERGENERATIONAL TIES

Numerous inquiries conducted from the mid-1950s have shown that in western industrial countries a close and strong network of ties between relatives is still maintained, and that those who marry, though they follow the rules of neolocal residence, maintain a strong relationship with their family of origin, particularly with their parents (Saraceno, 1988). A vast survey conducted at the beginning of the 1980s demonstrated that this also occurs in Italy (Istat, 1985; Sgritta, 1986).

We do not know, however, whether the strength of this trend has changed during the last thirty years[2], whether any differences exist between the various western nations, or if intergenerational ties are stronger in some countries than in others. For example, is the relationship between parents and adult children in Italy stronger than in other countries? Despite the importance of such questions, no answers to them appear in the existing sociological literature. Instead, the data we have allow us to carry out a firsthand comparison of two regions of Italy (Emilia-Romagna and Veneto) with other regions of Europe and North America, at least as far as parent-adult children relationships are concerned, on the limited basis of two indicators: residential proximity and frequency of interaction.

Research conducted at the end of the 1970s in Middletown, in the United States (Caplow, Bahr, Chadwick, & Modell, 1982), revealed that 43% of adult children with parents still living resided in the same locality as the latter. In France, according to Roussel (1976) and Gokalp (1978), 35–40% of adult children live in the same municipality as their mothers and fathers. In Veneto this proportion reaches 55% (La Mendola, 1991). Our investigation shows that in Emilia-Romagna the proportion of adult children over 30 years of age residing in the same municipality as their parents may be as high as 65–70% (Tables 6.1 and 6.2).

There seems therefore, to be a notable difference between these two regions of Italy and other areas of Europe and the United States for which we have comparable data. However, we must consider the second indicator before reaching sounder conclusions. In the mid-1950s in the traditionally working-class districts of London, characterized by extremely close intergenerational ties, 74% of adult children with parents still living saw them at least once a week (Young & Willmott, 1957; Townsend, 1957). Shortly after, in another district of London with a

Table 6.1. Proximity of Residence to Mother of People over 14 Years Old by Age in Emilia-Romagna

Those Living in Relation to Mother	*Age of Son/Daughter*				
	15–19	*20–29*	*30–39*	*40–49*	*50–59*
Together	97	56	19	20	26
In the same bulding	1	5	9	8	6
In the same street	—	2	3	3	4
In the same district	—	3	6	6	6
In the same municipality	1	16	30	31	27
In a different municipality	1	18	33	32	31
Total (%)	100	100	100	100	100
N	911	1607	1502	1206	671

Table 6.2. Proximity of Residence to Father of People over 14 Years Old by Age in Emilia-Romagna

Those Living in Relation to Father	Age of Son/Daughter				
	15–19	20–29	30–39	40–49	50–59
Together	95	56	16	17	21
In the same building	1	5	9	8	7
In the same street	—	2	4	4	4
In the same district	—	3	6	6	7
In the same municipality	1	16	30	31	33
In a different municipality	3	18	34	34	33
Total (%)	100	100	100	100	100
N	860	1444	1193	708	277

similar strong middle-class presence, about 60% of adult children with living parents met them at least once a week (Willmott & Young, 1960). According to another inquiry conducted in Swansea, Wales, the proportion of adult children who saw their fathers and mothers with such frequency was 70% (Rosser & Harris, 1965).

Since then, various other inquiries have been conducted, but none revealed a particularly high frequency of interaction between parents and adult children—for example, Goldthorpe et al.'s (1969) analysis of settlements of workers in technically advanced businesses. Nor did those carried out in other countries. In Middletown in the 1970s, for example, 48% of adult children saw their parents at least once a week (Caplow et al., 1982). The proportion reached 40–45% in Boston in the 1980s (Rossi & Rossi, 1990) and 50% in France in the 1970s (Pitrou, 1977). According to our research in Emilia-Romagna, however, the proportion reaches 80% (Table 6.3). In Veneto it is 75% (La Mendola, 1991).

Table 6.3. Frequency with which People over the Age of 14 in Emilia-Romagna see their Mothers, by Age

Frequency of Maternal Visits	Age of Son/Daughter				
	15–19	20–29	30–39	40–49	50–59
Every day	98	72	43	42	46
A few times per week	1	11	20	20	15
Once a week	—	7	20	18	20
Once a month	—	4	7	10	10
Two or three times per year	1	5	9	8	8
Never	—	1	1	1	1
Total (%)	100	100	100	100	100
N	911	1607	1501	1204	671

Though only partial and in no way satisfying, these data demonstrate that ties between parents and adult children are stronger in the two recorded regions of Italy examined than in other regions of Europe and the United States.

THE INFLUENCE OF LIFE COURSE

Although always close, the relationship between parents and adult children is influenced by the particular phase of life in which both are living. In short, three different phases may be distinguished: the first, up to age 25, has the strongest ties; the second, between 26 and 40 or 45 years of age, is characterized by distancing of children from parents; and the third, from age 45 on, by strengthening of ties once again.

The division between the first and the second occurs through marriage, as is shown by a comparison of those who do not marry with those who do (Tables 6.4 and 6.5). The former nearly always (85%) remain in the same municipality as their parents as long as the latter stay

Table 6.4.   Proximity of Residence to Mother of Men over the Age of 14 in Emilia-Romagna, by Age and Marital Status

Those Living in Relation to Mother	Single Men				
	15–19	20–29	30–39	40–49	50–59
Together	97	91	83	85	86
In the same building	1	2	2	6	2
In the same street	—	—	1	—	—
In the same district	—	—	1	—	—
In the same municipality	—	3	3	4	2
In a different municipality	2	4	10	5	10
Total (%)	100	100	100	100	100
N	460	536	114	71	43
	Married Men				
Together	n/a	15	13	17	24
In the same building	n/a	16	14	11	8
In the same street	n/a	6	4	4	4
In the same district	n/a	6	6	5	5
In the same municipality	n/a	28	32	33	28
In a different municipality	n/a	29	31	30	31
Total (%)	n/a	100	100	100	100
N	n/a	238	598	508	295

Table 6.5. Proximity of Residence to Mother of Women over the Age of 14 in Emilia-Romagna, by Age and Marital Status

Those Living in Relation to Mother	Single Women				
	15–19	20–29	30–39	40–49	50–59
Together	99	86	60	77	81
In the same building	1	2	6	2	—
In the same street	—	—	—	—	—
In the same district	—	1	3	—	—
In the same municipality	—	6	8	14	—
In a different municipality	—	5	23	7	19
Total (%)	100	100	100	100	100
N	409	388	73	43	21
	Married Women				
Together	n/a	6	8	9	12
In the same building	n/a	7	7	6	6
In the same street	n/a	2	4	3	5
In the same district	n/a	8	7	8	8
In the same municipality	n/a	35	34	33	34
In a different municipality	n/a	42	40	41	35
Total (%)	n/a	100	100	100	100
N	n/a	410	656	527	258

alive, or, if they move to another municipality, they often are followed by their fathers and mothers. An extremely high proportion of those who do not marry (between 75 and 85%) live with their parents until death. This figure slightly diminishes between the ages of 30 and 39 before increasing again in successive age groups.

Of those who marry, about 10% stay at home with one or both of their parents, and another 10% stay in close contact with them, living in a different flat (a different household), but in the same building. Another 10% live in the same district. About 35% live in another district within the same municipality, and another 35% in a different municipality.

As the years go by, the proportion of married sons and daughters living in a different municipality from their parents or living in another apartment in the same building diminishes, while the proportion of those living with their parents increases, reaching the highest percentage between the ages of 50 and 59.

Like the data on interaction frequency, the data on residence show, therefore, that many sons and daughters live quite close to their parents even after marriage and are able to see them often. Further, in Emilia-Romagna, as in other countries (Willmott & Young, 1960; Gokalp, 1978), relationships of sons and daughters with parents become even closer when, with old age, the parents' health worsens. In this phase a growing number of sons and daughters take their parents in, in order to be closer to them and look after them.

GENDER AND LINES OF KINSHIP

Research conducted in various western countries has brought to light "the persisting importance of gender structures, that is, the different positions which the two sexes occupy within kinship systems" (Saraceno, 1988, p.75). Therefore, we consider two different questions that are closely linked, but, which should be kept analytically distinct.

The first issue is the gender of those involved in intergenerational ties. Research conducted in Europe and in the United States has shown that kinship relations are strongly "feminized," that is, that women overall are more concerned with relatives. (Saraceno, 1988).

The second issue is the female and the male lines of kinship and the possibly greater importance of one or the other. In theory, the nuclear family and bilateral or cognatic kinship system dominate in Western nations. Thus those who marry should expect to live on their own and give equal importance to both lines of kinship, maintaining the same relationship with the husband's relatives as with the wife's.

Research conducted in Great Britain, the United States, Holland, Sweden, and Finland has shown, however, that the actual tendency is toward matrilateral preference—priority is given to relationships with relatives in the female line of kinship.

Studies have revealed that in families where married couples live with their parents, the parents are more often those of the wife than those of the husband (Sweetser, 1966); second, they demonstrate that couples live closer to the wife's parents than to the husband's; and third, they reveal that mothers stay in contact with their daughters more often than with their sons. In the mid-1950s in a traditionally working-class district of London, 55% of daughters and 31% of sons saw their mothers every day, after marriage (Young & Willmott, 1957, p. 29). In Swansea, the situation was the same: 54% of daughters and 31% of sons met their mothers every day (Rosser & Harris, 1965, p. 219). In the mid-1980s in the Boston area, 23% of daughters, as opposed to 9% of sons, spoke with their mothers on the telephone every day, and 17% of daughters, as opposed to 11% of sons, saw them every day (Rossi & Rossi, 1990, p. 370).

It was thought for some time that matrilateral kinship was a characteristic of the working class produced by the typical working and living conditions of its members: long periods of unemployment, low salaries, and scarcity of economic resources. In order to handle this situation and reduce their sense of insecurity, powerlessness, and anxiety, workers' wives held on to their families of origin. In this sense, the working-class matrilateral extended family would simply be a kind of "trade-union organized in the main by women and for women" (Young & Willmott, 1957, p. 158).

Such hypotheses, however, have not withstood examination of the data. Inquiries conducted during the 1960s (Willmott & Young, 1960; Rosser & Harris, 1965) have in fact demonstrated that there is also a tendency toward matrilateral kinship among members of the middle class, despite the fact that their living and working conditions are better than those of the working class. Generally, according to current studies done in all social classes it is normal to live nearer to the wife's parents than to the husband's, and ties with the former are stronger than those with the latter. This trend occurs in Great Britain and the United States, as well as in other western nations (Sweetser, 1964, 1966; Gokalp, 1978; Déchaux, 1990; Bengtson, Rosenthal, & Burton, 1990).

Residential proximity and the frequency of contact and interaction are the dimensions of intergenerational relationships considered by all inquiries. Rossi and Rossi (1990), however, arrived at the same conclusions by studying two other aspects of such relationships: the sentimental importance given to various relations and the moral obligations people feel toward certain kin. A sample of residents in the Boston area were asked which grandparents and uncles/aunts they considered particularly important to their upbringing, and which of them they would feel more obliged to help in case of need. The replies indicated that what counts most in defining the closeness or distance of various relatives is their sex and the line of kinship to which they belong. One feels closer to female blood relations than to male blood relations, and to those belonging to the female line of kinship than to the male line. Thus, in terms of both sentiment and moral obligations, the maternal grandmother is considered more important than the maternal grandfather; yet the latter comes before the paternal grandmother, while the paternal grandfather occupies the fourth place in this hierarchy.

THE MOTHER-DAUGHTER RELATIONSHIP

The key relationship in this kinship pattern is between mother and daughter. According to the results of inquiries conducted in Great Britain, the United States, and other western nations, the behavior of mothers seems to be inspired by the old English proverb "My son's a son till

him gets a wife, my daughter's a daughter all her life" (Young & Willmott, 1957, p. 43). Even after her daughter has married and left home, "a
special emotional bond" remains between mother and daughter (Willmott & Young, 1960, pp. 74–75). When a daughter gives birth, the relationship becomes even closer (Fischer, 1981; 1983). Indeed, the daughter
turns above all to her mother for advice and moral support during this
phase (Blaxter & Paterson, 1982; Finch, 1989).

The mother-daughter relationship is characterized not just by more
frequent contact. It is also much more regular and stable than others,
and is less influenced by circumstances of life. The fact that conflict may
have occurred between parents and adolescent children negatively influences the father-son relationship, even after many years, but not the
mother-daughter one. Further the contact between father and son increases if the father is in ill health or if the son is married with children.
The frequency with which mother and daughter see each other remains
independent of marital status, age, the health of one or the other, or the
number of children the daughter has (Rossi & Rossi, 1990, pp. 383–387).

The mother-daughter relationship is also different from others with
regard to the frequency with which they help each other (Rossi & Rossi,
1990, pp. 393–408). First, this frequency is higher than in the father-son
or even mother-son relationship; second, the frequency varies with the
age of the parent. The amount of help given the mother by both sons
and daughters decreases as she grows older. However, the amount of
help increases again when the mother has reached the age of 80, in the
case of sons, and when she is over 65, in the case of daughters.

It seems "natural"—a duty imposed by the kinship pattern—that the
mother-daughter relationship is closer and more involved than others.
"At Christmas," said a woman in London in the 1950s, "I go to my
daughter's and my son goes to his wife's mother. She's got the right to
do that, hasn't she? You couldn't expect him not to, could you?" (Townsend, 1957, p. 45).

At the end of the 1980s it was possible to hear this dialogue between
two 60-year-old women in the Manhattan subway:

> "So tell me, Sadie, what's with your daughter Millie?"
> "Millie? Much better today. Now she thinks she'll stay on her job. Yester-
> day she was ready to quit."
> "And your son Sam?"
> "Sammy? Who knows what's with him? You would have to ask his wife's
> mother. She knows more than I ever do." (Rossi & Rossi, 1990, p. 365).

An inquiry conducted recently in Boston revealed that a mother feels
that she has more duties (help and support in case of need) toward her
son-in-law than toward her daughter-in-law, for the simple reason that

the former has married her daughter, the latter her son. In other words, as Rossi and Rossi (1990, p. 207) observed, "daughters-in-law are more closely tied to their own mothers, while sons-in-law are brought closer to their parents-in-law as a consequence of daughters' closer bonds with their own parents."

LINES OF KINSHIP IN ITALY

The relationship between parents and adult children in at least one Italian region—Sardinia—seems identical to that of England or the United States. In this region, though the kinship pattern is considered bilateral, in reality it is strongly matrilateral. When Sardinians marry, they make a home of their own but live closer to the wife's parents, brothers, and sisters than to the husband's. In the subsequent years, married couples maintain a closer relationship with their matrilateral kin than with their patrilateral kin. Half of them meet the wife's parents and sisters nearly every day, but only 10% see the husband's relatives with the same frequency. What is more, they usually spend weekends and holidays with the wife's relatives and collaterals (Oppo, 1991).

Although this may happen in other southern regions of Italy, we cannot say that in Italy, as in other western nations, the dominant pattern of kinship is matrilateral. It certainly is not the case in some regions of central and northern Italy: Massimo Paci (1980) suggested that during the 1970s there was a mainly patrilateral kinship pattern in the Marche. And recent data show that this is certainly the dominant system of kinship in Veneto (La Mendola, 1991).

Our data show that Emilia-Romagna, too, exhibits a dominant pattern of kinship that is patrilateral, not matrilateral. Tables 6.6 and 6.7 show that in Emilia-Romagna, from the age of 20 on, the sons, rather than the daughters, live near their parents and see them more often. Up to age 30 this pattern depends on whether the former marry a little later than the latter. However, after age 30 this difference is explained only by the presence of a patrilateral system.

Table 6.6. Percentage of People between the Ages of 15 and 59 Resident in Emilia-Romagna Living with their Mothers, by Sex and Age

Percent of	Age 15–19	Age 20–29	Age 30–39	Age 40–49	Age 50–59
Men	97	68	25	26	33
Women	96	46	13	15	19

Table 6.7. Percentage of People between the Ages of 15 and 59 Resident in Emilia-Romagna seeing their Mothers Every Day

Percent of	Age 15–19	Age 20–29	Age 30–39	Age 40–49	Age 50–59
Men	98	82	50	48	50
Women	97	63	37	37	41

This can be seen by considering the variable of marital status. The lower parts of Tables 6.4 and 6.5, reflect marital patterns. After marriage women live in a different municipality from their mothers more often than do men. Men, live with their mothers or live very close to them (in a different apartment in the same building) more often than women do. It is not surprising, therefore, that after marriage, and for the rest of their lives, men see their mothers more frequently than do women (Tables 6.8 and 6.9).

Thus, in Emilia-Romagna there is a clear tendency toward the patrilateral pattern of kinship. After their children have married, parents[3] stay closer to their daughters-in-law than to their daughters and see the former more often than the latter. This pattern continues for the rest of their lives, and as the parents grow older they move even closer to the family of their son and daughter-in-law, while their daughter's family moves closer to her parents-in-law.

This strong patrilateral kinship pattern also emerges in the relationship between parents and sons and daughters who do not marry. Research carried out in Great Britain (Finch, 1989) has shown that daughters who remain single look after their elderly parents, going to live with or near them or seeing them very often. However, this does not seem to be the case in Emilia-Romagna.

The upper parts of Tables 6.4 and 6.5 compare men and women who do not marry, revealing that unmarried sons over age 30 live with their

Table 6.8. Number and Percentage of People between the Ages of 15 and 59 Resident in Emilia-Romagna Living with their Mothers, by Sex and Age, Provincial Capital and Nonprovincial Capital Municipality

	Age 15–19		Age 20–29		Age 30–39		Age 40–49		Age 50–59	
Provincial Capital										
Men	173	97	289	72	249	23	229	21	122	28
Women	99	99	284	54	301	15	237	14	132	20
Nonprovincial Capital										
Men	299	97	500	65	490	25	367	29	226	36
Women	284	94	531	41	454	12	368	16	191	18

Table 6.9. Percentage of People between the Ages of 15 and 59 Resident in Emilia-Romagna seeing their Mothers Every Day, by Sex and Age, Provincial Capital and Nonprovincial Capital Municipality

	Age 15–19	Age 20–29	Age 30–39	Age 40–49	Age 50–59
Provincial Capital					
Men	98	81	41	37	38
Women	99	69	36	35	40
Nonprovincial Capital					
Men	97	82	55	55	57
Women	98	60	37	39	41

mothers more often than do unmarried daughters. In addition, the former live in the same municipality as their mothers much more often than do the latter.

The tendency toward patrilateral preference is not, however, equally strong among all sectors of the population. Tables 6.8 and 6.9 compare the situation of provincial capitals with other municipalities in Emilia-Romagna. Analysis of the frequency with which sons and daughters see their mothers, reveals that the patrilateral pattern of kinship exists only in municipalities that are not provincial capitals. If, on the other hand, we consider the frequency with which sons and daughters between the ages of 30 and 60 live with their mothers, the tendency toward patrilateral preference becomes evident in provincial capitals, though it is weaker than in other municipalities.

Data from the Istat inquiry, which show that in Italy, too, intergenerational ties function through women, do not contradict the fact that in Emilia-Romagna and Veneto, and probably in other regions of central and northern Italy, the pattern of kinship is patrilateral. Even if some confusion exists in the sociological literature over this point, it is evident that women facilitate intergenerational ties not only in a matrilateral system but also in a patrilateral one. The difference is that in the first case their significance is above all as mothers, daughters, and sisters[4], but in the second as mothers-in-law, daughters-in-law, and sisters-in-law.

In Emilia-Romagna and Veneto, as in Sardinia, it is the women who maintain contact with relatives, organize family meetings, and give and receive help. The difference is that in the first two regions, a woman by marrying, moves away from her mother and closer to her mother-in-law. As far as we know, this movement is not a change in sentiment but one of location. From the onset of marriage the woman lives closer to her mother-in-law than to her mother. She will see the former more often than the latter, and she will look after and dedicate more time to her mother-in-law than to her mother.

INTERPRETIVE HYPOTHESES

Young and Willmott (1957, pp. 156–158) claim that in the past, when a son did the same work as his father, the ties between the two were not as strong as those between mother and daughter. However, the relationship radically changed with industrialization. The father-son relationship weakened because intergenerational social mobility increased, while the mother-daughter relationship remained as strong as before because the daughter continued to carry out the same domestic tasks as the mother (looking after the house, taking care of the children) and both continued to have many interests in common.

This hypothesis was elaborated and reformulated by Dorrian Sweetser (1963; 1966; 1968; 1970; 1984). According to Sweetser, "where there is succession in male instrumental roles, solidarity will be greater between the nuclear family and the lineal relatives of males, and, where there is no succession, solidarity will be greater with the wife's family" (Sweetser, 1966, p. 156). In western countries, the first situation would have occurred before industrialization, when the family was an economic unit of production and the son took his father's place on the land or in the shop, doing agricultural or artisanal work. In such cases, at marriage the norms of patrilocal residence were followed. Daughters left home and were incorporated into their husbands' families. Sons, took their wives into their parents' home. Priority was thus given to kin relationships in the male line.

Industrialization dispersed the family as a unit of production and the line of economic succession between father and son was broken. The working relationship that had encouraged patrilocality and a patrilateral system of kinship disappeared. Since women continued to dominate domestic affairs, matrilateral ties became more important, according to Sweetser, because with industrialization a society was born "in which a relative is rarely useful to a man in his daily affairs while a relative may be of great help to a woman in her daily activities" (1966, p. 169).

Industrialization, therefore, provoked the transition from the patrilateral to the matrilateral kinship pattern. This trend also means that the patrilateral kinship pattern was once dominant in all the western nations, just as today the dominant pattern in these nations is matrilateral. This interpretative hypothesis is widely shared by sociologists concerned with the question of lines of kinship in western nations and has been represented in this form in manuals on family sociology for years (Segalen, 1981, pp. 82–83).

A HISTORICAL PANORAMA OF ITALY
AND THE OTHER WESTERN NATIONS

The results of research conducted on intergenerational ties in several Italian regions create some doubt about the validity of the theory that western industrialization provoked the transition from a patrilateral to a matrilateral system of kinship. These doubts stem from two conclusions from our research on kinship patterns. First, not all western industrialized societies have matrilateral patterns of kinship, and second, not all agricultural societies have a patrilateral system of kinship. The data presented do indeed show that in the two industrialized regions of Emilia-Romagna and Veneto the patrilateral system of kinship is dominant. The information presented in this chapter and other information we have obtained—though fragmentary and unsatisfactory (because it only concerns geographic proximity)—suggests that in eighteenth- and nineteenth-century Sardinia there was a bilateral or matrilateral system of kinship (Oppo, 1990, 1991).

It would be a mistake to view the present situations in Emilia-Romagna and Veneto or that of Sardinia one or two centuries ago as irrelevant exceptions. If analyzed in light of the research on the history of the family conducted over the last 20 years in various European countries and the United States, the apparently deviant cases of Italian regions may help us to better understand the fundamental differences between the patrilateral and matrilateral kinship systems and the conditions that encouraged one or the other.

The field of intergenerational ties is the most difficult to conduct historical research, so our knowledge in this area is still modest. However, if we add to this material the vast pool of data we have on the norms of residence after marriage in various geographical regions and among various social classes during different historical periods, it becomes possible at least to suggest several hypotheses about the varying importance of male and female lines of kinship.

For many centuries, in the rural areas of regions of northern and central Italy (as in those of Austria, southern France, northern Spain, and northern Portugal), patrilocal postmarital residence norms were followed (Barbagli, 1984). In Piedmont, Liguria, and Lombardy, often only one of the sons (the first-born) took his wife into his father's house, allowing the formation of a stem-household. In Veneto, Emilia-Romagna, Tuscany, Umbria, and the Marche, often more than one son took their wives into their parent's home, allowing the creation of a "joint" family.

The dominant kinship system in these areas normally was patri-lateral. When a woman married she was incorporated into her hus-band's family. She was expected to dedicate more time and energy to her new relatives than to her blood relations. Her children were expected to be emotionally closer to their father's relatives.

The southern Italian family, as that of England, Germany, northern France,[5] and the United States, was formed differently. In all these zones, the neolocal postmarital residence norms were practiced and the married couple went to live on their own. There were even areas of Sardinia, Puglia, and France in which matrilateral postmarital residence norms were observed and the husband transferred to the village or house of his wife (Oppo, 1990; Delille, 1985; Todd, 1990). It is probable, therefore, that though the tendency was toward a patrilateral system among the most elevated classes in these areas, the bilateral (Wrightson, 1984) or even matrilateral system was dominant among the majority of the population.

If all this is true, the hypothesis that industrialization provoked the passage from a patrilateral to a matrilateral system of kinship does not provide us with an adequate description or explanation of what hap-pened in the western nations. Among several classes of the populations of England, northern France, and the United States, there was probably no transition for the simple reason that even before industrialization the kinship pattern was not usually patrilateral.[6] If any change occurred over the course of time, it was the transition from a bilateral to a ma-trilateral system. This probably happened in Sardinia and perhaps in some other areas of southern Italy (although we have no data at all on the present situation there). As for the regions of central and northeast Italy, industrialization and urbanization probably weakened the preced-ing system of patrilateral kinship, but were unable to transform it into a matrilateral system.

NOTES

1. This was a secondary analysis of data from research conducted on social mobility in this region (Barbagli, Capecchi, & Cobalti, 1988). The research took place in 1983, and was based on a sample of 12,946 people of 4,493 families who resided in the 94 municipalities of Emilia-Romagna.

2. Several researchers (Mendras, 1988; Dirn, 1990) claim that over the last decades there has been a "strengthening of intergenerational ties." However, the data we possess do not permit us to verify this. The data available on the

United States (Caplow et al., 1991) show that from this point of view there has been no change.

3. The tables on distance from fathers, according to age, sex, and marital status, which are not reproduced here for lack of space, are not substantially different from those on distance from mothers (Tables 6.4 and 6.5).

4. In Great Britain, for example, if an elderly person needs help, there is the following hierarchy of obligations: The first person to deal with the problem is the spouse, followed by the daughter, the daughter-in-law, then the son, and finally the other relatives (Qureshi & Simons, 1987).

5. Historical research has demonstrated a notable difference in the norms of postmarital residence between Northern and Southern France. In the former, neolocal norms were observed, and in the latter, patrilocal norms were followed. Perhaps for this reason, the inquiries recently carried out in this country on the basis of national samples (Gokalp, 1978, p. 1088, n. 8) show that there is a bilateral system of kinship rather than a matrilateral one, as in Great Britain or the United States.

6. Sweetser (1984) demonstrated that in 1900 in the United States, married couples lived more often with the husband's parents if the husband was a farmer and with the wife's parents if he was employed in industry or the service sector.

REFERENCES

Barbagli, M. (1984). *Sotto lo stesso tetto: Mutamenti della famiglia in Italia dal XV al XX secolo.* Bologna: Il Mulino.

Barbagli, M., Capecchi, V., & Cobalti, A. (1988). *La mobilità sociale in Emilia-Romagna.* Bologna: Il Mulino.

Bengtson, V., Rosenthal, C., & Burton, L. (1990). Families and aging: Diversity and heterogeneity. In R. H. Binstock & L. K. George (Eds.). *Aging and the social sciences* (pp. 263–287). New York: Academic Press.

Blaxter, M. & Paterson, E. (1982). *Mothers and daughters: A three generation study of health attitudes and behavior.* London: Heinemann.

Caplow, T. S., Bahr, H. M., Chadwick, B. A., & Holmes, W. M. (1982). *Middletown families: Fifty years of change and continuity.* Minneapolis: University of Minneasota Press.

Caplow, T. S., Bahr, H. M., Chadwick, B. A., & Modell, J. (1991). *Recent social trends in the United States, 1960–1990.* Frankfurt: Campus.

Déchaux, J. (1990). Les échanges économiques au sein de la parentèle. *Sociologie du travail, 32,* 73–94.

Delille, G. (1985). *Famille et propriété dans le Royaume de Naples (XV-XIX siècle).* Roma: Ecole francaise de Rome.

Dirn, L. (1990). *La société française en tendences.* Paris: Puf.

Finch, J. (1989). *Family obligations and social change.* Oxford: Polity Press.

Fischer, L. R. (1981). Transitions in the mother-daughter relationship. *Journal of Marriage and the Family, 43,* 613–622.

————. (1983). Mothers and mothers-in-law. *Journal of Marriage and the Family, 45*, 187–192.

Gokalp, C. (1978). Le réseau familial. *Population, 33*, 1077–1093.

Goldthorpe, J. H., Lockwood, D., Bechhofer, F., & Platt, J. (1969). *The affluent worker in the class structure*. Cambridge: Cambridge University Press.

Istat (1985). *Indagine sulle strutture e sui comportamenti familiari*. Roma: Istat.

La Mendola, S. (1991). I rapporti di parentela in Veneto. *Polis, 5*, 49–70.

Mendras, H. (1988). *La seconde révolution française, 1965–1984*. Paris: Gallimard.

Oppo, A. (1990). "Where there's no woman there's no home": Profile of the agropastoral family in nineteenth-century Sardinia. *Journal of Family History, 15*, 483–502.

————. (1991). Madri, figlie e sorelle: Solidarietà parentali in Sardegna. *Polis, 5*, 21–48.

Paci, M. (1980). Introduzione: Struttura e funzioni della famiglia nello sviluppo industriale "periferico." In *Famiglie e mercato del lavoro in un'economia periferica* (pp. 9–69). Milano: Franco Angeli.

Pitrou, A. (1977). Le soutien familial dans la société urbaine. *Revue Française de Sociologie, 18*, 47–84.

Qureshi, H. & Simons, K. (1987). Resources within families: Caring for elderly people. In J. Brannen & G. Wilson (Eds.), *Give and take in families* (pp. 117–135). London: Allen & Unwin.

Rosser, C. & Harris, C. (1965). *The family and social change: A study of family and kinship in a South Wales town*. London: Routledge & Kegan.

Rossi, A. S. & Rossi, P. H. (1990). *Of human bonding: Parent-child relations across the life course*. New York: Aldine de Gruyter.

Roussel, L. (1976). *La famille après le mariage des enfants*. Paris: Ined.

Saraceno, C. (1988). *Sociologia della famiglia*. Bologna: Il Mulino.

Segalen, M. (1981). *Sociologie de la famille*. Paris: Colin.

Sgritta, G. B. (1986). La struttura delle relazioni interfamiliari. In Istat (Ed.), *Atti del convegno "La famiglia in Italia"* (pp. 167–200). Roma: Istat.

Sweetser, D. A. (1963). Asymmetry in intergenerational family relationships. *Social Forces, 41*, 346–352.

————. (1964). Mother-daughter ties between generations in industrial societies. *Family Process, 3*, 332–343.

————. (1966). The effect of industrialization on intergeneration solidarity. *Rural Sociology, 31*, 156–170.

————. (1968). Intergenerational ties in Finnish urban families. *American Sociological Review, 33*, 236–246.

————. (1970). The structure of sibling relationships. *American Journal of Sociology, 76*, 47–58.

————. (1984). Love and work: Intergenerational household composition in the U.S. in 1900. *Journal of Marriage and the Family, 46*, 289–293.

Todd, E. (1990). *L'invention de l'Europe*. Paris: Seuil.

Townsend, P. (1957). *The family life of old people*. London: Penguin.

Willmott, P. & Young, M. (1960). *Family and class in a London suburb*. London: Routledge & Kegan.

Wrightson, K. (1984). Kinship in an English village: Terling, Essex 1550–1700. In R. Smith (Ed.), *Land, kinship and life-cycle* (pp. 313–332). Cambridge: Cambridge University Press.

Young, M. & Willmott, P. (1957). *Family and kinship in East London*. London: Routledge & Kegan.

7

Equity between Generations in Aging Societies
The Problem of Assessing Public Policies

Anne-Marie Guillemard

The questions of equity between generations and of assessing welfare policies that redistribute money and goods between generations are not easy to handle. Few scientific investigations have been carried out, and these have produced contrasting results. Meanwhile, arguments about intergenerational equity have been tapped for political purposes in many countries. They serve to justify welfare reforms, to curb rapidly rising social expenditures, and to deal with the eventual aging of populations in developed countries. This mixture of scientific and political arguments makes it even harder to deal with such questions.

The first part of this chapter attempts to clarify what "intergenerational equity" means and identifies the redistributive policies to be assessed. The second part explores the distribution of work and free time between generations, a central problem that has not often been addressed. This concrete example of assessing intergenerational redistributive policies will illuminate both the difficulties of such research and the results to be expected.

INTERGENERRATIONAL EQUITY AND THE ASSESSMENT OF SOCIAL POLICIES: EQUITY BETWEEN AGE-GROUPS OR BETWEEN GENERATIONS?

A major source of confusion and contradiction in the assessment of intergenerational equity is that the conceptual distinction made between age groups and generations is inadequate. Several studies have confused or even conflated these two concepts. For example, widely available cross-sectional data are used to analyze intergenerational equity, although they can only indicate levels of resource distribution at a given moment between age groups—not generations. In fact, measuring intergenerational equity requires a longitudinal analysis that follows contributions from successive generations over the whole life course. It also means looking beyond welfare systems to take into account private, as well as public transfers, as parents invest in children's education and help them (through gifts and donations in advance of inheritance) set up their lives as adults, and, in turn, children render financial support to aging parents.

What, then, is being analyzed when equity is measured? Should we restrict the scope of inquiry to resources redistributed through welfare programs? This would cover only one part of intergenerational equity: institutionalized social transfers. Services and nonmonetarized forms of help would be omitted. For international comparisons, this is a crucial omission. The extent of protection provided by such monetary transfers, as well as the proportions of public and private "social protection," varies from country to country. For example, this public/private ratio in the United States differs significantly from that in Europe. Another notable difference appears between Germany—where transfers are primarily monetary—and France, where, besides such transfers, services have been widely developed for the aged. Such a development undoubtedly takes part of the daily responsibility for aging parents off younger generations.

Exemplifying the difficulty in distinguishing between age groups and generations, the heated American debate about intergenerational equity centers mainly on age groups. Samuel Preston set off this debate when he showed that the redistribution of public resources in the United States, during the 20 years preceding his 1984 study, had favored older people at the expense of families with young children. This study had a political impact: In 1986, Americans for Generational Equity (AGE) was organized. This pressure group has fought this trend in public policy. Such systematic monetary transfers from young people toward retirees supposedly lays the groundwork for "age warfare." Retirees, their ranks swelling, are accumulating more than their fair share of welfare, whereas more and more families with young children are sinking into poverty. According to this lobby, old people are gaining more political clout, thanks to their increasing demographic weight. AGE supports reducing pensions and welfare benefits for this allegedly privileged age group so as to increase public investments in education and welfare services for children and young people (Longman, 1987).

Daniels (1989) has pointed out that discussions generally confuse age groups with generations. He contends that the question of justice must be handled in terms of age groups: It is the only question that can be reasonably answered. A political settlement can thus be reached about how to equitably redistribute public resources between young and old. To operationalize the question of intergenerational justice in terms of generations would mean assessing what is, nowadays, owed to the oldest generation, given its history of contributions to, and benefits from, welfare programs compared with those of the following generation. This would be too complicated. Therefore, it is better to initially limit inquiry to equity between age groups. Given the current life expectancy, everyone stands a good chance of passing through all stages in the life cycle—of being young and then old.

However we disagree with Daniels, we can object that measuring equity between age groups at a given moment entails drawing up a balance sheet of what two successive cohorts, with different positions on the age scale, receive through public welfare transfers. Such a balance sheet provides a snapshot, a partial one, especially when used to debate intergenerational justice. For one thing, the flow of resources between generations necessarily varies depending on their positions with respect to each other as they move through the life course. As we know, our society has provided more care and financial support to the elderly than to children, for whom care, apart from matters of education, has been mainly left up to families. Second, successive generations do not necessarily obtain as much from the welfare state. Retirement systems now definitely deliver a higher ratio of contributions and benefits to today's young retirees than future generations of retirees can hope to receive, given slower economic growth, lower inflation, and the like.

Measuring intergenerational equity calls for both micro- and macrosocial approaches that focus both on successive generations within the family and on generations coexisting in society. In contrast, when this question is raised in terms of age groups, a macrosocial approach alone is adopted.

WHAT KIND OF EQUITY AND HOW TO MEASURE IT?

The concept of equity is as confusing as that of intergenerational relations. In today's aging societies, young and old generations seem to be competing with each other for ever smaller benefits distributed by the welfare state, itself in the throes of a crisis. The debate about intergenerational equity has arisen in this context. It centers on a principle for redistributing resources that has been strongly influenced by J. Rawls' (1971) theory of justice. Does the welfare state fairly redistribute benefits between generations? To answer this question, criteria and values must be brought into play. What is equity? How do we make this concept operational so that it can be assessed? What constitutes "a fair share" in the part of national wealth redistributed by the welfare state? Are we referring to the subjective feelings that persons in society (or an age group) may have about justice? Or to an objective meaning? What constitutes a fair share—equal transfers or equal proportions of transfers? Is it fair that retirement pensions amount to less than an actively working adult's income? Such questions are hard to settle.

Such questions have been operationalized in different ways. When equity is assessed with respect to age groups rather than generations, studies either compare the percentage of each age group living below the poverty level and changes therein over the past 20 years, or else focus on relative variations in age groups' average income levels. Preston (1984) and Johnson and Falkingham (1988) have based their studies on this sort of indicator. In contrast, Thomson (1989) has adopted a generational approach. His study of New Zealand took as an indicator the fluctuations in welfare state programs over the past 20 years. He showed that the young people's welfare state, which used to devote a big part of social expenditures to family allowances, housing, and education, has gradually become an old people's welfare state. As a consequence, a single generation, which he has named "the welfare generation," has been a "winner" during its whole life span, whereas subsequent generations will systematically lose out. Various researchers have reached a relative agreement about one point: The welfare state has not, overall, redistributed resources between the rich and poor so much as it has organized transfers between generations.

Nowadays, a major question crops up: Do the now social and demographic changes underway not make it less and less probable that the welfare state's resources will be shared fairly among generations? In parallel, doubts arise about the implicit, moral contract between generations that underlies the welfare state. Such doubts, undermine any stable consensus about welfare programs. Retirement systems lie in the eye of the storm, given the aging of the population. In a not too distant past, however, they did much to reestablish equity between age groups (and generations) by bringing the welfare benefits received by the elderly up to par with those given the young. This has been an indubitable success for modern societies and their welfare states.

STUDIES WITH CONTRASTING CONCLUSIONS

The very few studies that have tried to assess intergenerational equity have yielded quite different conclusions.

The aforementioned research in the United States (Preston) and New Zealand (Thomson) has concluded that welfare benefits are being less fairly redistributed between generations. This redistribution, now clearly favoring older people, is being carried out at the expense of the young. Other authors disagree with this conclusion. With regard to the United States, Binney and Estes (1988) and Easterlin (1987) argue that those who foresee intergenerational conflict over the sharing of welfare benefits fail to see differences in income levels and so on *within* each generation (or age group). Johnson and Falkingham have drawn similar conclusions about the imminence of intergenerational conflict over transfers in Great Britain.

According to Johnson and Falkingham (1988), transfers under British welfare programs have been neutral with regard to age criteria. Young and old have been treated fairly. These scholars have concluded that the interpretation proposed in the aforementioned studies does not hold: Generations do not compete with each other over access to welfare benefits. In Great Britain, inequality owing to social class and sex, within a single age group is more a significant issue than inequality between age groups.

Cribier's (1989) comparative analysis of two successive cohorts of retirees in France has produced similar findings: With regard to France, too, the conclusions drawn from Thomson's analysis must be modified as a function of social class. Whereas middle- and upper-class retirees in the younger cohort do resemble what Thomson has called "winners," working-class retirees paid for their share of public welfare benefits throughout their working lives: They worked long hours, paid into social security funds for a long time, and helped support their aging parents (who received few benefits). We cannot rightly call them "winners."

I have reservations about restricting the notion of intergenerational equity to equal monetary transfers between generations (or age groups) (Guillemard, 1990). Nonetheless, if we do so, we clearly observe that retirees in most developed countries have reached an average income level comparable with that of other age groups. This success is definitely attributable to the welfare state, particularly to retirement systems. But the price retirees have paid for being well-off turns out to be their marginal, dependent social status. To globally assess intergenerational equity, other parameters must be taken into account—static, synchronic ones based on age groups, as well as more dynamic, diachronic ones referring to generations.

When one assesses intergenerational equity, it is misleading not to take into account the ways work and free time—not just monetary resources—have been redistributed between generations. During the past 20 years in most developed countries, the labor force participation rate of persons over age 55 has dropped, and young people are entering the labor market later. Overall, we can conclude that the working life is contracting the middle age of persons. This trend, most clearly visible in

Europe, sheds new light on the debate about intergenerational equity. Employment policies, compensation for early withdrawal from the labor force, the integration of young people in both society and the world of work are the topics that should focus any analysis of intergenerational equity. "Winners" and "losers" in such a focus are not likely to be the same as those in studies that have addressed monetary transfers via the welfare state between generations.

THE DISTRIBUTION OF WORK AND FREE TIME OVER THE LIFE COURSE: LESSONS ABOUT INTERGENERATIONAL EQUITY

Lower Labor Force Participation Rates after the Age of 55: Implications

Table 7.1 clearly shows that over the past 15 years, the employment activity rates of men from 55 to 64 years old have plummeted.[1] This early exit trend can be observed in all the indicated countries except Sweden.

Such results seem paradoxical when we remember that the life expectancy, particularly of people over 60, has risen during this same period. Persons who exit from the labor force at age 55 still have about 25 years ahead of them. Life after work tends to be longer than the period (also longer than it used to be) devoted to the education and training of young people. Men and women, most of them fully apt, are now leaving the labor market, dispensed from working, usually in exchange for rather generous compensations.

At first sight, these remarks might lead us to the same conclusions as those drawn about the redistribution of welfare benefits. Aging cohorts in the population seem relatively privileged: They are exempt from holding jobs while being entitled to sizeable social transfers and enjoying free time. But they are also a financial burden since, in Western European countries, unemployment compensation and disability funds bear the cost of benefits to those who have exited early from the labor force. Meanwhile, younger cohorts have a less enviable position. They have a hard time entering the labor market, and the programs for helping them find work provide less generous allowances than the financial incentives aging workers receive when they leave their jobs. Economically and socially, young people have a quite uncertain future. They do not feel reassured about their own prospects for retirement and even if they will some day draw some retirement benefits, all current indicators suggest that these will be lower than those of their elders.

Table 7.1. Employment Activity Rates of Men From 55–64 Years Old

	1970	1972	1974	1976	1978	1980	1982	1984	1986	1988	1990
United States	78.5	76.6	74.3	70.2	70.3	68.8	66.4	64.5	63.8	64.1	64.5
France	74.0	71.5	69.3	65.7	65.8	65.3	56.6	47.2	45.7	43.7	43.0
Germany	78.9	74.4	70.6	64.7	63.2	64.1	60.9	54.6	54.9	52.5	—
Netherlands	—	76.8	72.7	69.2	67.5	61.0	51.6	43.7	41.5	44.5	43.9
Sweden	84.1	81.6	80.4	80.2	77.6	77.5	75.3	73.0	73.3	73.7	74.5
United Kingdom	86.6	82.2	82.8	79.9	77.4	73.9	62.4	60.4	57.6	60.1	63.4

Source: OECD, Labor Force Statistics (1992)

163

But we should not hasten toward conclusions such as these. We must scrutinize the institutional arrangements that have justified shifting the boundaries between work and definitive economic inactivity. By examining their qualitative implications, we can begin to understand how these arrangements have affected intergenerational transfers. Only in this way will we be able to assess whether or not these effects have been fair.

THE EARLY EXIT TREND'S IMPACT

In Europe[2], early exit arrangements developed in four phases, each characterized by overall conditions in the economy, by type of arrangement, and by its objectives. This fourfold division is, of course, a simplification. Each country evolved through these phases in its own way, but differences from this overall scheme can be pointed out.

During the first phase (from the mid-1960s until the mid-1970s), a policy was launched to modernize and restructure the economy. Heavy industry was trying to lay off redundant workers, while other branches of the economy were experiencing a labor shortage. Older workers, with the lowest occupational mobility, were the first to be cut from the work force. These cutbacks were overseen by government-financed preretirement programs that were widely implemented in certain branches, such as iron and steel or the mines. They were part of labor agreements, usually restricted to industries in difficulty or depressed localities. On the whole, these programs very generously compensated wage earners for lost jobs. At the same time, welfare benefits of all sorts (old-age, unemployment compensation, sickness and disability) were being significantly raised.

During the second phase, conditions in the labor market worsened. In the early 1970s, the average period of unemployment was lengthening. Age became a means to discriminate in hiring, older wage earners were increasingly threatened in the labor market. Employment problems were no longer limited to certain areas or industries, and welfare programs were adjusted accordingly. Benefits covered longer periods in order to aid persons who remained unemployed. The government began to intervene so that labor agreements about the dismissal of redundant aging workers were expanded to cover wage earners in other industries or localities. Seniority was no longer the rule ("last hired, first fired") when wage earners had to be trimmed from the work force.

During the third phase, which started in the late 1970s, programs were expanded to cover older workers who resigned voluntarily. The aim was clear: Provide incentives for them to stop working. Many of these programs stipulated that new hirings should be made to replace such departures. As the government's job policy pursued this objective, social policy followed suit. The intention was no longer simply to facilitate job cuts and improve coverage for the aging unemployed. Jobs had to be freed for jobless young people. Accordingly, jobs were to be "shared" between generations, as under the Job Release Scheme in Great Britain, solidarity preretirement contracts in France, or the preretirement act in Germany.

During the fourth phase, the terms of debate shifted. In the 1980s, attention focused on the aging populations in western countries and the prospects for retirement funds. Consequently, many preretirement programs, deemed too expensive, have been terminated. Lowering the retirement age is no longer an issue. In fact, the minimum age for entitlement to an old-age pension is rising. Entitlement less often entails giving up one's job immediately and definitively, as recent programs make it possible to withdraw gradually from the labor force. However, this flexibility is still determined mainly by the job market. Gradual retirement programs have not met with much success, mainly because they still stipulate that new hirings replace departures. Meanwhile, retirement savings plans, and private supplementary old-age funds have been growing.

We are obviously in a transitional phase. Trends will slowly become visible, somewhere between short-term worries about conditions in the labor market and long-term concern about the aging of the population and its effects. With respect to the problem of intergenerational equity, let us now examine the implications of the early exit trend in terms of the distribution of jobs and joblessness; the welfare system (particularly, entitlement to benefits and the individual's integration); and the reorganization of the life course.

ON THE INTERGENERATIONAL DISTRIBUTION
OF EMPLOYMENT AND UNEMPLOYMENT

Most institutional arrangements that have provided incentives for early exit have aimed to reduce unemployment and improve conditions in the labor market by replacing older with younger wage-earners. Everywhere, the results seem disappointing; and because they have usually been ephemeral, their impact is hard to measure.

Unemployment statistics have been affected: Rising joblessness among older wageearners has been hidden provision of coverage to those who exit early. Even when these new arrangements are set up under unemployment funds, these "definitively unemployed" persons no longer count as job seekers.

Further, getting rid of older wage earners has not created many openings for younger workers. During the second phase, eliminating aging workers was, for companies, a way to trim the work force without hiring. In the third phase, when early exit arrangements provided for replacing departing workers, the effect on job openings was greater, but it soon petered out. Therefore, the age of eligibility for these programs has been repeatedly lowered in order to renew the positive effect on job openings. The "intergenerational sharing" of employment has had a very low yield.

Besides this positive effect on employment, these programs were intended to help firms modernize and restructure, as old workers with their obsolete know-how were replaced with young, more qualified, and efficient wageearners. It is difficult to evaluate early exit's impact on productivity. With the arguments currently being used in all countries, neither governments nor firms any longer advocate early exit on a large scale. Almost everywhere, preretirement programs are being phased out.[3]

Employers have discovered that systematically eliminating wage earners upsets personnel's age pyramid and thereby obstructs the normal progression of careers. Older employees lose all motivation as they near the early exit age. At 45, they turn "precociously old." They can no longer hope for any job training, since their firm cannot amortize the investment. Nor do they have any real chances for promotion. In addition, recently recruited young people, many with high-level diplomas, also have lost motivation. Given the skewed age pyramid, they have few chances for promotion, so many are looking for better openings elsewhere.

In the past few decades, the middle-aged generation seems to have cornered jobs for themselves—to the detriment of young and old. The demographic profile of personnel in firms, shows a bulge in this age group.

When comparing positive effects to costs, we are forced to draw a bleak conclusion about early exit arrangements.

ON THE WELFARE SYSTEM AND
ENTITLEMENT TO BENEFITS

Bloated Expenditures

Quite visibly, expanding early exit has swollen the costs of the welfare programs most frequently used to this end. For instance, the cost of disability insurance has become a major concern in the Netherlands and in Germany; and in France, the government, employers, and unions are preoccupied with financing the Unemployment Compensation Fund.

The Retirement System's Loss of Power to Regulate Definitive Exit. Comparing points of convergence between different countries yields a major result: Everywhere, a significant number of wage earners now quit the labor force well before they receive a public old-age pension. Definitive exit no longer systematically corresponds to direct admission into a public retirement system: Definitive exit and retirement no longer fully overlap. Out of the six countries under study, only Sweden, thanks to a program for part-time retirement by age 60, has been able to maintain the retirement system's power over definitive exit. Elsewhere, the eligibility requirements for retirement (age and number of years worked) no longer mark the threshold between work and rest. Public retirement systems are no longer the central means of regulating definitive withdrawal from the labor market (Guillemard, 1989, 1991).

Intermediate Programs between Work and Retirement. Early exit arrangements in the countries under study share a common characteristic: They are intermediate programs, providing a substitute income between the time when a wage is no longer paid and the time when a public old-age pension will be drawn. Each country has tapped the many possibilities resulting from adjustments made in its welfare system—usually in the unemployment compensation or disability insurance subsystems. In addition, ad hoc temporary arrangements often have been made, such as preretirement programs themselves. There has been much "tinkering," but little actual planning. Welfare systems have been manipulated, their rules loosened or adapted to open new pathways for definitive early exit. Considered redundant in the labor force and now superfluous in the labor market, older people are unemployed or "unemployable." These adjustments have deflected these welfare subsystems from their original duties.

This "tinkering"—these successive, circumstantial adjustments in welfare subsystems—accounts for the flexibility of early exit arrangements. Each of the countries under study has made adjustments again and again to substitute one definitive exit pathway for another. When a preretirement program shuts down, a new early exit pathway opens up. France ended solidarity preretirement contracts in 1985, and a new definitive exit pathway opened up under the unemployment compensation fund. As a result, the long-term jobless rate of persons over 55 shot up. When, in 1985, Germany attempted to close down the much overused early exit arrangement under disability insurance, the pathway through the unemployment compensation fund was broadened, as eligibility requirements were slackened for older wage earners. In general, these intermediate programs for covering early exit have come out of the interplay among social actors, as costs have been shifted between programs and from one actor onto another as one pathway closes down and another opens up (Kohli et al., 1991, p.366 ff.).

More and More Intermediate Statuses and Shifting Coverage.   Given the many arrangements for covering the period between definitive exit and admission into a retirement system, individuals often move through several intermediate statuses on their way from work toward retirement. Depending on the country, they may first be covered under disability insurance (for long-term illness), and then later retire; or they may first be assigned the status of unemployed person, then of preretiree and, finally, of retiree. Welfare policies define and then manipulate administrative categories, which become statuses. Thus, policy itself affects the identity of the thus defined social group, and determines its chances of reaching a given "status" (Schnapper, 1989).

In the European countries in the survey, where various welfare subsystems have covered early exit, the increasing number of intermediate statuses apparently corresponds to a change in entitlement. First of all, the older wageearner's right to a job has been restricted. Second, the eligibility requirements for welfare benefits have changed. For instance, social security systems provide general coverage for universal risks. After contributing the required number of years and reaching a certain age, one is entitled to a pension. All French citizens know that they will automatically have a full pension, once they have contributed to the Old-Age Fund for 37.5 years and reached the age of 60. In contrast, the conditions for admission to the intermediate statuses between "wageearner" and "retiree" are neither universal nor stable. Fluctuating with the circumstances, they are continually modified. For instance, the status of "unemployed" does not inevitably lead to retirement. In all countries, the length of time a person can draw long-term unemployment benefits has been continually modified by both conditions in the labor market and the job policy objectives. To cite one example, the arrangement has been abolished that allowed unemployed Germans to quit the labor force at 55 and receive benefits till retirement at the normal age of 60.

Under these intermediate early exit arrangements, beneficiaries have very restricted "rights" in comparison with entitlement under social security. A person who falls victim to the covered risk is not necessarily eligible right away, but only if society decides to provide coverage. This trend in welfare makes us doubt whether today's young retirees are "winners." At least, they pay for this period of nonwork through their precarious status. These fluctuating intermediate statuses have set off an identity crisis. Few "early exiters" think of themselves as retirees. Instead, they claim to be jobless or, in many cases, "discouraged wage earners," with no hope of finding an opening in the labor market (Guillemard, 1986; Laczko, 1987; Casey, & Laczko, 1989).

ON THE ORGANIZATION OF THE LIFE COURSE

Welfare systems have been based on the postulate of a permanent, stable, long-term relationship between wage earner and employer. They have, in turn, helped stabilize both this model of the employment relationship, as well as the threefold model of the life course into which it fits. Under the latter model, which has gradually developed with industrialization, the life course comprises three periods: education during youth; continuous work during adulthood; and rest during old age, marked by the threshold of admission into a retirement system. However, modifications in early exit arrangements and welfare programs are linked to in-depth changes in both the life course and the wage-earning relationship.

The causes of the early exit trend are a mystery. Although it was provoked by economic factors (the job crisis and growing unemployment), opposite factors (the economic recovery signaled in certain countries and a predicted shortage of skilled labor) do not seem to be reversing this trend. In my opinion the business cycle does not fully explain this trend. Early exit has wrought deep changes in welfare systems, in group as well as individual conceptions of the life course, and in social definitions of age and old age. Cultural factors are also at work.

Comparative analysis of definitive exit pathways brings to light the shifting boundaries between work and retirement. Thus, we gain insight into the social construction of old age as the transition between work and retirement is modified. Do changes in definitive exit merely represent a change in the *timing* of retirement? Accordingly, retirement occurs even earlier; but ages (or stages) in the life course still follow each other in the same way, and the threefold model is still intact. I advocate another interpretation. The shifting boundaries between work and retirement are evidence that the threefold model of the life course is no longer an institution. The boundaries between economic activity and inactivity are shifting, not only because the retirement logic is being applied to younger age groups, but because the link between the welfare system and the life course is changing to undermine the threefold model itself. Under the impact of adjustments in welfare systems, the life-course model has undergone two major changes: The new early exit arrangements and their eligibility requirements have "dechronologized" and "destandardized" the life course. These arrangements have blurred temporal boundaries and disrupted the orderly succession of education, work and rest.

From Chronological Milestones to Functional Criteria for Defining Stages in the Life Course. In many countries, disability insurance has largely taken the place of public old-age funds in providing coverage for definitive exit. This finding is crucial. This substitution of one arrangement for another has brought along new eligibility requirements. The latter are no longer based on the age of entitlement to a pension. Now a function of the applicant's "fitness" for work, these requirements have nothing to do with age-based criteria as such. Admission under disability insurance is based on purely functional criteria: Benefits are paid out when an applicant is deemed unfit for work. For this reason, changes in the definitive exit trend can be interpreted as the emergence of a new way of staking out the life course. Instead of chronological age-based criteria, functional ones more often mark off phases in the life course, and are now marking the boundary between work and definitive exit. The end of the life course is being "dechronologized," and this entails a "destandardization" of the life course. Since people's fitness for work as they grow older depends upon their occupations, each socioeconomic category undergoes "differential aging." Adoption of functional eligibility requirements introduces more variability in the beginning of stages in the life course.

This functional redefinition of definitive exit under disability insurance leads to a new social construction of stages in the life course and modifies the linkage between age and work. The aging worker is no longer primarily considered as someone nearly ready for entitlement to an old-age pension, but is now defined as unfit for work or even "unemployable." When almost half of those who go on retirement have already left the labor force through disability insurance (as happened in Germany and the Netherlands), the phase of definitive inactivity comes to be seen not as a time of entitlement to rest but rather as a period when one is—or is classified as being—unfit for work.

In countries where unemployment compensation covers early exit, the eligibility requirements introduced in favor of older wage earners often set up age criteria where none existed before. Coverage under these funds rarely were associated with age. This introduction of age requirements might indicate that chronological criteria remain a major means of marking off phases in the life course, at least in the case of early exit arrangements under unemployment compensation. But we must be able to differinate between these age requirements and those under public old-age funds. The former fluctuate; they are constantly reset. They cannot, therefore, serve as a standardized chronological reference mark (like the retirement age) for the transition toward inactivity. They do not mean that the right to rest has been advanced, but rather that older wage earners have an ever less secure position. In fact, their job security varies widely depending on the industry where they work, their qualifications and training, and their occupational backgrounds.

Underlying these fluctuating, ad hoc age requirements define older wage earners' fitness for work. No boundary with fixed age limits any longer clearly separates work from rest at the end of the life course. The new boundaries shift, depending on conditions in the labor market and the social constructions of age. Other evidence can be found for this interpretation in the United States, where unemployment compensation and disability insurance have not been overused to cover early exit, a 1986 Federal act abolished age discrimination in employment. This act suggests a different way of organizing the life course, one based on the individual's ability and efficiency—the only criteria American employers can invoke to justify the layoff, dismissal, or forced retirement of older wageearners.

The many preretirement programs in Europe were launched mainly in response to the business cycle. Intended to improve conditions in the labor market, these programs often contained clauses for replacing departures through new hirings. Age-based requirements were basic, and older wage earners had room for choice. Although age requirements were continually modified according to conditions in the labor market, these preretirement programs have regulated the transition from work to rest in much the same way as retirement funds. Their beneficiaries have not been assigned successive, precarious statuses beyond their control—as has happened under the other early exit arrangements.

These preretirement programs, under both public arrangements and labor agreements, are ending. This fact cannot be interpreted as a mere lowering of the age for definitive exit. Instead, it is evidence that the last stages in the life course are being "dechronologized." The retirement system has lost the power to regulate definitive exit—to set the boundary between work and rest. And now, preretirement programs, which, by age-based criteria, constructed a bridge spanning the period between withdrawal from the labor force and admission to retirement, are being shut down. Here too, we see that chronological criteria are losing importance.

Much evidence shows the end of the life course as being "dechronologized" and that, as a result, the organization of the life course is being "destandardized. The statistical dispersion of the age of definitive exit is widening, and the long-term unemployment of persons over 50 is rising. The social construction (closely associating old age and retirement) of the third stage of life is coming apart. Old age, retirement, and definitive exit no longer coincide. Occupational old age begins with definitive exit—well before retirement. When retirement no longer determines the meaning of the last phase of life, the threefold life-course model itself comes undone.

Disorganization of the Life Course.   Nowadays, people can less easily foresee when they will enter the last stage of the life course. The chronological milestone of retirement has been overturned and, with it, the principle of an orderly, regulated transition from work toward rest. The life course is becoming more flexible, its organization more closely tied to conditions in both the labor market and company personnel policies. In each of the countries studied, early exit arrangements under disability and unemployment compensation funds have been adjusted to conditions in the labor market. And, similarly, the life course is becoming variable, imprecise, and contingent.

Nowadays, no one in the private sector knows at what age and under what conditions they will exit from the labor force. Retirement as a social situation and a system of transfers no longer constitutes the path that workers will one day take out of the labor force toward old age. The reforms now being proposed (in the United Kingdom and Spain) or adopted (in the United States, Germany, Italy, and France) are pushing the prospects of retirement farther away. Meanwhile, the working life is being shortened, prematurely suspended. As a consequence, the new, long period between definitive exit and retirement is left undefined.

Stages in the life course no longer follow each other in orderly succession. Exit from the working life is no longer a regulated transition toward retirement. Nor is entry into the working life any longer an orderly transition from the educational system into the labor market. Sociologists who have studied youth have described this disorganization: Once out of school, young people are unemployed. Many of them enroll in training programs and hold "small jobs" that, instead of leading to a true occupation, often combine unemployment and training. Uncertainty abounds. This bears close resemblance to the previously described early exit arrangements! The end of the working life also comprises intermediate phases in which people have no full-fledged status, being not exactly jobless, employed, or retired. Many older wageearners are being dismissed and then going on unemployment; some of them benefit from special arrangements. They may find an unstable job, and then go back on unemployment before being admitted into the retirement system. If benefits are reduced and the retirement age is retarded, as is now happening, then "preretirees" will fully join young people in the role of "welfare recipient" or in the even more precarious position of being ineligible for any public support.

We might think that the life course is being "individualized," as individuals dispose of more room for choice. But early exit is more often forced upon than chosen by individuals (Guillemard, 1986; Casey & Laczko 1989). This new "flexibility" at the end of the life course comes from factors related to the job market and companies' labor strategies. The passage toward economic inactivity is no longer a transition, but a sudden break over which the individual has little control. Moreover, early exit arrangements, as set up under disability insurance and unemployment compensation, have eroded older people's right to a job. In effect, early exiters are entitled to benefits only if they abstain from exercising their right to employment. In contrast, the principles underlying old-age funds usually separate the right to a job from the right to a pension; and the retiring wageearner does not have to give up the first right in order to exercise the second.

CONCLUSION: DEINSTITUTIONALIZATION OF THE LIFE-COURSE MODEL AND INTERGENERATIONAL TRANSFERS

Deinstitutionalizing the end of the life course not only keeps people from foreseeing how their lives will evolve, but it also upsets the system of reciprocity between generations. Uncertainty encompasses both retirement and the underlying long term contract. What are the prospects for this long-term contract, which binds *successive* generations together? One cannot count on the reciprocity of commitments across generations in a society where the life course no longer has a long run marked by standard chronological milestones. People still working are beginning to doubt whether the coming generation will pay for their pensions as willingly as they are now paying for current retirees' pensions. The temporal strategy underlying this transfer implies delaying compensation for the alienation of work in exchange for the right to rest at a later stage. But the motivations behind this strategy are weakening, because the life course no longer places individuals in a foreseeable continuum.

For younger generations, it is no longer evident that retirement will continue to organize the life course and regulate social transfers. Youth are less likely than older or middle-aged people to be able to foresee a continuous career that ends in retirement. They also have the least secure position in the labor market; therefore, they see more keenly than other generations the contradictions between organizing social transfers on the basis of a stable wage-earning relationship and an immutable life course and increasing flexibility, both in the life course and in labor management (in response to changes in the labor market).

The intergenerational retirement contract should not be reduced to a mechanized demographic/economic explanation for arguing that the current system is too costly to sustain. As seen, cultural changes in perceptions of time and of the future are just as important in explaining the prospects of this intergenerational contract. They also help us to understand why questions about the retirement system's future are now being raised in such bold terms. In the United States and Great Britain, framing this debate in terms of intergenerational equity has come out of the determination to cut back the welfare state and curb its expenditures—rather than out of the desire to balance transfers between generations. To back up this affirmation, it suffices to observe that the debate about intergenerational equity has not produced any concrete political measure in favor of younger generations (Quadagno, 1989).

The distribution of jobs between generations does not support arguments about intergenerational injustice. Although early exit has often been based on the principle of redistributing work as older wage earners "make room" for unemployed youth, such policies have yielded meager results. The middle-aged have fared best in the labor market, whereas more and more of the young and old are precariously covered under diverse welfare programs.

Measuring intergenerational equity is much more complicated than imagined. It cannot be reduced to the simplistic dichotomy of "winners and losers." The "winners" are certainly not young retirees. Although this group has "won," it has also "lost"—by being assigned precarious statuses and by being deprived of certain rights. Are working, middle-aged wage-earners the "winners"? It is hard to answer a question put in such terms. Although these persons are better placed in terms of jobs, they do not have very clear retirement prospects—even though they have had to pay steep raises in contributions to old-age funds in order to cover today's retirees. If, in order to reduce the cost of retirement, the number of years of contributions for entitlement to an old-age pension is increased, this generation risks being "sacrificed." Although it has made heavy contributions to old-age funds, it is at the risk of receiving lower pensions. To prevent this from happening, older wageearners will have to be given the chance to continue working or remain active. This calls for an active public employment policy.

ACKNOWLEDGMENT

This article has been translated from French by Noal Mellott, CNRS, Paris.

NOTES

1. Employment activity rates, based on the actively working population, are a better indicator than labor force participation rates, based on both wageearners holding jobs and those enrolled in unemployment. Since the persons in the age group under study herein have few chances, once unemployed, of finding jobs again, they should be counted as early definitive withdrawals from the labor force.

2. This is based on results from two international research projects. The first one, headed by Kohli, Rein, Guillemard, and Van Gunsteren, was published in 1991. It concentrated on the six countries in Table 7.1. The second project, linked to the *Observatoire Européen des Politiques de Vieillesse*, focused on the 12 EEC nations (Guillemard, 1993). For a general review of studies about retirement, see Guillemard and Rein (1993).

3. Except in France (where the FNE program covers aging wage earners dismissed for "economic reasons," i.e., redundancy), the Netherlands (which has maintained its VUT program), and Denmark.

REFERENCES

Binney, E., & Estes, C. (1988). The retreat of the state and its transfer of responsibility: The intergenerational war. *International Journal of Health Services, 18,* 83–96.

Casey, B., & Laczko, F. (1989). Early retirement or long-term unemployment? The situation of non-working men aged 55–64 from 1979 to 1986. *Work, Employment and Society, 3,* 505–526.

Cribier, F. (1989). Changes in life course and retirement in recent years: the example of two cohorts of Parisians. In P. Johnson, C. Conrad, & D. Thomson (Eds.), *Workers versus pensioners: Intergenerational justice in an ageing world* (pp.181–201). Manchester: Manchester University Press.

Daniels, N. (1989). Justice and Transfers Between Generations. In P. Johnson, C. Conrad & D. Thomson (Eds.), *Workers versus pensioners: Intergenerational justice in an ageing world* (pp. 57–79). Manchester: Manchester University Press.

Easterlin, F. (1987). The new age structure of poverty in America: Permanent or transient? *Population and Development Review, 1,* 195–208.

Guillemard, A. M. (1986). *Le Déclin du social: Formation et crise des politiques de la vieillesse.* Paris: Presses Universitaires de France.

————. (1989). The trend toward early labor force withdrawal and the reorganization of the life course: A crossnational analysis. In C. Conrad, P. Johnson, & D. Thomson (Eds.), *Workers versus pensioners: Intergenerational justice in an ageing world* (pp.164–180). Manchester: Manchester University Press.

————. (1990). Les paradoxes des politiques de la vieillesse. *Revue Française des Affaires Sociales, 3,* 127–152.

————. (1991). International perspectives on early withdrawal from the labor force. In J. Myles & J. Quadagno (Eds.), *States, labor markets and future of old-age policy* (pp. 209–226). Philadelphia: Temple University Press.

————. (1993). Emploi, protection sociale et cycle de vie: Résultats d'une comparaison internationale des dispositifs de sortie anticipée d'activité. *Sociologie du Travail, 3,* 257–284.

Guillemard, A. M., & Rein, M. (1993). Comparative patterns of retirement: Recent trends in developed societies. *Annual Review of Sociology, 19,* 469–503.

Johnson, P., & Falkingham, J. (1988). *Intergenerational transfers and public expenditures on the elderly in modern Britain.* Discussion paper CEPR (London), 254, 27.

Kohli, M., Rein, M., Guillemard, A. M. & van Gunsteren, H. (Eds.). (1991). *Time for retirement: Comparative studies of early exit from the labor force.* Cambridge: Cambridge University Press.

Laczko, F. (1987). Older workers, unemployment and the discouraged worker effect. In S. di Gregorio (Ed.), *Social gerontology: New directions* (pp. 239–251). London: Cromm Helm.

Longman, P. (1987). *Born to pay: The new politics of aging in America.* Boston: Houghton-Mifflin.

Preston, S. (1984). Children and the elderly: Divergent paths for America's dependents. *Demography, 21,* 435–457.

Quadagno, J. (1989). Generational equity and the politics of the welfare state. *Politics and Society, 17,* 353–376.

Rawls, J. (1971). *A theory of justice.* Cambridge, MA: Harvard University Press.

Schnapper, D. (1989). Rapport à l'emploi: protection sociale et statuts sociaux. *Revue Française de Sociologie, 30,* 3–29.

Thomson, D. (1989). The welfare state and generation conflict: winners and losers. In P. Johnson, C. Conrad, & D. Thomson (Eds.), *Workers versus pensioners: Intergenerational justice in An ageing world* (pp. 32–56). Manchester: Manchester University Press.

II

EAST ASIA

8

Types of Supports for the Aged and Their Providers in Taiwan

Albert I. Hermalin, Mary Beth Ofstedal, and Ming-Cheng Chang

INTRODUCTION

In periods of relative stability, societies tend to develop cultural, socioeconomic, and political institutions that define, with more or less clarity, the nature and mechanisms of major life transitions, such as the passage to adulthood, marriage, and parenthood, or to old age. Rapid social change may cause shifts in these long-standing arrangements, which engender greater uncertainty for certain groups in securing a spouse, a means of livelihood, or an assured source of physical and material support in old age.

Rising interest in the status of the elderly in many parts of Asia stems in part from the convergence of rapid demographic and socioeconomic change. The former is leading to an increase in the number—and, in many cases the proportion—of the population in the higher age groups, while the socioeconomic changes call into question the persistence and strength of family arrangements that generally have been the source of support of the elderly in these societies.

This chapter presents an introductory analysis of the supports needed and received by the elderly in Taiwan, and the individual and institutional providers. Taiwan is an excellent laboratory for studying many of the emerging issues concerning the status of the elderly in Asia. A predominantly Chinese culture, it shares with many countries in East Asia a tradition that views the multigenerational extended family as ideal. At the same time, it has undergone rapid demographic change in the last 25 years, manifest in sharply lower fertility, increasing life expectancy, and continued urbanization, and a dramatic economic trans-

formation from a fairly poor agricultural country to a prosperous industrialized society. In addition, the existence of two distinct groups among
the elderly—the native Taiwanese and their descendants and the Mainlanders, the approximately one million Chinese who arrived after 1949
in the aftermath of the Chinese Civil War—provides interesting contrasts that may help reveal emerging trends.

The following section discusses the trends in living arrangements in
Taiwan, and presents some of the key demographic and socioeconomic
indicators that measure the nature and pace of change. This is followed
by a discussion of some of the methodological issues involved in a study
of support, and the types of data used in this analysis. Differences
between Taiwanese and Mainlanders in living arrangements and other
characteristics, as well as the type of support needed and received by
each group, form the core of the analysis.

THE DEMOGRAPHIC, CULTURAL, AND SOCIOECONOMIC
CONTEXT OF SUPPORT

The Chinese who settled Taiwan from the seventeenth through the
nineteenth centuries brought with them the patriarchal/patrilineal family system that had as its ideal large joint and extended households of
parents with married sons and their families. Authority mainly resided
in senior male members, though it was shared to some extent by a senior
female as long as the husband was alive (Fricke, Chang, & Yang, 1994;
Cohen, 1976). As is well known, mortality patterns and economic circumstances actually limited the size and generational scope of families; a
sizable proportion of families at any one time were either nuclear (husband, wife, and unmarried children) or stem (husband, wife, and one
married son—often the oldest) rather than joint (parents with more than
one married son) (Lang, 1946; Taeuber, 1970).

Here we focus on potential and actual sources of support of the elderly, and note some complexities of the Chinese household and family
structure. In addition to coresident units, Chinese also recognize the
"economic family (chia) i.e., the unit consisting of members related to
each other by blood, marriage, or adoption and having a common budget and common property" (Lang, 1946, p. 13). The chia, although a
relative term with various uses, signifies a collective economy that receives the earnings of all members, provides for their support, and
maintains property that upon partition will be divided (fen-chia) among
those entitled to share (Cohen, 1976, pp. 57–59). Members of a chia may
or may not be coresident, and a variety of economic activities can be

included. Dependent members (the ill, young, students, and elderly) are provided for through the chia's income and resources, and there is active management of the chia economy—often, but not necessarily, by the oldest male of the senior generation (Cohen, 1976). Greenhalgh (1982) claims that the chia is a more appropriate economic unit in Taiwan than the household, on the basis of her analysis of the degree of interdependency among chia households.

Another relevant corporate unit in Chinese society is the lineage, most common in Southeast Asia (including Fukien, the province from which many immigrants to Taiwan originated), which incorporates all males descended from a common ancestor, who know their links to that ancestor. Members of a lineage often live together in a single settlement, own some land in common, maintain ancestral halls and schools for the benefit of their members, and provide other forms of mutual assistance and support.[1] A given individual in Chinese society therefore might have rights and obligations in a widening circle of kinship-based units, starting with the conjugal family and extending through the household (those coresiding), the chia (the family economic unit), and the lineage.

Also relevant from the standpoint of potential mutual support is the existence of associations based on common surnames (clans) and the tendency in some places for married brothers to live near each other—often in the same compound with separate kitchens and living quarters—even when not coresiding. Social and economic ties also frequently develop between the wife's relatives and her husband, and these affinal relations can also be a source of various types of support (Cohen, 1976, pp. 40–41).

The occupation of Taiwan by Japan from 1895 to 1945 did little to change basic family organization or to alter the basic structure of rural society (Barclay, 1954; Cohen, 1976; Hermalin, 1976). The Japanese improved agricultural production and invested in public health, rail, and other infrastructures, but educational and occupational opportunities for the Taiwanese were extremely circumscribed. For example, the proportion of the Taiwanese population that was agricultural decreased only slightly from around 60% early in the century to about 50% in 1940 (Hermalin, Freedman, & Lin, 1994).

In 1949 and for several years thereafter, Taiwan experienced a migration of approximately one million Nationalist military and civilian supporters from the Mainland. The Mainlanders, as they are often called, were mostly young males, and though the total migration was about 13% of the population, it was a much higher percentage of the young adult population. Accordingly, as these cohorts have aged, the Mainlanders represent a significant proportion of the current elderly, and their special history needs to be considered in any investigation.

During the past 40 years, Taiwan has undergone several demographic and socioeconomic changes that have transformed many aspects of Taiwanese life but left other dimensions relatively intact. These changes have introduced both opportunities and constraints in the level and nature of support for the Taiwanese elderly.

Table 8.1 presents indicators that help gauge the direction and magnitude of these changes. Of the demographic changes, fertility levels have decreased dramatically. The total fertility rate dropped from 5.9 children per woman in 1949 to the replacement range of 1.9 in 1988. As a result of these patterns, the ratio of adult children to older parents is currently quite high in Taiwan, but in the future the average number of adult children available to the elderly will diminish substantially. Mortality levels dropped throughout the period, as witnessed by the 23-year improvement in life expectancy. The net result of the fertility and mortality changes has been a sharp reduction in the rate of growth of the population and a shift in age structure, with the proportion under 15 declining to under 30% and the proportion 65 and over more than doubling to nearly 6%. The population has grown more urban, with the proportion in cities advancing from less than one-quarter in 1949 to nearly three-quarters by 1988. The slowing of population growth and the migration patterns has led to a 25% reduction in average household size, from 5.6 in 1949 to 4.1 in 1988. The postwar period was also marked by a sharp advance in the average age at marriage. The proportion of women 20 to 24 years of age who are married has declined from about 70 to 28% in a little over 30 years.

The middle bank of this table presents several economic indicators that illustrate the rapid industrialization of Taiwan and its improvement in living standards. Gross national product in constant Taiwan dollars increased 22 times between 1952 and 1988, which translated into a ninefold improvement in per capita income. Industrial production increased 68 times in the same period, compared to a fourfold increase in agricultural production, with a concomitant rapid shift away from a predominantly agricultural labor force (56% in 1952 to 14% in 1988) to one mostly engaged in industry and services.

Some of the accompanying social indicators appear in the third bank of the table. There was a rapid increase in people's access to communication with the outside world, suggested by the availability of television, and with one another (via telephones). Particularly noteworthy is the rapid rise in educational attainment and the diminishing gender gap. By 1988 about three-quarters of senior high age youth were attending high school and about 30% of college-age youth were attending college. Attendance rates for females, which were traditionally much lower than males', advanced very quickly through the 1960s and 1970s, and by the

Table 8.1. Demographic and Socioeconomic Indicators

	1949	1952	1958	1964	1970	1976	1982	1988
Demographic Indicators								
Population (1000s)	7397	8,128	10,039	12,257	14,676	16,508	18,458	19,904
Average household size	5.55	5.45	5.56	5.60	5.60	5.19	4.58	4.14
% of population: 0–14	41.1	42.4	44.6	45.5	39.6	34.7	31.2	28.2
65 or over	2.5	2.5	2.8	2.6	3.0	3.6	4.6	5.6
Rate of natural increase	29.2	36.7	34.1	28.8	22.3	21.2	17.3	12.1
% of population in cities of 50,000+	24.9	27.4	37.9	45.7	55.5	60.9	68.8	72.9
Total fertility rate	5900	6615	5990	5100	4000	3080	2320	1850
Life expectancy at birth	51.0	58.6	64.2	66.5	68.2	70.0	72.4	73.6
% women 20–24 married	—	—	70[c]	59	50	43	38	28
Economic Indicators								
Per capita income index[a]	—	100.0	126.9	172.7	259.9	390.0	528.2	894.8
GNP index[a]	—	100.0	155.3	257.7	454.1	770.2	1190.4	2171.4
Industrial production index	—	100.0	187.4	400.0	1105.9	2481.1	4017.8	6829.0
Agricultural production index	—	100.0	144.7	182.4	245.5	312.7	362.3	437.7
Avg. No. of people per farm	6.25	6.26	6.34	6.77	6.81	6.39	5.99	5.16
Avg. size farm (hectares)	1.39	1.29	1.15	1.06	1.03	1.06	1.09	1.22
% labor force in agriculture	—	56.1	51.1	49.5	36.7	29.0	18.9	13.7
Social Indicators								
TV sets per 1000 households	—	—	—	14.3	371.0	931.1	1028.7	1100.0
Telephones per 1000 households	13	17	25	40	95	310	801	1105
School attendance rates (%)[b]								
senior high (15–17)								
males	—	11.7	21.8	29.4	47.8	63.1	63.8	72.5
females	—	3.6	8.9	17.6	35.1	54.9	63.5	79.7
college (18–21)								
males	—	2.1	5.5	11.3	21.5	22.1	23.8	29.2
females	—	0.3	1.5	4.8	16.3	19.0	25.3	32.7
Percent women in labor force	—	41	37	34	35	38	39	46

[a] At 1986 prices

[b] Number of students at each level divided by number in each age-sex group

[c] Refers to 1967

Source: Hermalin et al., 1994.

early 1980s equaled or exceeded the enrollment rates for males. The data on the percentage of women in the labor force, which show only a modest upward trend since 1964, do not capture several important changes. One is the shift from agricultural work on the farm to manufacturing and service positions outside the home; the other is the rapid increase in the proportion of married women employed, which reached 42% in 1990 and was even higher among the married women in the prime adult years, 25–50 (Thornton, Chang, & Sun, 1984; ROC, 1991).

These rapid demographic, social, and economic changes have manifold implications for current and future patterns of living and support arrangements of the elderly. For example, from the standpoint of living arrangements, higher income allows parents and children to achieve more privacy via separate households insofar as this is desired, while at the same time the increasing industrialization and migration of children from rural to urban jobs make coresidence difficult. The increasing age at marriage means that unmarried children are likely to be in the parental home for longer periods. From the standpoint of support arrangements, the growing labor force participation of married women outside the home may limit the amount of support daughters-in-law can provide their in-laws even when parents coreside with one or more married sons. Attention must also be paid to the implications for both the working-age population and the elderly population of the rapidly developing social welfare measures that Taiwan, along with other industrialized countries, is implementing.

We will expand on several of these themes later. There is little evidence that the changes described above have dramatically affected the living arrangements of the elderly to date, although changes are clearly underway. Long-term trend data on household composition are not available, but Table 8.2 presents an overview of the pattern since 1976, based on two sources: the household data collected as part of the Survey of Income and Expenditures (Lo, 1987) and the 1989 Survey of Health and Living Status of the Elderly (Taiwan Provincial Institute et al., 1989), which is the source of the analyses to be presented here.[2] Despite the limited range and lack of complete comparability in the sources, the strong trend to independent living on the part of the elderly (either alone or with a spouse only) is clear, concomitantly, the proportion of elderly residing with one or more married children has declined from about two-thirds to a little over a one-half. The trend of living with an unmarried child is less clear. The Survey of Income and Expenditure data suggest an upward trend, but the proportion obtained in the 1989 Survey of Health and Living Status is substantially lower than that of the 1985 Survey of Income and Expenditures. Several definitional issues may be at play here.[3] Before turning to a more detailed analysis of the

Table 8.2.   Percentage Distribution of Living Arrangements of the Elderly 65 and Older, Select Years, 1976–1989

Living Arrangements	1976	1978	1980	1982	1984	1985	1989
Alone or with spouse only	08.8	08.9	12.8	12.8	15.4	17.3	22.8
With married children	66.9	64.5	60.6	59.6	56.8	55.3	56.6
With unmarried children	16.8	20.6	21.0	22.3	22.4	23.0	14.1
Other arrangements	07.5	06.0	05.6	05.3	05.4	04.4	06.6
Total	100.0	100.0	100.0	100.0	100.0	100.0	100.0

Note: Data for 1976–1985 are from the *Survey of Income and Expenditures;* data for 1989 are from the *Survey of Health and Living Status of the Elderly.* The two sources may not be totally comparable (see text).
Sources: 1976–1985 from Lo, 1987
1989 from special tabulation of the *Survey of Health and Living Status of the Elderly.*

1989 cross-section, we address several methodological and conceptual issues.

CONCEPTUAL AND METHODOLOGICAL ISSUES IN ANALYZING SUPPORT ARRANGEMENTS AND A DESCRIPTION OF THE DATA

A study of the levels and types of support received by the elderly is often predicated on a complex set of assumptions that rarely are tested or made fully explicit. First and foremost is the assumption that a set of needs exists, some of which at least are difficult or impossible for the elderly to meet alone. Clearly, two individuals may differ in the amount of support they receive in total or of a particular type, because they have different needs or differ in their ability to meet these needs from their own resources. If needs are to be measured, which areas are to be included and how are they to be assessed? The importance of assessing needs is well recognized, and various measuring instruments have been developed for different dimensions, ranging from rather broad indicators of socioeconomic status—such as education or income—to detailed assessment protocols (for a review of several measures on different dimensions see George & Bearon, 1980; see also Manton & Soldo, 1985, on health service needs). Despite those efforts we are still at some distance from a broad typology and a set of widely accepted measuring instruments. Besides these basic considerations there are several more subtle issues. First, emphasis on the needs of the elderly, and the supports they receive, may inadvertently portray the elderly as passive recipients and overlook the support they may be extending to others through their financial resources, their authority and advice, and through a wide range of services. Any typology of needs must also wrestle with the possibility that the lack of a certain type of support (e.g., emotional) may dampen the expression of that need, and with the problem of how to combine different types of needs and supports into a composite measure (on the use of latent structures, see Hogan & Eggebeen, 1991).

In addition to a careful enumeration of needs, an assessment of support must also consider the number and nature of potential support providers, and their propensity to provide support. Given equal needs, individuals may differ in the amount of support received because they differ in the number of potential providers or in these providers' ability or willingness to extend support. Again, several factors are involved. The perceptions of need on the part of the potential provider must be taken into account, as well as his or her ability and willingness to assist. The location of potential providers vis-à-vis the potential elderly recipient can be critical. Certain forms of support require close proximity; others can be performed at a distance. Those coresiding with the elderly may be more aware of the full range of needs, yet reluctant to provide beyond those requiring daily or frequent attention.

Ideally, therefore, a study of support arrangements would include an assessment of needs across several dimensions; an inventory of potential providers (ranging from the older person, through family and kin, to community resources and governmental programs) and their characteristics (for example, for individuals: location, family status, education, and income); as well as the nature and magnitude of the specific items of support provided by each provider. Few studies attempt to obtain this full array of data and there is little agreement at present on the requisite data collection procedures. Considerable variation exists in the range of potential providers covered (the degree of relationship; their location— coresident or nonresident or both; the nature of the supports covered; and the means of assessing frequency and magnitude of support, to name some of the most obvious factors).

The questionnaire employed in the 1989 Taiwan Survey of Health and Living Status of the Elderly, although it collected considerable data on each of the major elements (needs, providers, and support) was far from exhaustive on all these dimensions. The information is based on a national probability sample of more than 4,000 men and women 60 years or older residing in the nonaboriginal areas of Taiwan, including those in institutions as well as regular households.[4] (For details on the sampling plan, field operations and the questionnaire employed, see Taiwan Provincial Institute et al., 1989.) Of major relevance to this analysis, detailed information was collected on the characteristics of all those residing in the same household as the elderly respondent; the characteristics, location, and frequency of contact with close relatives not in the household; and the exchanges that took place between the respondent and others on several dimensions. More specifically, the respondent was asked separately whether he or she received assistance with activities of daily living (bathing, dressing, toilet); with certain instrumental activities (household chores, shopping, meal preparation, transportation, or managing finances); by receipts of money; and by receipts of food, clothing, or other goods. In each case the respondent was asked to identify all persons who provided any support as well as the most important provider. Those receiving any support were asked to characterize the adequacy of that support, and those not receiving any were asked if they needed this type of assistance. Given the assumption that those who receive support do need it, this structure provides an estimate of overall needs as well as supports.

Since respondents might overlook provisions of support from local or national agencies in favor of individuals, specific questions were included to record whether support of this type was received, and the nature of the organization and the type of support.

In addition to this elaborate support matrix (which was also asked of the support *provided by* the elderly respondent), other sections of the questionnaire went into considerable detail on health and health care utilization, finances and financial management, occupational and residence histories, recreational activities, and a wide range of attitudes and background characteristics. Many of these sections also contain items that are related, more or less explicitly, to questions on the nature and sources of support.

Table 8.3 presents the major characteristics of the elderly; because of the special history of the Mainlanders, many of their demographic and socioeconomic characteristics differ sharply from those of the Taiwanese, so the two groups are shown separately here and in many of the subsequent tables.

There are rather dramatic differences in the demographic composition of Taiwanese versus Mainlander elderly—differences that have important implications for the resources (i.e., either family or other individuals, or formal resources) available to these individuals for meeting support needs, as well as the degree of need itself. Mainlanders are overwhelmingly male, and the magnitude of this group (22% of all elderly respondents) results in a sex ratio of 1.3 among all elderly in Taiwan. This substantial excess of elderly males in Taiwan is quite different from the sex composition of most other developed or newly developed countries.

Another important distinctive feature of the two groups is that al-

Table 8.3. Percent Distribution of Respondents across Selected Characteristics, by Ethnicity

Demographic Characteristics	Taiwanese	Mainlander
Sex		
Male	49.7	84.0
Female	50.3	16.0
Marital status		
Married	64.4	63.8
Widowed	32.6	14.8
Separated or divorced	01.7	08.2
Never married	01.2	13.2
Age		
60–64	34.1	42.4
65–69	27.5	32.2
70–74	19.5	14.3
75–79	11.7	08.1
80+	07.1	03.0
Type of residence		
Large city	23.9	45.9
Urban township	37.3	33.2
Rural	38.8	20.9
Family and Household Characteristics		
Mean number of children		
Married	4.35	1.55
Unmarried	0.77	1.14
Living arrangements		
Alone	05.4	21.3
With spouse and/or unmarried children	29.1	50.0
With married children (w/ or w/o spouse)	59.5	20.8
Other	06.0	07.9
Health and Socioeconomic		
Health status		
Very good	14.4	27.7
Good	21.4	23.2
Fair	40.5	30.4
Not so good	19.5	15.4
Very bad	04.2	03.3
Work status		
Working	25.9	34.9
Not working	74.1	65.1
Income		
<NT$ 3,000	22.7	03.2
NT$ 3,000–9,999	36.9	26.8
NT$ 10,000–19,999	26.2	38.4
NT$ 20,000+	14.2	31.6

(*continued*)

Table 8.3.   (Continued)

Demographic Characteristics	Taiwanese	Mainlander
Education		
Less than primary	49.4	13.4
Primary	39.9	39.0
Jr. high and above	10.7	47.6
House ownership		
Self or spouse	54.0	54.0
Child	37.9	12.0
Housing provided	02.3	25.7
Renting	05.8	08.3
Division of property		
All divided to children	18.8	01.5
Part divided to children	11.2	03.5
Have not divided	41.5	50.0
No property	28.6	45.0
Total *N*	(3158)	(891)
(%)	(78.0)	(22.0)

though roughly equal proportions are currently married, the marital status composition among those who are not currently married is quite different. Whereas the vast majority of unmarried Taiwanese are widowed, Mainlanders tend more to be either never married or else separated or divorced. Their status has important implications for their current family structures and potential sources of support.

Mainlanders also are substantially younger than Taiwanese on average; roughly 75% of Mainlander elderly are age 60–69, compared to 62% of Taiwanese elderly. Finally, geographic distribution is quite different for the two groups. Mainlanders tend to be concentrated in urban areas, especially large cities, relative to the Taiwanese elderly.

With respect to the availability of family, there are sharp differences between Taiwanese and Mainlanders. Mainlanders on average have substantially fewer married children than Taiwanese, but more unmarried children (because Mainlanders are younger, as are their children, and less likely to be married). The excess of unmarried children for Mainlanders, however, does not make up for their relative lack of married children, so that, overall, Mainlanders have just over one-half the number of children than Taiwanese. In addition, Mainlanders and Taiwanese are distributed differently across living arrangements. Note that 21% of Mainlanders live completely alone (not even with spouse), compared to only 5% of Taiwanese—and Taiwanese are more likely to live with a married child (almost always a son) than are Mainlanders.

Finally, Mainlanders are healthier, more likely to be working (largely because they are predominantly male), and tend to be somewhat advantaged relative to Taiwanese with respect to socioeconomic indicators (income, education). However, Taiwanese are more likely to have, or at some point to have had, assets in terms of property and house.

THE NATURE OF SUPPORTS RECEIVED
AND SUPPORT PROVIDERS

This section presents a preliminary analysis of the complex support matrix previously described. In a series of tables we describe the reported level of need and sufficiency of support received with regard to ADL, IADL, financial support, and material support, the providers of this support, and several interrelationships. The receipt of support and the likely provider are highly conditioned by living arrangements, and because Mainlanders and Taiwanese differ so sharply on characteristics relevant to the need or provision of support, we will frequently control on one or another of these characteristics.

Table 8.4 presents a broad overview of the needs and sufficiency of support for each type, by living arrangement and ethnicity. In reading this table it is well to recall that respondents were asked if they were receiving each type of support; if so, they were asked if it was adequate ("could use more help," "receiving about right amount," "receiving more than would like"); if they were not receiving any, they were asked if they needed this type of assistance. For each type of support in Table 8.4, therefore, the first row represents those who said they neither received nor needed support, the second row those who needed and received none or an insufficient amount, and the third row those who received an adequate amount of support. The first three rows sum to 100%, and the fourth row is the ratio of row 3 to the sum of rows 2 and 3.

With respect to ADL assistance, a very high proportion claim that they do not need or receive this type of support. Mainlanders are slightly less likely to need or receive this type of support than are Taiwanese, as are those who live either alone or in a nuclear unit compared to the other living arrangements. In general, however, the variation across living arrangements and ethnicity is quite small.

Although we must be cautious about the small base numbers for these proportions, some variation appears across both living arrangements and ethnicity in terms of the sufficiency of ADL support that is received. In general, Taiwanese are more likely than Mainlanders to receive a sufficient amount of support. In addition, among the Taiwanese, those living either with a spouse and/or unmarried/or married child are more likely to receive sufficient ADL support than are those living alone or

Table 8.4. Proportion of Respondents Receiving Support and Sufficiency of Support Received for Four Types of Support, by Ethnicity and Living Arrangement

| | Ethnicity and Living Arrangement | | | | | | | |
| | Taiwanese | | | | Mainlander | | | |
Type and Sufficiency of Support	Alone	R/U/S*	R/M/S*	Other	Alone	R/U/S*	R/M/S*	Other
ADL:								
Does not need or receive support	92.9	95.1	91.8	89.2	97.3	96.6	96.2	95.6
Need and/or receive support								
• Support received - insufficient	05.3	01.7	02.4	06.4	02.2	01.6	02.2	01.5
• Support received - sufficient	01.8	03.2	05.8	04.4	00.5	01.8	01.6	02.9
Proportion receiving sufficient amount	25.4	65.3	70.7	40.7	18.5	52.9	42.1	65.9
IADL								
Does not need or receive support	68.6	38.3	17.9	27.6	87.8	31.4	29.5	60.9
Needs and/or receives support								
• Support received - insufficient	15.3	04.5	04.5	07.9	06.4	02.6	04.0	05.8
• Support received - sufficient	16.1	57.2	77.6	64.5	05.8	66.0	66.5	33.3
Proportion receiving sufficient amount	51.3	92.7	94.5	89.1	47.5	96.2	94.3	85.2
Financial Support								
None needed or received	22.0	19.0	15.1	21.2	75.1	52.0	26.6	62.3
Needs and/or receives support								
• Support received - insufficient	29.8	21.0	11.2	25.2	15.8	13.1	07.8	06.3
• Support received - sufficient	48.2	60.0	73.7	53.6	09.1	34.9	65.6	31.4
Proportion receiving sufficient amount	61.8	74.1	86.8	68.0	36.5	72.7	89.4	83.3
Material Support								
None needed or received	49.7	60.7	46.1	52.7	87.2	81.2	62.8	82.9
Needs and/or receives support								
• Support received - insufficient	20.8	08.9	05.6	12.3	05.9	05.5	03.0	05.5
• Support received - sufficient	29.5	30.4	48.3	35.0	06.9	13.3	34.2	11.6
Proportion receiving sufficient amount	58.6	77.4	89.6	74.0	53.9	70.7	91.9	67.8
Total Ns	618	900	1845	184	189	442	184	69

* R/U/S = Respondent with unmarried child and/or spouse only.
R/M/S = Respondent lives with married child (spouse may or may not be present).

with others. Among Mainlanders, those living with others are most likely to receive a sufficient amount of support (but based on a small number of cases), followed by those living with a spouse and/or unmarried child.

With respect to IADL assistance, the proportion who either need or receive this type of support is much higher than that for ADL. In addition, substantial variation occurs across both living arrangements and ethnicity in terms of the likelihood of receiving this type of support—but less variation in terms of the sufficiency of IADL support (except for those living alone). For both ethnic groups, the elderly are most likely to receive (or need) IADL support when living with a married child, and least likely when living alone. Mainlanders are also quite unlikely to receive (or need) support when living with others.

Within categories of living arrangements, Mainlanders generally are less likely to receive (or need) support than Taiwanese, except among those who are living with a spouse and/or unmarried children only. This is probably due, in large part, to the fact that Mainlanders are disproportionately male and that the IADL support provider tends to be female (in this case primarily a wife). In general, both Taiwanese and Mainlanders tend to receive a sufficient amount of IADL assistance, except among those who live alone.

In considering the receipt of and/or need for financial support, we see substantial variation by ethnicity and, among Mainlanders only, substantial variation by living arrangement. A very high proportion of Taiwanese, regardless of living arrangement, receive and/or need financial support. Mainlanders are significantly less likely to need or receive financial support than Taiwanese across all living arrangements. Among Mainlanders, those living with a married child are more likely than those in all other living arrangements to receive (and need) financial assistance. Sufficiency of financial support varies across living arrangements, with those living alone least likely to receive a sufficient amount (especially for Mainlanders), and those living with married children most likely to receive sufficient support.

In the case of material support, again Taiwanese are more likely than Mainlanders to receive and/or need this type of support across all living arrangements. For both ethnic groups, those living with a married child are most likely to receive this form of assistance. However, unlike Mainlanders, Taiwanese who live alone are also quite likely to receive material support (30% receive a sufficient amount versus only 7% of Mainlanders). Sufficiency of material support varies according to living arrangement in much the same way as sufficiency of financial support.

Overall, although Mainlanders are less likely to need support currently, those who are living alone or with a spouse and/or unmarried children (a strong majority of Mainlanders) are fairly consistently less likely to receive a sufficient amount of support (at least from individuals). In addition, although data are not shown here, Mainlanders are less optimistic than Taiwanese regarding the extent to which their future support needs will be met. This gives rise to some concern about the adequacy of support for Mainlanders as their needs increase in the future.

Tables 8.5–8.8 focus on the individual support providers (as distinct from formal service providers), and examine how provision of support is distributed across these providers. Unlike Table 8.4, Table 8.5 is restricted to those who received each type of support. The left panel of this table presents the proportion of respondents who receive support from each type of individual according to living arrangement. Because more than one person may be providing support to any given respondent, and because supports from formal services are excluded, the proportions may add to more or less than 100%. The panel on the right side identifies the most important provider of each type of support, also by living arrangement. Total Ns (i.e., the number of support recipients) are given in the last row of the panel for each type of support separately.

The most common providers of ADL are spouse and daughter-in-law. The daughter-in-law is the most prominent provider when she is proximately available (i.e., living in the household), and the spouse when the daughter-in-law is not in the household. Children are less, but still somewhat, important providers of ADL.

A similar pattern exists with IADL, in that the daughter-in-law and spouse are most common providers (in that order). Children (sons and daughters) are quite a bit less likely to provide IADL than ADL assistance, and most of their portion of the responsibility seems to fall onto the daughter-in-law. Even among those who are living alone and receiving IADL support (albeit a fairly small number), the daughter-in-law has an important role as provider.

With respect to financial support, children, especially sons, emerge as the most common (and most important) providers. Daughters are more important when respondents live with spouse and/or unmarried children than they are when respondents live with a married child (most often a son), but even in these cases the son is the more important provider. Daughters-in-law also tend to provide when they are in the household, but are rarely identified as the most important provider.

Children are also the most common providers of material support, but, in contrast to financial support, daughters play a much more prominent role as providers. Daughters are particularly important when the elderly respondent is living either alone or with spouse and/or unmarried children, the sons more so when the respondent lives with a mar-

Table 8.5. Proportion of Respondents with Specific Kin as Providers and most Important Providers of Four Types of Support, among Support Recipients, by Living Arrangement

	Living Arrangements							
	Specific Kin is Provider				Specific Kin is Most Important Provider			
Type of Support and Specific Kin	Alone	R/U/S	R/M/S	Other	Alone	R/U/S	R/M/S	Other
ADL:								
Spouse	—	77.1	23.1	34.6	—	75.6	21.6	33.5
Child	00.0	33.3	49.3	41.8	00.0	22.3	33.6	28.2
• Son	00.0	18.8	37.0	28.8	00.0	06.7	22.4	16.2
• Daughter	00.0	20.8	13.8	15.4	00.0	15.6	11.2	12.0
Other kin	60.0	02.1	59.4	44.7	60.0	00.0	43.2	33.5
• Daughter-in-law	40.0	02.1	48.6	34.6	40.0	00.0	37.6	26.7
• Son-in-law	00.0	00.0	03.6	02.4	00.0	00.0	00.0	00.0
• Other	20.0	00.0	14.5	13.0	20.0	00.0	05.6	06.8
Friends, neighbors, other nonkin	40.0	00.0	00.7	01.9	40.0	00.0	00.0	01.6
Nurse, maid, other paid help	00.0	02.1	02.2	03.4	00.0	02.2	01.6	03.1
(Total N)	(5)	(48)	(139)	(208)	(5)	(45)	(125)	(16)
IADL								
Spouse	—	86.3	25.3	44.4	—	88.2	19.4	41.4
Child	27.7	12.5	23.3	19.3	36.4	09.5	13.3	12.0
• Son	19.1	06.4	16.6	12.8	21.2	04.4	07.8	06.6
• Daughter	12.8	07.5	07.9	07.8	15.2	05.1	05.5	05.4
Other kin	29.8	02.5	76.7	50.8	36.3	01.4	66.8	45.0
• Daughter-in-law	27.7	01.9	73.8	47.0	33.3	01.2	64.7	42.0
• Son-in-law	00.0	00.0	00.9	00.6	00.0	00.0	00.2	00.2
• Other	04.3	00.6	04.6	05.0	03.0	00.2	01.9	02.8
Friends, neighbors, other nonkin	14.9	00.5	00.1	01.0	12.1	00.2	00.0	00.7
Nurse, maid, other paid help	08.5	00.5	00.7	00.9	12.1	00.6	00.6	00.9
(Total N)	(47)	(843)	(1634)	(2680)	(33)	(804)	(1610)	(2586)

Financial Support

Spouse	—	15.3	05.7	08.3	—	09.9	03.6	05.4
Child	88.2	92.3	97.3	94.1	94.1	88.7	93.3	90.8
• Son	75.2	80.7	91.8	86.1	75.7	73.1	85.0	79.8
• Daughter	36.6	41.8	31.3	34.7	18.4	15.6	08.3	11.0
Other kin	05.9	03.5	15.8	12.4	03.6	01.1	03.1	03.6
• Daughter-in-law	02.0	01.4	11.0	07.5	00.7	00.2	01.5	01.2
• Son-in-law	00.0	00.7	02.2	01.6	00.0	00.0	00.7	00.4
• Other	04.6	01.8	03.6	04.4	02.9	00.9	00.9	02.0
Friends, neighbors, other nonkin	02.6	00.2	00.0	00.3	02.2	00.1	00.0	00.2
Nurse, maid, other paid help	00.0	00.0	00.1	00.0	00.0	00.1	00.0	00.0
(Total N)	(153)	(866)	(1696)	(2870)	(136)	(848)	(1675)	(2802)

Material Support

Spouse	—	16.5	04.4	07.4	—	13.9	02.9	05.7
Child	78.6	85.9	89.4	85.9	82.2	83.9	81.4	80.3
• Son	39.3	49.2	63.2	56.8	39.7	40.8	52.7	47.9
• Daughter	59.5	66.0	51.3	54.6	42.5	43.1	28.7	32.4
Other kin	20.2	07.7	34.8	28.0	16.4	02.0	15.5	13.6
• Daughter-in-law	10.7	06.1	30.8	22.8	08.2	01.7	14.2	10.5
• Son-in-law	00.0	00.5	02.0	01.5	00.0	00.0	00.4	00.3
• Other	09.5	01.6	03.6	05.1	08.2	00.3	00.9	02.8
Friends, neighbors, other nonkin	09.5	01.3	00.4	01.3	01.4	00.3	00.1	00.8
Nurse, maid, other paid help	00.0	00.0	00.1	00.1	00.0	00.0	00.0	00.0
(Total N)	(84)	(376)	(1026)	(1572)	(73)	(360)	(985)	(1499)

Table 8.6. Selected Characteristics of Daughters-in-Law, among Those Living with Respondent, by Daughter-in-Law's Caregiving Status[*]

Characteristic	Caregiving Status[**]	
	Most Important Provider	*Not Most Important Provider*
Mean age	37.7	35.4%
Education		
no formal education	11.3	08.3
primary	45.6	40.1
junior or Senior High	37.2	40.6
college and above	05.9	11.0
Work status		
works full-time	40.4	56.0
works part-time	08.2	07.5
does not work	51.4	36.5
Total *N*	768	1300
(%)	36	64

[*] Analysis is restricted to daughters-in-law living with respondents who are currently receiving some type of support.
[**] A daughter-in-law is identified as most important provider here if the respondent reports her as such for at least one of the four types of support.

ried child. Daughters-in-law show up again as fairly active providers, especially when there is coresidence with a married child.

In general, very little support of any type is provided by nonkin or paid individuals, although when it does occur, it is usually among those who live alone. Spouses drop out of the picture for financial and material support, probably because respondents do not consider sharing of these resources between spouses an exchange of support, as we imply in our questions.

Table 8.5 shows that daughters-in-law are important as providers of support (particularly for ADL and IADL, and somewhat for material support). In Table 8.6, we look at the characteristics of those daughters-in-law who are identified as important providers of support, in order to get some sense of her position in the family and of the extent to which she has competing demands on her time. This table focuses on daughters-in-law who live with the respondent, and compares those identified as most important providers of any of the four types of support with those who are not so identified. In order to be included in this table, the respondent with whom the daughter-in-law coresides must be receiving at least one type of support.

As the data indicate, daughters-in-law who are identified as most important providers tend to be older on average, somewhat less educated, and less likely to be working than those in the household who are

Table 8.7. Matrix of Supports Received and Distribution of Providers (%)[*]

	Physical Care	IADL	Financial	Material
Physical care	—	04.6	03.8	3.3%
IADL assistance	63.1	—	48.5	28.8
Financial assistance	16.8	09.2	—	34.0
Material assistance	29.5	24.6	40.4	—

[*] Figures above the diagonal represent proportions receiving both types of support; figures below the diagonal represent the proportion of those receiving both types that receive them from the same person.

not the most important providers. But even among the daughters-in-law who are the most important providers, 40% work full-time. Nevertheless, the differentials suggest the possibility that in the future, as daughters-in-law are increasingly educated (especially relative to the older parents for a period of time) and increasingly likely to be working, they may not be available (and/or willing) to provide the support that previous generations of daughters-in-law have.[5]

Tables 8.7 and 8.8 (from Hermalin et al., 1990, p.21) attempt to capture the extent to which responsibility is diffused across different family members. Figures above the diagonal in Table 8.7 reflect proportions receiving the specific pairs of support; on this point, the data suggest that the most frequent support combination received is assistance with IADL and financial assistance (49%), followed by the combination of financial and material assistance (34%). Figures below the diagonal represent the proportion of those receiving this combination for whom the most important provider of each type of support is the same person. For example, among those receiving both IADL and financial assistance, the most important provider is the same person in only 9% of the cases, compared to 40% for the combination of financial and material support. The provider is the same most often for those receiving both IADL and physical care (ADL) assistance, although the proportion receiving this combination of support is quite small (less than 5%).

Another perspective on the distribution of support received is provided by Table 8.8, which shows the number of different types received and their distribution across providers, controlling for the presence or absence of the respondent's spouse in the household. Consistent with the results in Table 8.5, which suggested a distribution of support across certain people for different types, these figures also suggest that primary responsibility is diffused among a number of different providers. For example, for those respondents who report receiving two or more types of support, at least two main providers are involved a minimum of 75%

Table 8.8. Number of Types of Supports Received and Distribution across Providers by Presence of Spouse in Household

Number of Supports/ Distribution of Providers	Spouse Present		Spouse Not Present	
No. support received	07.1		20.1	
One support received	30.9		21.2	
Two supports received	36.4		27.4	
• same main provider		16.8		24.9
• different main provider		83.2		75.1
Three supports received	23.2		26.3	
• same provider		07.5		10.8
• two providers		47.3		53.7
• three main providers		45.2		35.5
Four supports received	02.4		05.0	
• same main provider		09.4		16.2
• two main providers		47.2		47.0
• >2 main providers		43.4		36.8
Total (%)	100.0		100.0	
(N)	(2492)		(1535)	

Source: Hermalin et al., 1990, Tables 4 and 5.

of the time. The percentages representing involvement of three or more main providers are somewhat more modest, but nevertheless support the suggestion that responsibility for care of the elderly tends to be distributed among several family members, rather than resting solely in one person.

Table 8.9 focuses on the contribution of formal services to each of the four potential areas of need (ADL, IADL, financial, and material). As noted earlier, a specific question asked whether the respondent received "any support we just mentioned from government, religious or other private services." Those who responded "yes" were asked the name of the service and the type of support received. The types of services used varies by type of support, but those most often mentioned include government or other public institution; public nursing home; public or private hospital; and other religious institutions.

The figures in this table represent the proportion of respondents who receive each type of support from a formal service, among those who receive the specific support. The respondents may also be receiving assistance from individuals as well, and the formal source may or may not be the most important source.

We have excluded formal support for ADL because only about one percent of recipients obtained this type of assistance from a formal service. The data are subdivided by Taiwanese and Mainlander because of their differential reliance on formal agencies.

Table 8.9. Proportion Receiving Specific Type of Support from Formal Source, among those Receiving each Type of Support, by Ethnicity and Selected Sociodemographic Characteristics

| | \multicolumn{6}{c|}{Ethnicity and Type of Support} |
| Characteristics | \multicolumn{3}{c|}{Taiwanese} | \multicolumn{3}{c|}{Mainlander} |
	IADL	Financial	Material	IADL	Financial	Material
Sex						
Male	00.2	03.8	06.8	04.3	52.1	19.8
Female	00.7	02.7	06.3	01.9	09.3	05.9
Age						
60–69	00.3	02.4	04.2	02.4	41.5	12.3
70+	00.6	04.3	09.3	08.3	42.9	22.2
Marital Status						
Married	00.0	02.1	05.6	00.5	32.2	10.1
Not married	01.2	05.1	07.8	22.4	60.1	27.6
Place of residence						
Large city	00.6	04.5	03.6	05.9	42.6	09.4
Urban township	00.5	03.0	04.9	00.6	40.6	19.0
Rural	00.2	02.6	09.0	05.5	42.7	27.6
Work status						
Working	00.2	04.0	04.5	01.6	57.0	18.9
Not working	00.5	03.0	07.0	05.6	36.9	15.0
Income						
<NT$ 3,000	01.5	05.9	10.7	10.0	14.3	16.7
NT$ 3,000–9,000	00.1	02.7	07.7	14.4	59.7	25.8
NT$ 10,000–19,999	00.0	01.5	02.0	01.2	43.3	09.5
NT$ 20,000+	00.0	02.8	02.7	00.6	24.6	08.8
Education						
Illiterate	00.3	02.9	08.2	12.5	36.0	20.0
Can read or primary	00.6	03.3	04.6	05.1	52.0	21.7
Jr. high and above	00.4	04.5	04.1	01.6	35.2	10.7
Health status						
Very good	00.0	02.0	04.8	01.6	46.5	10.4
Good	00.4	01.6	08.7	02.1	33.9	21.1
Fair	00.5	02.6	04.6	05.3	42.1	17.0
Not so good	00.7	04.6	07.5	03.4	43.5	13.8
Very bad	00.0	08.2	16.0	14.3	45.0	22.2
Living arrangements						
Alone	22.6	19.5	24.3	55.6	83.1	47.6
Spouse or unmarried child(ren) only	00.0	03.7	07.9	00.3	37.8	12.2
Married child(ren)	00.0	00.8	04.2	00.0	14.6	03.1
Other	01.6	11.8	13.6	25.8	70.5	46.7
Total (%)	00.4	03.2	06.5	04.0	41.3	15.8
(Base *N*)	(2184)	(2507)	(1436)	(472)	(491)	(177)

For each type of support, the proportions of recipients receiving support from a formal source are consistently higher for Mainlanders than Taiwanese, and in the case of financial support the difference is marked (41% Mainlander vs. 3% Taiwanese; see last row of Table 8.9). Most of the Mainlanders receiving financial support are male and they exceed females in the other types of formal support as well. By contrast, very little sex differential appears in formal support among the Taiwanese. It should be kept in mind that many of the Mainlander males are or were career military officers or enlisted men or civilian government officials, and therefore eligible for benefits and services not yet available to the population at large, this will be discussed later.

With few exceptions, the differential in formal support in favor of Mainlanders holds within the categories of the other characteristics presented in Table 8.9. For several characteristics, the patterns across categories are similar for Taiwanese and Mainlanders. The proportion receiving support from a formal source increases with age for both ethnic groups, and is lower among those who are married compared to those not married. For both groups, the proportion receiving *financial* support from a formal source is higher for those working versus not working; and the proportion receiving *material* support is highest among rural residents in both cases. The patterns by living arrangement are also consistent by ethnic group: Those living alone are the most likely to receive each type of support from a formal source, and the proportion of those recipients benefiting from such sources is substantial, ranging from 20 to 25% among the Taiwanese, and from 50 to 80% among the Mainlanders. Those in "other" living arrangements are the second most likely category to use formal sources, while those living with a spouse and/or children were least likely to derive such assistance.

Among Taiwanese, the likelihood of receiving formal support of any type shows a negative relationship with income (with a slight upturn at highest income for financial and material support). In contrast, Mainlanders, in the second income group are consistently most likely to receive formal support of each type; and those in the lowest income group are the least likely to receive financial support from a formal source.

These patterns suggest that the existing formal support sources in Taiwan are functioning, in part at least, as a "safety net" for those outside the traditional familial arrangements (e.g., those living alone) and for those at the lower end of the income scale. Among the Mainlanders, those at intermediate levels seem to benefit most, probably because they are most affiliated with the formal programs associated with their military or civilian government careers.

MULTIVARIATE ANALYSIS OF FACTORS
AFFECTING SUPPORT

To this point we have focused on the nature of the supports received and the providers, and examined differentials on a bivariate basis. Many of the factors affecting the receipt of support are, of course, interrelated, and it is of interest to study their relative importance in a multiple regression context.

Modelling the receipt of support presents several challenges, and the results presented must be viewed as tentative. In keeping with the earlier discussion, the two broad conceptual factors affecting levels of support are need, on the one hand, and number, location, and willingness of potential providers, on the other. At the current stage of analysis we do not have an independent measure of need, since the support module assumes that all those who receive a type of support need it.[6] As an alternative, we use a series of background characteristics of the elderly generally associated with differential levels of need, including: age, sex, work status, education, and health status. (Although we also have measures of the incomes of the elderly, these include receipts from children and thus are not independent of support received.) As measures of the potential support environment, we include the living arrangements of the elderly, the number of children they have, and place of residence of the elderly.[7]

Since the previous tables reveal sharp differences between the Taiwanese and Mainlanders, the analyses were carried out separately for each. The results of the logistic regressions appear in Tables 8.10 and 8.11, respectively. The tables present the effects of being in the specified category of the independent variable (versus the omitted category) or of a one-year increment in age or a one-level increment in health status on the log-odds of receiving the type of support indicated. These analyses focus on support that is received from individuals, as opposed to formal service providers. Receipt of support for ADL is omitted because the proportion receiving this type of support was very small.

Table 8.10, for the elderly Taiwanese, reveals similarities and differences in the factors affecting the different types of support. Increasing age and poorer health increase the likelihood of respondents' receiving each type of support; being male enhances the probability of receiving assistance with IADL, but lowers the probability of financial or material assistance. Those not living with married children are less likely to receive each type of support, confirming the patterns of Table 8.4; the disadvantage is particularly marked with respect to IADL and material

Table 8.10. Estimated Effects of Demographic, Socioeconomic, and Health Factors on the Log Odds of Receiving each Type of Support, among Elderly Taiwanese

Explanatory Variables	Assistance with IADL	Financial Support	Material Support
Constant	−2.36***	−.95*	−3.16***
Age	.04**	.02**	.04***
Sex			
female	—	—	—
male	1.69***	−.32**	−.20**
Place of residence			
large city	.10	−.57***	−.67***
urban township	.41***	−.54***	−.76***
rural township	—	—	—
Work status			
currently working	—	—	—
retired/not working	−.13	1.19***	.37***
Education			
no formal education	—	—	—
up to primary education	−.10	−.14	.04
jr. high education or more	−.18	−.77***	.11
Self-reported health			
(#1 = very good . . . #5 = very poor)	.09**	.10**	.08**
Number of children in Taiwan			
0	−.10	−.48	−.45
1–2	—	—	—
3+	.15	.62***	.21*
Living arrangements			
live alone	−3.60***	−.39*	−.52***
live with spouse only	−1.18***	−.14	−.50***
live with unmarried children (w/ or w/o spouse)	−1.27***	.01	−.57***
live with married children (w/ or w/o spouse)	—	—	—
live with others (w/ or w/o spouse & unmarried children)	−.77***	−.43**	−.37**

* Significant at 10.0% level
** Significant at 5.0% level
*** Significant at 0.5% level

support. Interestingly, those without children in Taiwan are not at a disadvantage with respect to those with one or two children, but larger numbers of children do contribute to the probability of support. Educational differentials are quite muted, except for the sharp decrease in financial support among those with junior high or more education. The likelihood of receiving financial or material support is higher for those retired or not working and for those in rural areas, but work status has

Table 8.11. Estimated Effects of Demographic, Socioeconomic, and Health Factors on the Log Odds of Receiving each Type of Support, among Elderly Mainlanders

Explanatory Variables	Assistance with IADL	Financial Support	Material Support
Constant	−5.22***	−4.23***	−2.16
Age	.07***	.07***	.02
Sex			
female	—	—	—
male	1.63***	−1.46***	−.63**
Place of residence			
large city	.70**	.42*	−.13
urban township	.70**	.25	.12
rural township	—	—	—
Work status			
currently working	—	—	—
retired/not working	−.64***	.94***	.45*
Education			
no formal education	—	—	—
up to primary education	−.30	.39	.07
jr. high education or more	−.18	.17	.07
Self-reported health			
(#1 = very good . . . #5 = very poor)	.19**	.02	.02
Number of children in Taiwan			
0	.02	−1.04**	−1.19**
1–2	—	—	—
3+	.03	.69***	−.25
Living arrangements			
live alone	−4.51***	−1.32***	−.85*
live with spouse only	.04	−1.21***	−.47
live with unmarried children (w/ or w/o spouse)	−.36	−.48**	−.88***
live with married children (w/ or w/o spouse)	—	—	—
live with others (w/ or w/o spouse & unmarried children)	−1.30***	−.89**	−.91*

* Significant at 10.0% level
** Significant at 5.0% level
*** Significant at 0.5% level

no effect on IADL; and the elderly in urban townships are more likely than those in rural townships to receive IADL assistance.

These similarities and differences in the patterns of coefficients suggest that the underlying dynamics may be quite specific by type of support and that analyses of overall levels of support can be misleading. Table 8.11, for Mainlanders, reinforces the apparent distinctions. Age and health status and gender show effects among the Mainlanders similar to those for the Taiwanese, although some of the coefficients for age and health do not achieve statistical significance. The effect of living arrangements is broadly similar in the sense that those not living with married children are generally disadvantaged, but the magnitudes and patterns across types of support differ noticeably. Unlike Taiwanese, Mainlanders without children are less likely to receive financial or material support than those with one or more children. The effects of work status are similar for the two groups of elderly, although retired Mainlanders are significantly less likely to receive IADL assistance than are those who work, and the residence pattern for Mainlanders is quite distinct from that of Taiwanese.[8]

The preliminary analysis suggests that needs, availability of support providers, and, possibly established traditions concerning the timing and appropriate recipient of specific types of support (mothers versus fathers, before or after retirement, etc.) all contribute to the patterns of support received. Subsequent analyses will investigate these patterns in more detail in terms of location and characteristics of the potential providers and the characteristics of the elderly.

USE OF MEDICAL SERVICES AND SOURCES OF SUPPORT FOR MEDICAL EXPENSES

We noted at the outset that besides the four areas of potential need and sources of support obtained via the social exchange schedule analyzed in the previous section, several other questions are relevant to understanding the needs of the elderly and the extent to which they are being met. Taiwan, like many industrializing countries, has been assembling an array of health and welfare measures for both the working population and the elderly. Not surprisingly, the provision of health care and coverage of health care costs is a prime component of these efforts. Taiwan has had a strong health infrastructure for a long time. In 1986, the number of people per physician was 1,077, and per hospital bed 238 (ROC, Department of Health, 1986, Table 11). Starting in 1950, the government has sponsored a number of social insurance programs that provide medical care and other benefits to specified groups of workers and in some cases their dependents (including, in some instances, parents as well as spouses and unmarried children) (ROC, Bureau of Statistics, 1988). In 1988, the government promulgated a broad set of senior welfare measures that include in the area of health an expanding number of free health examinations, free or subsidized medical treatment to needy elderly, improved geriatric facilities, an expanding program of household nursing service, and promotion of health awareness (Taiwan Provincial Government, 1988).

With this as backdrop, Tables 8.12 and 8.13 explore the use of health facilities by the elderly and the means of covering medical expenses, respectively. Table 8.12 presents the proportion of the elderly who used a government hospital or clinic or a private hospital or clinic for medical care or medication in the past year, as well as the proportion who ever went to the emergency room of a hospital or clinic in the same period. Respondents may have visited more than one type of facility and/or had multiple visits to each type; the purpose of the visit was not restricted, so it could range from routine matters to serious illnesses. As before, the data are presented for each ethnic group and by various characteristics.

Overall, about two-thirds of Mainlanders used a government hospital or clinic in the year preceding the interview, more than twice the proportion of Taiwanese. For private hospitals and clinics, the pattern was reversed: 60% of the Taiwanese used these facilities, compared to 31% of Mainlanders. Use of emergency rooms was much lower for both groups and slightly more prevalent among Mainlanders.

The strong differentials by ethnic group hold within each of the characteristics examined, and the differences by category are generally muted. Females tend to use private facilities more than males, with the situation reversed for government hospitals and clinics. The use of private sources is greater in rural areas and to some extent among the lower income and the less educated. Surprisingly little variation occurs in proportions using services or the source of services by living arrangement. As expected, use of all facilities is higher among those in poor health.

Table 8.13 displays the proportion of the elderly who covered the past year's medical expenses from one of these sources: insurance; self (or spouse); child. Respondents could indicate more than one source, and several other possible supports—friends, other relatives, and the social service department, which were reported infrequently—are not included. Consequently, the percentages in any one row can add to more or less than 100.[9]

Given the differential affiliations of Taiwanese and Mainlanders with governmental organizations, it is not surprising to find that overall over 50% of Mainlanders were assisted by insurance, compared to only 16% of Taiwanese (last row of Table 8.13); reliance on self or spouse was very similar (40 to 46%); but children provided medical care cost assistance to 37% of Taiwanese, compared to only 7% of Mainlanders.

This broad pattern held across the characteristics examined, with some interesting variations. Males of both ethnic groups were more likely to use insurance than females, while females relied much more frequently on children. Similar patterns are observed by income and

Table 8.12. Proportion of Respondents who used Hospital or Clinic Services in Year Preceding Interview, by Ethnicity and Selected Sociodemographic Characteristics

| | Ethnicity and Source of Support | | | | | |
| | Taiwanese | | | Mainlander | | |
Respondent Characteristics:	Government Hospital/Clinic	Private Hospital/Clinic	Emergency Department	Government Hospital/Clinic	Private Hospital/Clinic	Emergency Department
Sex						
male	31.4	53.7	08.9	66.6	30.6	12.0
female	27.0	66.1	05.6	60.8	35.0	10.8
Age						
60–69	29.1	58.2	08.0	66.2	34.2	12.4
70+	29.4	62.8	05.8	64.2	22.7	9.8
Marital status						
married	31.3	58.2	07.7	66.6	32.4	12.2
not married	25.7	63.2	06.3	64.0	29.2	10.9
Place of residence						
large city	34.6	50.5	07.2	66.4	24.1	9.3
urban township	28.5	61.0	07.0	64.9	34.7	13.6
rural	26.5	64.8	07.3	65.2	41.4	13.9
Work status						
working	27.6	53.6	06.0	58.0	28.4	07.6
not working	29.8	62.2	07.5	69.7	32.9	14.0

Income						
<NT $3,000	27.4	62.6	07.0	57.1	32.1	08.7
NT $3,000–9,999	27.1	61.5	06.1	65.8	32.1	15.7
NT $10,000–19,999	31.4	57.8	06.1	69.3	32.2	11.8
NT $20,000+	33.9	53.6	07.7	61.7	31.5	08.6
Education						
illiterate	25.1	64.8	07.2	55.1	36.8	09.8
can read or primary	29.7	58.4	06.3	63.8	37.5	10.5
jr. high and above	46.5	43.2	10.2	70.3	24.0	13.5
Health status						
very good	22.4	39.4	01.7	60.2	22.3	05.0
good	21.4	52.7	03.4	56.7	30.7	05.1
fair	28.9	63.1	04.6	66.2	34.6	11.8
not so good	37.7	72.7	11.1	81.5	42.5	22.5
very bad	51.2	70.4	23.4	89.7	31.0	40.7
Living arrangements						
alone	31.4	56.2	03.5	63.5	28.0	11.6
spouse or unmarried child(ren) only	31.0	56.5	07.8	67.4	33.2	12.7
married child(ren)	28.0	61.8	07.5	60.1	34.1	10.7
other	29.7	62.0	04.3	76.8	22.9	09.5
Total (%)	29.2	59.9	07.2	65.7	31.3	11.8

Table 8.13. Proportion of Respondents Receiving Help with Medical Expenses from Specified Sources, by Ethnicity and Selected Sociodemographic Characteristics

| | Ethnicity and Source of Support | | | | | |
| | Taiwanese | | | Mainlander | | |
Respondent Characteristics:	Insurance	Self	Child	Insurance	Self	Child
Sex						
male	23.5	47.9	24.8	56.6	39.6	03.2
female	09.2	43.7	48.8	35.0	41.3	24.5
Age						
60–69	19.9	50.4	28.8	54.7	41.8	05.0
70+	10.6	38.3	49.9	48.2	34.1	11.5
Marital status						
married	19.1	51.0	29.6	53.2	42.1	05.8
not married	11.4	35.8	50.0	52.9	35.9	08.0
Place of residence						
large city	16.1	40.7	33.0	52.8	28.6	09.3
urban township	17.1	48.1	36.3	55.4	43.9	05.7
rural	15.7	46.6	39.9	50.0	58.1	02.2
Work status						
working	24.3	58.5	11.3	51.6	41.0	01.0
not working	13/5	41.3	45.9	54.0	39.1	09.7

Income					
<NT $3,000	11.8	31.9	55.6	21.4	25.0	21.4
NT $3,000–9,999	14.2	49.1	38.1	48.3	40.2	11.5
NT $10,000–19,999	19.5	52.6	24.6	57.7	41.4	04.5
NT $20,000+	26.2	54.0	19.5	54.0	39.5	02.5
Education					
illiterate	09.9	41.4	47.1	40.7	44.9	16.9
can read or primary	19.1	51.2	30.2	48.5	47.1	07.8
jr. high and above	36.3	45.0	15.1	60.2	31.9	02.9
Health status					
very good	15.4	38.0	20.7	48.8	31.0	01.7
good	16.0	46.0	27.4	47.8	41.4	05.4
fair	16.9	49.7	38.6	57.9	42.5	07.5
not so good	17.0	51.6	45.4	56.3	48.1	14.8
very bad	19.2	38.4	56.0	62.1	41.4	10.3
Living arrangements					
alone	17.8	54.4	25.4	54.5	40.2	01.1
spouse or unmarried child(ren) only	21.9	54.4	22.0	56.7	40.0	03.4
married child(ren)	13.8	40.7	45.8	42.9	37.5	20.1
other	12.4	47.0	31.4	54.3	47.1	07.1
Total (%)	16.3	45.8	36.9	53.2	40.1	06.7

education, and higher levels are associated with greater use of insurance and less reliance on children, largely reflecting differential enrollment and access to social insurance programs. Aside from the tendency of those residing with married children to show more assistance from a child, there was relatively little difference across living arrangements within ethnic groups.

This brief overview of two aspects of health care use and costs reveals the emergence of government-sponsored facilities and government-promoted social welfare mechanisms, which are differentially used by Taiwanese and Mainlanders and by several other characteristics. In general, those who are less tied to long-standing familial arrangements and those in higher socioeconomic categories are more likely to seek medical attention from government hospitals or clinics and to rely on insurance for a portion of their medical costs.

SUMMARY AND CONCLUSIONS

The major goal of this chapter has been to present a broad descriptive overview of the current support patterns of the Taiwanese elderly, taking advantage of the relatively rich detail of the 1989 Survey of Health and Living Status of the Elderly. This survey obtained extensive information on the sources of support, both formal and informal, on four dimensions; on characteristics of the individual actual and potential providers of support; and on the sufficiency of support, including its absence despite a perceived need on the part of the elderly respondents.

A major axis of differentiation among the current elderly is the division between the Taiwanese and Mainlanders, arising from the large-scale immigration of Chinese Nationalists shortly after World War II. The Mainlanders currently comprise 22% of all elderly and are very different from the Taiwanese in their sex composition, marital status, size of families, living arrangements, and occupational distribution. The Mainlanders are much more likely to live alone or with spouse and/or unmarried children than are the Taiwanese. As a result of this and their position among the elderly, they are a significant factor in the apparent trend in Taiwan away from the more traditional extended or stem family (i.e., residence with at least one married son). As the Mainlanders move out through the age structure, the overall trend away from extended coresidence may slow for a time, but other socioeconomic and demographic factors—such as rising incomes (facilitating more independent living), smaller family sizes, and increased urbanization and educational level—point to less coresidence among the elderly in the future.

Living arrangements greatly condition the expressed level of support needed and received, and indeed the need for support often influences the mode of living arrangement. Even after living arrangement is controlled, Mainlanders often express a lower level of need and tend more often to receive an insufficient amount of support (see Table 8.4). The overall patterns are as follows:

	Taiwanese	Mainlanders	Total
ADL			
% Needing and/or receiving	7.3	3.4	6.4
% Receiving sufficient	4.7	1.6	4.0
Proportion sufficient	64.4	47.1	60.6
IADL			
% Needing and/or receiving	72.8	54.4	68.7
% Receiving sufficient	67.5	50.3	63.7
Proportion sufficient	92.7	92.5	92.7
Financial			
% Needing and/or receiving	83.0	47.5	75.1
% Receiving sufficient	67.1	35.3	60.0
Proportion sufficient	80.8	74.3	79.9
Material			
% Needing and/or receiving	49.0	21.4	42.9
% Receiving sufficient	41.3	16.3	35.7
Proportion sufficient	84.3	76.2	83.2

If we assume that those who receive support also need that type of support, for all elderly Taiwanese, needs for assistance with money and instrumental activities of daily living (shopping, meal preparation, etc.) are most often voiced and sufficient help is reported by 80 to 90% of respondents; the need for assistance with material goods is expressed less often, but appears to be well met. Although only a small proportion express a need for assistance with activities of daily living (bathing, dressing, etc.), this is also the area with the lowest proportion reporting sufficient assistance. The general patterns for Taiwanese and Mainlanders are similar, except that on each dimension a much smaller percentage of Mainlanders express a need or receive sufficient support.

Which individuals are critical in meeting these needs? The analysis suggests that there is considerable diffusion of responsibilities and a degree of specialization. For those who received two or more types of support, it was relatively uncommon for the main provider to be the same person (Table 8.8). For those living with married children, the daughter-in-law is a major provider for those needing assistance with ADLs or IADLs, with spouse also important; for financial assistance, the son is critical; and for material goods both sons and daughters are highly active. From the standpoint of the future elderly, this division of labor suggests that needs could be met with smaller family size, if the children (and daughters-in-law) are available and filial. Nevertheless, given the shortfalls in needed assistance already apparent in the current larger family environment, we expect that coverage of needs from family members will decline in the future, given the competing demands faced by the smaller cohorts of educated and occupationally mobile children.

What is the likelihood that formal programs will pick up the slack? The experience of the Mainlanders may be instructive if not conclusive in this regard. Significant proportions of Mainlanders are receiving support (especially financial) from formal sources (see Table 8.9); are using government hospitals and clinics to a high degree (Table 8.12); and are meeting their medical bills through insurance (Table 8.13). There is also some evidence that the formal programs are acting in part as a "safety net" for those without other means of assistance, regardless of ethnicity.

To the extent that the Mainlander profile becomes the dominant pattern in the future—more educated elderly with occupational histories in government or large industry and smaller families—we can expect to find support increasingly balanced between family and formal mechanisms. The exact nature of that balance, and the degree to which it will resemble patterns now observed in other industrialized countries, cannot be discerned clearly at present. Taiwan's experience in developing programs well adapted to Mainlanders should stand it in good stead in meeting future needs.

ACKNOWLEDGMENTS

This paper was prepared for the Conference on Aging and Generational Relations in Historical and Cross-cultural Perspectives, October 10–13, University of Delaware, Newark, Delaware. The authors greatly appreciate the research assistance of Lora Myers and the assistance of Ingrid Naaman in preparation of the manuscript.

NOTES

1.   Lineages were slow to develop in Taiwan because of its recent settlement and because government regulations prevented entire lineages or villages to migrate from the mainland (Fricke et al., 1994).

2.   The Survey of Health and Living Status of the Elderly covered everyone above age 60. For purposes of comparison with the Survey of Income and Expenditures, only those 65 and over are included in Table 8.2.

3.   For some years, the marital status of the children was not directly ascertained in the Survey of Income and Expenditures and had to be inferred from the presence of grandchildren, which might lead to misclassification of married children who were childless. Also, the definition of household might vary slightly between the Income and Expenditures Survey and the Elderly Survey since the objectives and procedures were quite different.

4.   The very small proportion of the elderly population living in institutions is excluded from the analyses presented in this paper since the meaning of support for this group is quite different.

5.   Data on the characteristics of daughters-in-law not in the household are not available. Insofar as these women are likely to be younger and better educated (since the parents-in-law will tend to be younger and less in need), the differences portrayed in Table 8.6 tend to be conservative. That is, inclusion of all daughters-in-law would probably show a sharper difference between those who are main providers and others.

6.   We plan to develop independent measures of need in several categories from questions on functional ability and financial resources, and these will be used to analyze the relationship of needs to supports received, with appropriate controls.

7.   The effect of residence on support can take different forms. For example, since most of the elderly grew up in rural areas, some of those still residing there may be well situated with regard to a support network but others may be relatively isolated because children have moved away. In subsequent analyses details on kin availability and their proximity will be introduced as explicit measures of potential support.

8.   These observations on differences between Taiwanese and Mainlanders are not based on formal statistical tests. By combining Mainlanders and Taiwanese in the same equation it would be possible to test for the significance of interaction terms and thereby determine whether the patterns for a given independent variable differ between the groups. Such tests will be reserved for the final specification of the model.

9.   It should be noted that some respondents will have had insurance, but no medical expenses, over the previous 12 months, so the data presented do not indicate the proportion with coverage.

REFERENCES

Barclay, G. W. (1954). *Colonial development and population in Taiwan*. Princeton: Princeton University Press.

Cohen, M. L. (1976). *House united, house divided*. New York: Columbia University Press.

Fricke, T., Chang, J. S., & Yang, L. S. (1994). Historical and ethnographic perspectives on the Chinese family. In A. Thornton and Hui-Sheng Lin (Eds.), *Social change and the family in Taiwan* (Chapter 2). Chicago: University of Chicago Press.

George, L. K. & Bearon, L. B. (1980). *Quality of life in older persons: Meaning and measurement.* New York: Human Sciences Press.

Greenhalgh, S. (1982). Income units: The ethnographic alternative to standardization. In Y. Ben-Porath (Ed.), Income distribution and the family. *Population and Development Review, 8* (Suppl.), 70–91.

Hermalin, A. I. (1976). Empirical research in Taiwan on factors underlying differences in fertility. In A. J. Coale (Ed.), *Economic factors in population growth.* (pp. 243–266). New York: John Wiley & Sons.

Hermalin, A. I., Chang, M.-C., Lin, H.-S., Lee, M.-L., & Ofstedal, M. B. (1990). Patterns of support among the elderly in Taiwan and their policy implications. *Comparative study of the elderly in Asia: Research Report No. 90–4.* Ann Arbor: Population Studies Center, University of Michigan.

Hermalin, A. I., Freedman, D., & Liu, P. K. C. (1994). The social and economic transformation of Taiwan. In A. Thornton and Hui-Sheng Lin (Eds.), *Social change and the family in Taiwan* (Chapter 3). Chicago: University of Chicago Press.

Hogan, D. P. & Eggebeen, D. J. (1991). *The structure of intergenerational exchanges in American families.* (unpublished).

Lang, O. (1946). *Chinese family and society.* New Haven: Yale University Press.

Lo, J. C.-C. (January 6–8, 1987). *The changing patterns of household structure and economic status of the elderly: 1976 to 1985.* In Conference on Economic Development and Social Welfare in Taiwan (I), The Institute of Economics, Academia Sinica, Taipei, Taiwan, 375–401.

Manton, K. G. & Soldo, B. J. (1985). Health status and service needs of the oldest old: Current patterns and future trends. *Milbank Memorial Fund Quarterly/ Health and Society, 63,* 286–319.

ROC, Department of Health, Executive Yuan. (1986). *Health statistics,* Vol. 1. General Health Statistics.

ROC, Bureau of Statistics, Directorate General of Budget, Accounting and Statistics, Executive Yuan. (1988). *The social insurance system in the Taiwan area of the Republic of China.* National Conditions of the ROC, Spring, 27–38.

ROC, Directorate General of Budget, Accounting and Statistics, Executive Yuan. (1991). *Report on the manpower utilization survey,* Taiwan area, ROC, 1990.

Taeuber, I. B. (1970). The families of Chinese farmers. In M. Freedman (Ed.), *Family and kinship in Chinese society.* Stanford: Stanford University Press.

Taiwan Provincial Government. (1988). *Taiwan Province planning for elderly—Concerning senior citizen welfare measures.* Taiwan Provincial Government Bulletin, Winter, No. 65 (in Chinese).

Taiwan Provincial Institute of Family Planning, Population Studies Center and Institute of Gerontology, University of Michigan. (1989). *1989 survey of health and living status of the elderly in Taiwan: Questionnaire and survey design.* Comparative Study of the Elderly in Four Asian Countries: Research Report No. 1.

Thornton, A., Chang, M.-C., & Sun, T.-H. (1984). Social and economic change, intergenerational relationships, and family formation in Taiwan. *Demography, 21,* 475–499.

9

Familial Support and the Life Course of Thai Elderly and Their Children

John Knodel, Napaporn Chayovan, and Siriwan Siriboon

Thailand's people generally expect that the elderly will be taken care of by their children and that at least one child will coreside with them (Cowgill, 1972; Knodel, Havanon, & Pramualratana, 1984; Pramualratana, 1990; Tuchrello, 1989). Results of a recent survey in the rural areas of two different regions indicate almost universal agreement among adults that "it is the children's responsibility to take care of their parents when the parents get old" (Wongsith, 1990). Evidence from earlier surveys makes clear that such responsibility typically is perceived to include some form of coresidence (Knodel, Chamratrithirong and Debavalya, 1987). National estimates of the extent to which elderly parents actually live with children and the nature of intergenerational exchanges of types of support, however, have been lacking.

The present study examines several aspects of the living arrangements and material support of Thai elderly in relation to their children, with special attention given to the influence of the life course of the elderly and their children on these phenomena. The data come primarily from a survey conducted in 1986 by the Institute of Population Studies, Chulalongkorn University, as part of the Socio-economic Consequences of the Aging Population in Thailand (SECAPT) project, which in turn was part of the ASEAN Population Program sponsored by the Australian government. The survey interviewed a national probability sample of 3,252 respondents age 60 and over living in private households, and covered a wide range of topics. Overall nonresponse was 25%, almost half of which was attributable to hearing problems or illness. Thus the SECAPT sample overrepresents elderly who are in better physical and mental health (Chayovan, Wongsith, & Saengtienchai, 1988). Nevertheless, it represents a unique source of detailed data on Thailand's elderly population.[1]

In accordance with the SECAPT survey, elderly are defined as the population aged 60 and over. In Thailand, age 60 has traditionally been the legally required age of retirement for government officials, and as such has gained some currency in popular thought especially for men, as the start of old age. Moreover, 60 marks the end of the fifth cycle and the beginning of the sixth in terms of the 12-year traditional animal calendar; this may also reinforce the popular view that old age starts at 60 (Cowgill, 1968).

When examining the situation of the elderly population in Thailand or elsewhere, one must recognize that the elderly age span, especially if defined to start as early as age 60, includes persons at different stages of their lives. Important life-course transitions—including marital dissolution, disengagement from economic activities, and the onset of chronic health problems and functional impairments—often occur during this period of life. As data presented in Table 9.1 indicate, the likelihood of having a spouse present declines rapidly with age among Thai elderly, as mortality renders increasing numbers of widows or widowers. The percentage who reported that they worked recently also declines rapidly

Table 9.1.   Indicators of Marital Status, Economic Activity, Functional Impairments and Health of the Population Age 60 and Older, by Age and Sex

	% Married & Living w/Spouse	% Working		% Rating Health as Poor	% Having a Problem w/		
		Last Week	Last Year*		Seeing	Hearing	Walking
Men							
60–64	90	55	70	33	35	12	20
65–69	82	43	54	37	40	19	27
70–74	66	29	37	42	55	32	43
75+	56	22	27	45	60	32	58
Total	75	40	51	38	45	21	34
Women							
60–64	53	35	47	39	45	12	29
65–69	40	29	34	41	52	16	44
70–74	29	15	16	41	62	20	54
75+	13	8	9	52	67	38	70
Total	36	23	30	43	55	20	47
Both Sexes							
60–64	66	43	56	36	41	12	26
65–69	59	35	43	39	47	17	36
70–74	43	21	24	41	59	25	50
75+	30	13	16	50	64	36	65
Total	52	30	38	41	51	21	41

Note: * includes last week
Source: 1986 SECAPT Survey

during this age span. The far lower level of economic activity among the older compared to the younger elderly, has important implications for both their need for material and financial support and their ability to provide it to others. Likewise, the decline in health and the increase in functional impairments with age—evident from the percentages reporting poor health and difficulties in seeing, hearing, and walking—has important bearing on differences between younger and older elderly in their ability to live without help from others in the activities of daily living.[2]

We recognize that any particular living arrangement or system of supports typically involves both advantages and disadvantages for each generation. Viewing such arrangements only in terms of the needs of the elderly and the benefits they receive ignores potentially important contributions that the elderly make to the welfare of their adult children. These include access to living quarters (when coresidence occurs in the elderly's house), access to income-producing assets owned by the elderly, and the share of household income and services the elderly provide, such as child care and housekeeping. Nevertheless, as Table 9.1 illustrates, as the end of the life course nears, the elderly's need for support and assistance from their children is likely to increase as their ability to contribute to their children's welfare wanes.

LIVING ARRANGEMENTS

Given that the SECAPT survey is restricted to elderly who lived in private households as well as those able and willing to be interviewed, it is of some interest to compare results based on the SECAPT sample with a full tally of elderly based on data from the one percent sample of the 1980 census. The census, at least in principle, covers the entire elderly population including both those living in collective households and those unable to respond to an interview because of such problems as hearing loss, illness, or senility (since the census questionnaire can be filled out by any responsible member of the household and did not require a separate interview with the elderly). As previously noted, the SECAPT survey received substantial nonresponse.

One limitation common to the census and the SECAPT survey is a tendency to treat dwelling units with separate addresses (house numbers) as separate households, following the government's household registration system. As a result, households are likely to be equated with dwelling units and coresidence can only be examined in terms of living together in the same dwelling unit. Typically, nothing explicitly indicates whether a household is part of a compound or cluster of dwelling units that are in some degree linked together. Thus instances where the elderly live in their own dwelling unit with its own registration number, but in close proximity to their children or other family members, cannot be detected from the data provided by the census or SECAPT survey. Such living arrangements clearly occur in Thailand, especially in rural areas, and can meet many of the same needs of the elderly as does a more narrowly defined coresidence (Cowgill, 1972; Tuchrello, 1989). Thus to define coresidence as living together within the same officially designated household (i.e., usually a dwelling unit), as necessitated by the census and most surveys, is likely to understate somewhat the extent to which the living arrangements of elderly and their families are intertwined.

Descriptions of the living arrangements of the elderly that can be derived from the census are also restricted by the amount of information that is collected and coded. Nevertheless, some insight can be gained by examining the distribution of the elderly through the number of members of the household in which they live, combined with information on their marital status and relationship to head, and whether the person lives in a private or collective household.[3] Table 9.2 shows the distribution of the elderly population by sex, according to a combined classification of size and type of household for the 1980 census and according to household size for the SECAPT sample. In both sets of results, one may distinguish elderly persons living alone as well as elderly in two-person households who live with a spouse only. These two groups, along with elderly who live in collective households, are of particular interest given

Table 9.2. Percent Distribution of the Population Age 60 and Older According to the Type and Size of Household, by Sex, based on the 1980 Census and the 1986 SECAPT Survey

Number of Members and Type of Household	All Persons 60+		Men 60+		Women 60+	
	1980 Census	1986 SECAPT	1980 Census	1986 SECAPT	1980 Census	1986 SECAPT
Private Household						
one person	3.8	4.4	2.5	3.6	4.9	5.0
two persons						
spouses only	6.6	6.7	8.1	9.3	5.5	4.9
nonspouses	4.1	5.1	1.8	2.6	5.9	6.8
three persons+	83.7	83.7	84.5	84.6	83.1	83.2
Collective	1.7	—*	3.1	—*	0.6	—*
Total (%)	100	100	100	100	100	100

* Collective households were excluded from the sample frame for the SECAPT survey
Note: The 1980 census results are based on original tabulations from the 1 percent sample tape.

the norm in Thailand that the elderly should be taken care of by the family and reside with children or other family members.

In the census, collective households refer to institutional living quarters, including temples, hospitals, prisons, welfare homes, and hotels. The census results show that less than two percent of the elderly live in such households, although the phenomenon is considerably more common for men than women. Examination of detailed data (not shown) in which collective households are divided according to specific type reveals that the vast majority (94%) of persons age 60 or over who live in such households live in temples, and that most of them (85%) are males who presumably are Buddhist monks. Even among the small number of women living in collective households, three-fourths live in temples (presumably in many cases as Buddhist nuns). Thus the collective household category for the elderly primarily represents cases in which a religious institution serves as an alternative to familial living arrangements. Unlike in some western countries, however, virtually no elderly reside in nursing homes or special facilities for the elderly.[4]

Since living in a collective household is more common for men than women, their exclusion from the SECAPT sample produces a slight exaggeration of the extent to which elderly men coreside with children or other family members, relative to women. However, since the proportion of elderly living in collective households is quite low, the overall picture of living arrangements provided by the SECAPT data is unlikely to be seriously distorted by the omission of such households from the sample.

Generally, the distribution of private households is consistent between the census and SECAPT results. Both sources show that very few elderly live alone and only a small proportion live with their spouse only. In the vast majority of cases, the elderly person lives with someone in addition to or other than a spouse. The results are also quite consistent in indicating several differences between elderly men and women in the distribution of living arrangements. Both the census and SECAPT results show that elderly men are less likely than women to live alone, less likely to live in a two-person household with someone other than a spouse, more likely to live with a spouse only, and about equally likely to live in a three-person or larger household.

Table 9.3 provides a more detailed breakdown of the Thai elderly population according to with whom they live, by age and sex of the elderly respondent based on the SECAPT survey. In particular, the presence of a spouse as well as the respondent's children (including step and adopted children) is distinguished from that of any other coresident members. The results show that very few Thai elderly of either sex at any age live alone, although the tendency to live alone does increase

Table 9.3. Living Arrangements of the Population Age 60 and Older, by Age and Sex

Living Arrangements	Both Sexes	Men					Women				
		Total	60-64	65-60	70-74	75+	Total	60-64	65-69	70-74	75+
Alone	4.3	3.6	1.6	4.0	5.9	4.1	4.8	2.4	5.8	5.0	7.6
Spouse only	6.7	9.3	7.0	9.2	11.1	11.6	4.9	5.5	5.9	5.4	2.6
Children only	4.9	2.8	1.6	3.0	4.2	3.0	6.3	6.2	5.1	6.9	7.3
Others only	6.8	3.7	2.2	2.5	1.4	9.5	9.0	7.0	7.4	10.1	12.7
Spouse, children	11.6	18.8	26.9	22.2	10.0	8.5	6.6	12.4	5.0	4.8	1.1
Spouse, others	5.3	6.8	4.8	7.3	10.5	6.2	4.3	5.8	3.7	4.1	2.6
Children, others	31.8	14.7	8.7	7.8	22.1	27.6	43.8	31.8	42.0	49.3	59.2
Spouse, children, others	28.6	40.4	47.3	44.0	34.7	29.5	20.3	28.9	25.0	14.3	6.9
Total	100.0	100.0	100.0	100.0	100.0	100.0	100.0	100.0	100.0	100.0	100.0
Total with children	76.9	76.7	84.5	77.0	71.0	68.6	77.0	79.3	77.1	75.3	74.5
Total with spouse	52.2	75.3	86.0	82.7	66.3	55.8	36.1	52.6	39.6	28.6	13.2
Total with others	72.5	65.6	63.0	61.6	68.7	72.8	77.4	73.5	78.1	77.8	81.4

Note: Household composition is inferred from information on number of household members, marital status (including specification of living with spouse), and number of children (including step and adopted) reported as coresident. A small number of cases in which this information was inconsistent are omitted. Results are weighted.
Source: 1986 SECAPT Survey.

with age, reaching almost 8% of women 75 and older. In addition, only modest proportions of Thai elderly live only with their spouse. The likelihood, however, is almost twice as high for men as for women, undoubtedly reflecting the strong tendency for women to outlive their husbands (both because of higher male mortality and the fact that men tend to marry younger women) and probably a greater tendency for widowed older men to remarry. While over half (52%) of the total elderly population live with a spouse (besides others who might be coresident), the reasons just mentioned lead to a very large gender difference (75% of men compared to only 36% of women).

Over three-quarters of the elderly (77%) live with at least one child (including step and adopted children), with virtually no difference evident between men and women overall. The percentage living with children, however, declines steadily with age for both sexes. Moreover, the decline is sharper for men than for women, so that despite the lack of a gender difference in the overall proportion living with children, at the younger elderly ages men are more likely than women to do so, while at the older elderly ages the reverse is true. As discussed in more detail below, the decline by age in the proportion of those who live with children chiefly reflects differences in the life-course stage of the children. Those in their sixties are far more likely to have children who still live in their parental home. That this is particularly true for men reflects the fact that the children of male elderly are younger than those of their female counterparts. For this reason, a more thorough examination of gender differences among elderly with respect to coresidence needs to control for the age of their children.

The low proportion living alone or with only their spouse and the high proportion living with at least one child among Thai elderly are not unusual for other Asian countries, but contrast sharply with those of developed countries in the West. For example, it is not uncommon to find 25 to 40% of the total population age 65 and above in western countries living in solitary households, and substantially higher percentages of women 75 and older in this situation (Kinsella, 1990). Likewise, living only with one's spouse is far more common in the West. For example, among Americans age 65 and over in 1975, 42% lived only with a spouse, in addition to the 33% who lived in one person households (calculated from DeVos & Holden, 1988). Thus fully three-fourths of American elderly (age 65 and over) lived either alone or only with a spouse, compared to only about one-tenth of the elderly Thai population (age 60 and over). In contrast, only 14% of Americans age 65 and over lived with one or more of their children, while the large majority of Thai elderly live with their children.

As Table 9.3 demonstrates, the most prominent feature of the living arrangements of the Thai elderly is coresidence with at least one of their children. Indeed, this is probably the most crucial aspect of the familial system of support and assistance, since many of the elderly's needs can be met through shared residence in a household with adult children. Since the possibility of coresiding with a child is obviously restricted to those elderly who have at least one child, further analysis of coresidence is restricted to those elderly with children. In any event very few Thai elderly are without living children.

As Table 9.4 shows, only 6% of Thai elderly have no living natural child. Moreover, a substantial proportion (44%) of those who have no natural child of their own have a step or adopted child, further reducing the proportion with no child available to less than 4% of the elderly. There is virtually no difference between men and women in this respect. Among those elderly who have no living child at all, almost a third (29%) had never been married, while the remainder either were in an infertile marriage or had lost all their children through death. In the present study, coresidence refers to living together with any child, whether natural, step, or adopted, since there are no prior grounds for expecting the nature of coresidence to differ on this basis.[5]

A more thorough exploration of coresidence of elderly parents and their children also requires recognition that living arrangements are likely to be affected by the life-course stage of both. As previously discussed, the elderly age span includes elderly's who themselves are at

Table 9.4. Indicators Relating to Childlessness among the Population Age 60 and Older, by Sex

Percent	Total	Male	Female
With no living natural child	6.3	5.6	6.7
With at least one step or adopted child among elderly who			
• never married	17	16	17
• married but had no live-born child	58	54	61
• had live-born children but all died	32	18	41
• have no living natural child for any of above reasons	44	40	46
With no living child (including biological, step, and adopted children)	3.5	3.4	3.6
Distribution of elderly with no living natural, step, or adopted children because			
• never married	29	19	35
• married but had no live-born child	42	49	38
• had live-born children but all died	19	32	27
Total percent	100	100	100

Source: 1986 SECAPT Survey

Table 9.5. Percent Distributions of All Children and of Youngest Child, Percentage of Children Single, and Percentage of Children Economically Active, by Age and Sex of Parent

	Men				Women			
Percent Distribution	*Total*	*60–64*	*65–69*	*70+*	*Total*	*60–64*	*65–69*	*70+*
Age of all children								
under 15	3	6	2	1	0	0	0	0
15–17	3	5	3	1	1	1	0	0
18–24	14	24	15	5	7	15	5	1
25–29	17	22	19	10	13	21	15	4
30+	63	44	61	83	79	62	79	05
Total	100	100	100	100	100	100	100	100
Age of youngest child								
under 15	10	19	9	3	1	2	2	0
15–17	9	15	10	3	2	6	1	0
18–24	30	43	37	15	24	49	19	5
25–29	20	13	24	24	23	25	40	11
30+	31	10	20	56	50	18	39	94
Total	100	100	100	100	100	100	100	100
Single among all children	22	32	23	12	14	22	12	8
Economically active among all children	13	17	13	9	10	11	9	9

Source: 1986 SECAPT Survey

different stages of their own lives. At the same time that parents age, however, their children also proceed through different stages—completing school, entering the labor force, and forming families of their own. Indeed, each transition has important bearing on the costs and benefits of coresiding with parents, the need for different types of assistance from the parents, and the ability to provide different types of support to the parents. Moreover, normative expectations associated with coresidence and support exchanges, some of which may be gender and/or birth order-specific, often change with these transitions.

Differences in the life-course stages of the children of younger and older elderly can be quite pronounced. As Table 9.5 shows, some of the younger elderly and especially men (whose wives are likely to be even younger) have children who are not yet adults. In some cases the children are still attending school and are likely to be totally dependent on their parents. Interpreting their presence in the household as part of a support system for their parents can thus be misleading, overstating the extent to which coresidence entails support for the elderly.[6] Table 9.5 also shows that while the children of the older elderly are more likely to have entered the labor force than the children of the younger elderly,

Table 9.6. Percentage Coresident among Children of Elderly Parents, by Age and Marital Status of the Child

| Age of Child | Total | Marital Status | |
		Single	Ever-married
Under 15	93	90	—
15–17	77	79	55
18–24	56	71	35
25–29	32	56	23
30+	17	61	13
Total	25	66	16

Source: 1986 SECAPT Survey

they are also more likely to have married and to be raising families of their own.

That the age and marital status of the child are related to coresidence in the parental household is clearly illustrated in Table 9.6, which refers to the children of the elderly interviewed in the SECAPT survey.[7] Among the children of elderly parents, the percentage coresident decreases rapidly with age, from over 90% of those under 15 to only 17% of those age 30 or older. In addition, at every age, single children are far more likely to be coresident than their married siblings. This is consistent with the customary practices regarding postnuptial residence whereby newlyweds temporarily coreside with one set of parents, preferably the wife's, and then move to their own house, often nearby or even in the same compound. Only the last child (or last daughter) to marry will remain coresident indefinitely (Limanonda, 1989). Thus differences in the life-course stages of children are likely to exert an important influence on the living arrangements of elderly parents at different stages of the elderly's life course. Moreover, the effect is likely to differ for elderly men and women in the same age group, since the men's children will be younger on average than the women's.

Table 9.7 indicates the percentage of elderly parents (i.e., elderly with at least one living child, whether natural, step, or adopted) who coreside with at least one of their children, according to the age and sex of the elderly parent. Results are presented based both on coresidence with any child regardless of age and on coresidence with at least one child age 18 or older. The significance of the latter results is that they focus on coresidence with children who are likely to be economically active adults and thus relatively certain to be contributing to the economic well-being of the household. For example, as reported in the SECAPT survey, almost four-fifths (79%) of the elderly respondents' children age 18–24

Table 9.7. Percentage of Elderly Parents Coresident with a Child, Unadjusted and Adjusted for the Age of the Youngest Child, by Age and Sex of an Elderly Parent

Form of Results and Age of Elderly Parents	With a child of any age			With a child age 18 or older**		
	Total	Men	Women	Total	Men	Women
Unadjusted Results						
60–64	84	86	82	81	81	82
65–69	80	80	81	79	77	81
70–74	76	74	78	76	74	78
75+	75	72	77	74	70	77
All ages	80	79	80	78	76	80
*Adjusted Results**						
60–64	79	78	79	78	75	79
65–69	79	75	81	78	73	81
69–74	80	75	83	78	74	81
75+	83	77	89	79	74	85
All ages	80	77	82	78	74	81

Notes: * Statistical adjustment made through linear regression. Cases in which the age of the youngest child is unknown are excluded.
** Results limited to elderly parents with at least one child age 18 or over.
Source: 1986 SECAPT Survey

were economically active, compared to less than two-thirds (64%) of children 15–17 and only 16% of children under 15. In addition, to take more fully into account the influence of differences in life-course stage of the elderly's children on coresidence, we have made a statistical adjustment for the age of the youngest child. This measure serves as a convenient proxy indicator for the ages and hence life-course stages of the entire sibship of the elderly respondent's children. Both sets of results appear in unadjusted and adjusted form.

Overall, exactly four-fifths (80%) of elderly parents coreside with a child. The figure is slightly lower if we consider only coresidence with a child age 18 and older. The unadjusted results show almost no difference in the extent of coresidence among elderly men and women if we consider coresidence with any child, but show a slightly higher proportion of elderly women than men coresident when children under 18 are excluded from consideration. An inverse association between age of the elderly parent and coresidence with children is apparent in the unadjusted results even when we consider only coresidence with children who are 18 or older. Therefore, despite the presumed greater need for assistance as the elderly age, their chances for living with a child declines. It is necessary to turn to the adjusted results, however, to gain an appropriate perspective for interpreting these findings.

Once differences in the age of the elderly's youngest child (and hence differences in the life course stages of all the elderly's children) are taken into account, the relationship between age of the elderly respondent and coresidence essentially disappears for men and reverses in direction for women. This finding indicates that decline in coresidence with age observed in the unadjusted results derives from the fact that as elderly parents age, their children enter stages where coresidence with parents competes with other social mandates. Once this is taken into account, it no longer appears that coresidence is discouraged by the greater burden posed by an older, compared to a younger, elderly parent for a coresident child. Once the changes in pressures to live outside the parental household created by shifts in the children's life course are controlled, coresidence seems to respond to the life course situation of the elderly, at least in the case of elderly mothers. Life-course events after 18, particularly marriage, are important in influencing children to depart from the household. Merely considering coresidence to children who are 18 and older is not sufficient (i.e., without adjusting for age of the youngest child) to reverse the direct association between age of the elderly parent and coresidence.

Loss of a spouse is one of the important life-course transitions that frequently occurs after persons enter the elderly age span. Presumably such an event increases the need for assistance and support from adult children. Table 9.8 shows that marital status, defined as whether or not the elderly respondent lives with a spouse, influences the chances of coresidence with children age 18 or older. The results are statistically

Table 9.8. Percentage of Elderly Parents Coresident with at least One Child Age 18 or Over, Unadjusted and Adjusted for the Age of the Elderly Parent and the Age of the Youngest Child, by Sex and Marital Status of the Elderly Parent

	Adjusted	Adjusted for Age of Elderly Parent	Adjusted for Age of Elderly Parent and Youngest Child*
Men			
Married, live with spouse	76	76	73
Other marital status	76	78	77
Women			
Married, live with spouse	75	74	75
Other marital status	82	83	86

Notes: Results are limited to elderly parents with at least one child age 18 or over. Statistical adjustment made through linear regression.
* Cases in which the age of the youngest child is unknown are excluded.
Source: 1986 SECAPT Survey

adjusted first for the respondent's age, in order to control for other features of the life course that might influence coresidence, and then adjusted also for the age of the youngest child to take into account the influence of the life-course stage of the respondent's children. Unadjusted results are also shown for comparison.

If neither the age of the elderly respondent nor the age of the youngest child is taken into account, coresidence with an adult child is more common for women who no longer live with their spouse than for those who still do, but seems unrelated to marital status for elderly men. Results presented above indicate that, when age of the youngest child is not controlled, age of the elderly is negatively related both to coresidence with a child and to living with a spouse. Thus after statistically adjusting for the age of the elderly respondent, the difference in the percentage coresiding with an adult child increases slightly between elderly women who live with a spouse and those who do not, and a small difference in coresidence associated with marital status emerges in the same direction among the men. When results are also adjusted for the age of the youngest child, the difference becomes more pronounced. This probably reflects the fact that elderly who have lost their spouse are more likely to have older children who already have married and started their own families (thus lowering the chance of coresidence). Once this is taken into account, being without a spouse for an elderly person—and thus presumably in greater need of assistance—increases the chance of receiving such assistance in the form of coresidence.

MATERIAL SUPPORT FROM NONCORESIDENT CHILDREN

While coresidence is undoubtedly the most comprehensive type of support exchange between elderly parents and their adult children in Thailand, noncoresident children are typically expected to share in the support of their parents to at least some degree. Such support can be critical for the parents' well-being when parents do not live with others who help keep the household, and presumably eases the burden of coresident children when elderly parents do live with one or more children. The SECAPT survey provides some limited information on the support provided by each of the elderly's children. Every respondent who reported having at least one living child was asked a series of questions about each of them. These questions included whether or not the child had ever provided regular support, and if so, what kind of support was provided during the past year. Given the responses to these questions, we can examine the extent to which elderly parents received material support in the form of food and/or clothes as well as money from noncoresident children.[8]

There are several limitations to the data derived from the responses about support provided by individual children. First, while the question about the type of support provided was open-ended and permitted multiple responses, there were no systematic probes about types of support not spontaneously mentioned. Also, respondents sometimes reported that a child provided everything, without specifying what was encompassed.[9] Second, the frequency with which specific types of support are provided cannot be ascertained.[10] Finally, the questions referred only to regular support, and did not inquire about support received on an irregular basis from those children who were reported as never having provided regular support.[11] Despite these limitations, the information obtained should suggest at least general patterns, if not noncoresident specific levels.

Whether or not a noncoresident child provides material support to an elderly parent household is clearly associated with the life course of the child. Obviously, such support can be provided only after the child moves out of the household. In addition, as Table 9.9 shows, the type and probability of such support is influenced by whether or not the child lives nearby (in the same village, town, or district of Bangkok) and whether or not the child has married. Provision of food and/or clothes is far more likely from noncoresident children who have married than from those who are still single, and far more common from those who live in the same locality as the parents than from those who live further

Table 9.9. Percentage of Noncoresident Children Reported to have Provided Material Support to Elderly Parents during the Prior Year, by Residence Relative to their Parents, Sex and Marital Status

Residence Relative to Parents and Marital Status of Child	% Provided Food and/or Clothing			% Provided Money		
	Total	Sons	Daughters	Total	Sons	Daughters
Live in same locality as elderly parents*						
total	55	50	59	32	31	34
ever married	56	51	60	33	31	34
single	26	25	27	27	21	34
Live in other place						
total	30	28	33	41	39	42
ever married	32	29	34	40	39	41
single	17	15	20	48	42	57
All noncoresident children	39	35	43	38	36	39

* The same locality refers to the same village, town, or district of Bangkok.

away. Provision of money is more likely from children who live away, and, among them, single children are somewhat more likely to provide money than married ones. Although single noncoresident children who live in the same locality as their parents are less likely than their married counterparts to provide money, they constitute a very small group, since most noncoresident single children live away from the parents' locality. Although daughters are more likely to provide either type of support than sons, generally the same pattern in marital status and residence relative to the parents characterizes both sexes.

Despite the association between provision of material support to elderly parents from outside the household and the life-course stage of their children, the availability of noncoresident children to provide such support is not systematically related to the life- course stage of their elderly parents. Thus, as Table 9.10 shows, the vast majority of elderly parents at all ages have at least one noncoresident child. Moreover, the age of elderly men and women is not related to the number of noncoresident children in a consistent direction. In part this probably results from tendencies operating in opposite directions. While increased age of an elderly parent is likely to be associated with a greater chance that any particular child will have left the household, mortality also takes its toll by reducing the total number of children still alive.

Clear associations are also lacking between the age of the elderly and the availability of noncoresident children to provide specific types of support. For example, the probability of having at least one child living outside the parents' locality, which is particularly important for the provision of money, as well as the mean number of children living outside the locality, shows an irregular relationship to the age of elderly men and actually declines with the age of women. Likewise, the probability of having at least one married child living in the same locality as the parents, which is particularly important for the provision of food and clothes, as well as the mean number of such children, is not related in a consistent direction with the age of the elderly parent. Thus despite the apparent influence of certain life-course events on the likelihood of providing material support from outside the household to elderly parents, the interface between the relevant aspects of the children's life course and that of the elderly parents is sufficiently complex that little net effect can be expected on the relationship between receipt of such support and the age and sex of the elderly parent.

Table 9.11 indicates the percentage of elderly parents (including those with no noncoresident children) who received food and/or clothes and who received money from at least one noncoresident child during the past year, according to the age and sex of the elderly parent. In addition, results are shown statistically adjusted for the availability of children at

Table 9.10. Indicators of Availability of Noncoresident Children with Respect to Selected Characteristics Related to Provision of Material Support to Elderly Parents, by Age and Sex of Elderly Parent

	Men				Women			
Percentage of Elderly with at Least One Child	*Total*	*60–64*	*65–69*	*70+*	*Total*	*60–64*	*65–69*	*70+*
Noncoresident	94	92	96	94	92	93	92	92
Residing outside parents' locality	81	80	84	81	78	81	77	77
Married and noncoresident	92	89	94	92	90	91	90	90
Married and residing inside parent's locality	61	57	62	64	64	60	67	66
Mean Number of Children								
Total (including coresident)	5.6	5.7	5.8	5.3	5.0	5.5	5.1	4.6
Noncoresident	4.1	3.7	4.2	4.3	3.9	4.1	4.0	3.7
Residing outside parents' locality	2.6	2.4	2.8	2.6	2.4	2.7	2.3	2.1
Married and noncoresident	3.5	3.1	3.6	3.9	3.4	3.5	3.6	3.2
Married and residing inside parent's locality	1.4	1.2	1.3	1.5	1.4	1.3	1.5	1.4

Table 9.11. Percentage of Elderly Parents who Received Material Support during the Prior Year from at Least One Noncoresident Child, Unadjusted and Adjusted for Selected Indicators of the Availability of Noncoresident Children, by Age and Sex of the Elderly Parent

Form of Results and Age of Elderly Parents	Received Food and/or Clothes			Received Money		
	Total	Men	Women	Total	Men	Women
Unadjusted results						
60–64	61	56	64	69	64	71
65–69	60	61	60	67	65	68
70–74	64	61	66	71	67	74
75+	55	58	52	62	64	61
All ages	60	59	61	67	65	69
Adjusted results·						
60–64	61	57	63	68	65	71
65–69	60	59	60	66	64	68
70–74	64	60	67	71	67	75
75+	56	56	55	62	64	62
All ages	60	58	62	67	65	69

Notes: Results refer to all elderly parents regardless of whether or not any children are coresident.
· Statistical adjustment made through linear regression. In the case of receipt of food and/or clothes, adjustment is made for the total number of noncoresident children and number of married noncoresident children living in the same locality (village, town, or district of Bangkok) as the elderly parents; in the case of receipt of money, adjustment is made for the total number of noncoresident children and the number of children living outside their parents' locality.
Source: 1986 SECAPT Survey

those stages of their life course that are particularly pertinent to the provision of such support. In the case of receipt of food and/or clothes, we adjusted for both the total number of noncoresident children and for the number of noncoresident married children living in the same locality as the parents. In the case of receipt of money, we adjusted the results for both the total number of noncoresident children and the number of noncoresident children (regardless of marital status) living away from the parents' locality.[12]

In general, statistical adjustment for the availability of adult children at the pertinent stage of their life course has little effect on the results. Moreover, no consistent relationship appears between the elderly parent's age and receipt of material support through either food and/or clothes or money. Thus the association that exists between the life-course stage of children and their tendency to provide different types of material support, has minimal influence on the relationship between the

Table 9.12. Percentage of Elderly Parents who Received Material Support during the Prior Year from at least One Noncoresident Child, Unadjusted and Adjusted for the Age of the Elderly Parent and Selected Indicators of the Availability of Noncoresident Children, by Sex and Coresidence Status of the Elderly Parent

	Unadjusted		Adjusted for Age of Elderly Parent		Adjusted for Age of Elderly Parent and Availability of Noncoresident Children[*]	
	Received Food/Clothes	Received Money	Received Food/Clothes	Received Money	Received Food/Clothes	Received Money
Men						
Coresident with adult child	57	64	57	64	57	64
Not coresident	68	68	68	68	63	66
Women						
Coresident with adult child	58	68	58	68	59	68
Not coresident	72	72	73	73	71	72

Notes: Results refer to all elderly parents with at least one child age 18 or older, regardless of whether any children are not coresident. Statistical adjustment made through linear regression.

[*] In the case of receipt of food and/or clothes, adjustment is made for the total number of noncoresident children and the number of married noncoresident children living in the same locality (village, town, or district of Bangkok) as the elderly parents; in the case of receipt of money, adjustment is made for the total number of noncoresident children and the number of children living outside their parents' locality.

elderly parent's life-course stage and whether or not the parents receive material support from noncoresident children.

The need for material support from noncoresident children is presumably greater among elderly who are not coresident with another adult child than among coresident elderly. Table 9.12 indicates the percentage of elderly men and women who received food and/or clothes and the percentage who received money during the prior year, according to whether or not they were coresident with an adult child (age 18 or older), among elderly who have at least one adult child. Results are both unadjusted and adjusted, first for the age of the elderly (as an indication of the elderly's life-course stage), and then for the availability of children at those stages of their life course that are particularly pertinent to the provision of such support. The unadjusted results indicate that both noncoresident elderly men and women are somewhat more likely to receive both types of support than are those who coreside with an adult child. Adjustment for the age of the elderly has virtually no effect on the results, while additionally adjusting for availability of children at the relevant life-course stages modestly reduces the association of coresidence for men and women, particularly the former.

For both men and women, adjusted and unadjusted results indicate that the influence of the elderly's coresidence status is greater on the receipt of food and/or clothes than on the receipt of money. The magnitude of the difference is modest, however, and may be at least partly an artifactual effect of an overly narrow definition of household when defining coresidence, as discussed above. For example, elderly who reside in separate dwelling units within the same compound or related cluster of houses may be sharing resources, including food, as well as responsibilities, such as cooking, in the same way elderly and coresident children who are living together in the same dwelling units. However, since technically they do not coreside in the same dwelling unit, they are defined as living separately. Thus the receipt of food and/or clothes from children in dwelling units within the same cluster appears to be provided by noncoresident children, even though those children are actually quasi-coresident.

CONCLUSIONS

The foregoing analysis underscores the importance of the life course of elderly parents and their children for understanding support systems for the elderly in a third world setting. The familial support system for elderly in Thailand relates in many ways to the life course of both the elderly themselves and their adult children. As elderly parents, they experience important life-course transitions, such as disengagement from work, loss of spouse, and deterioration of health. All of these have important implications for both their need for different types of support and assistance from their children and their ability to provide support and assistance to their children. At the same time as parents pass through the elderly age span, their children experience important life-course transitions, such as entering the labor force, moving out of the parental home, and forming conjugal families of their own. These transitions also have important implications for their support relationships with their parents.

In the present study, we have examined the association between the life course of Thai elderly and their children, as well as two important aspects of the familial support system for the elderly—namely, coresidence with children and the receipt of material support from noncoresident children. In particular, we have focused on the extent to which the life course of the adult children affects how much the support they provide responds to the increasing needs of their parents as the latter grow older. The results demonstrate that while both types of support are related to the life-course stage of the children, the extent to which this relationship influences the association between life course of the elderly parent and receipt of such support differs according to the type of support being considered.

In Thailand, for example, there is an inverse association between the age of elderly parents and the proportion who live with children. If this is viewed solely in terms of the life course of the elderly, it might appear that children become less responsive as their parents' need for coresidence increases and ability to contribute to their children's welfare decreases. That this impression is misleading becomes apparent once differences in the life course stages of children are taken into account. It is important to recognize that older elderly are more likely than younger elderly to have older children, who in turn will likely be at stages where separate residence is more common and coresidence more problematic. Our analysis suggests that it is changes in life-course stage of the children, rather than of the parents, that account for lower coresidence among older than younger elderly parents. Once the life-course stage of the children is considered, older elderly parents appear at least as likely as their younger counterparts to coreside with adult children. The fact that adult children in Thailand respond to their parents' need for coresidence is further illustrated by the association between coresidence and marital status of the parent. Thus parents who are divorced, separated, or widowed are more likely to coreside with children than are parents who live together as spouses.

The life-course stage of noncoresident children is clearly associated with the provision of at least two types of material support provided to their elderly parents. Married children living near their elderly parents are more likely than other noncoresident children to provide food and/or clothes, while single children living outside the locality are more likely than other noncoresident children to provide money. Nevertheless, the availability of adult children to provide either type of material support does not appear to relate to the life-course stage of their parents in any simple manner. Thus in contrast to coresidence, examination of the life-course stages of adult children has little effect on the observed relationship between the life-course stage of their parents and the receipt of material support from noncoresident children. That provision of such support is in part a response to the needs of elderly parents, however, is suggested by the somewhat greater likelihood for elderly parents who are not coresident with adult children to receive both types of material support than elderly parents who do live with an adult child. The magnitude of these differences is admittedly rather modest.

While the life courses of the elderly and their children undoubtedly exert some influence on the relationship between the two generations, the importance of life-course transitions as the determinants of support patterns that currently exist in Thailand should not be overstated. In particular, the role played by cultural values that underlie the current familial support system needs to be explicitly recognized. The pervasive nature of coresidence of elderly parents and adult children and the common provision of material support to elderly parents from noncoresident children, especially when contrasted the western traditions, underscores the strength of the normative imperatives that underlie the support system. As elsewhere, life-course transitions affect living arrangements and other aspects of support of the elderly only within a context of cultural values that dictate the overall pattern. It is in interaction with this broader framework of normative expectations that life course influences can be best understood.

ACKNOWLEDGMENTS

This chapter was prepared for presentation at the Conference on Aging and Generational Relations in Historical and Cross-cultural Perspectives, October 10–13, 1991, University of Delaware, Newark, Delaware. Helpful comments from John Casterline and Susan De Vos on an earlier version of this paper are gratefully acknowledged.

NOTES

1.   Although the sample was intended to be representative and self-weighting, a variety of circumstances affecting fieldwork resulted in a sample that was disproportionately urban. To obtain more representative results, we applied a set of case-weights (normalized to 1.00) (Chayovan, Wongsith, & Saengtienchai, 1988).

2.   The level of hearing impairment is likely to be substantially underestimated in the data from the SECAPT survey, since hearing problems were one of the chief reasons for nonresponse (Chayovan, Wongsith, & Saengtienchai, 1988).

3.   A more thorough analysis of living arrangements based on the 1980 census data is provided by Chayovan, Knodel and Siriboon, 1990.

4.   In 1989, there were 2,150 elderly living in twelve government operated homes for the elderly. The number living in private sector homes for the aged also appears to be small (Pichyangkura & Singhajend, 1991). Thus as a proportion of the total number of elderly, the numbers are negligible.

5.   Adopted and stepchildren cannot be distinguished from each other in the present version of the SECAPT survey data set. It is likely, however, that the majority of such children are stepchildren resulting from a remarriage. In other cases, however, children may have been adopted specifically with the idea that they would be responsible for the adopting parents during old age (Rubenstein, 1987).

6.   Of course, such a coresident youngster could eventually become a coresident adult child and contribute significantly to the support of the elderly parents in the future. The problem is that it is not possible to distinguish which among those dependent children who are present in the household at the time of the survey will remain coresident as adults.

7.   Information was collected from each elderly respondent about each child, resulting in information for a total of approximately 16,000 children. However, since all elderly in each sample household were included in the survey, in cases where both a husband and wife were interviewed, their children are represented twice in the set of data referring to the children of the elderly.

8.   Although questions about support provided were asked in relation to every child of the respondent, we limit our analysis to noncoresident children only. Respondents often simply indicated the fact that they were coresident with the child, rather than mentioning specific types of support. This probably reflects the fact that in cases of coresidence the elderly and their coresident children share income and other resources, and thus it is difficult to specify who gives what to whom.

9.   In such cases it is assumed that both food and money are provided.

10.   Respondents were in fact asked how frequently the child provided support. However, in the substantial number of cases where a child was reported to provide more that one type of support, it is not possible to know to which type of support the respondent's reply referred.

11.   Although the question specifically referred to regular support, this was

interpreted in some cases as including support provided as infrequently as once a year. For example, in about 6% of the (unweighted) cases where a child was reported as providing some sort of support (including "visiting"), the elderly respondent indicated support was provided once a year.

12. Because of the way the data file has been constructed, the number of noncoresident married children living in the same locality refers to children who are currently married rather than ever married.

REFERENCES

Chayovan, N., Knodel, J., & Siriboon, S. (1990). *Thailand's elderly population: A demographic and social profile based on official statistical sources.* Comparative study of the elderly in Asia (Research Report No. 90–2). Ann Arbor: University of Michigan, Population Studies Center.

Chayovan, N., Wongsith, M., & Saengtienchai, C. (1988). *Socio-economic consequences of the ageing of the population in Thailand: Survey findings.* Bangkok: Chulalongkorn University, Institute of Population Studies.

Cowgill, D. O. (1968). The social life of the aged in Thailand. *The Gerontologist, 8,* 159–163.

———. (1972). The role and status of the aged in Thailand. In D. O. Cowgill & L. D. Holmes (Eds.), *Aging and modernization* (pp. 91–101). New York: Appleton-Century-Crofts.

DeVos, S., & Holden, K. (1988). Measures comparing living arrangements of the elderly: An assessment. *Population and Development Review, 14,* 688–704.

Kinsella, K. (1990). *Living arrangements of the elderly and social policy; A cross-national perspective* (CIR Staff Paper, No. 52). Washington, DC: U.S. Bureau of the Census, Center for International Research.

Knodel, J., Chamratrithirong, A., & Debavalya, N. (1987). *Thailand's reproductive revolution.* Madison: University of Wisconsin Press.

Knodel, J., Havanon, N., & Pramualratana, A. (1984). Fertility transition in Thailand: A qualitative analysis. *Population and Development Review, 10,* 297–328.

Limanonda, B. (1989). *Analysis of postnuptial residence patterns of Thai women.* In Institute of Population Studies, Chulalongkorn University, Health and Population Studies Based on the 1987 Thailand Demographic and Health Survey (pp. 223–252). New York: Population Council.

Pichyangkura, C., & Singhajend, M. (1991, 15–22 July). *Thailand national review on the elderly.* Paper presented at the Workshop on Population Aging, ESCAP, Bangkok, Thailand.

Pramualratana, A. (1990). *Support systems of the old in a rural community in Thailand.* Unpublished Ph.D. thesis. Australian National University, Canberra.

Rubenstein, R. L. (1987). Childless elderly: Theoretical perspectives and practical concerns. *Journal of Cross-Cultural Gerontology, 2,* 1–14.

Tuchrello, W. P. (1989). The society and its environment. In B. L. LePoer (Ed.),

Thailand: A country study, (6th Ed.) (pp. 55–120). Washington, DC: U.S. Government Printing Office.

Wongsith, M. (1990, October 20–24). *Attitudes towards family values in Thai society.* Paper presented at the Nihon University International Symposium on Family and the Contemporary Japanese Culture: An International Perspective, Tokyo.

10

Intergenerational Support in Sri Lanka
The Elderly and Their Children

Peter Uhlenberg

In Sri Lanka, as in most societies, a vital relationship is formed between parents and their offspring. As both child and parent age over the life course, the nature of their relationship changes. But at each stage of life, this relationship remains socially significant. This study explores aspects of this intergenerational relationship when parents are old and their children are adults. The setting is a rural area of Sri Lanka in 1990.

Three questions related to intergenerational relationships in later life direct this inquiry. The first concerns patterns of intergenerational coresidence. Which older persons share a household with one or more of their children? Which children coreside with their elderly parents? And what are the attitudes of the young and old regarding coresidence? The second question involves the giving and receiving of other forms of support between generations. How widespread are exchanges of money, goods, and services across generations? And who participates in these types of exchanges? Third, what is the basis for continuing support in later life? Do relationships involve reciprocity, with valued support flowing in both directions? Is support of elderly parents viewed as a burden upon their children?

There are both theoretical and policy reasons for being interested in current patterns of intergenerational support in Sri Lanka. The population of Sri Lanka is on the threshold of experiencing a dramatic transition in its age structure. Study of intergenerational relationships at this time can establish a baseline evaluating the effects of subsequent demographic change. And an understanding of existing mechanisms for supporting the elderly may allow policy planners to prepare for challenges to the well-being of the elderly that loom on the horizon. Currently, there are still relatively few old persons in Sri Lanka—in 1990 only eight percent of the population was over age 60. But in response to declining

241

fertility that has occurred over the past several decades, a rapid aging of the population can be anticipated. According to United Nations projections, the proportion over age 60 will more than double over the next 35 years, reaching 17.2% by 2025 (United Nations, 1989). Any discussion of how this new demographic regime will affect intergenerational relationships must begin with a clear understanding of how these relationships are currently structured.

This chapter begins with a brief overview of the sociodemographic situation in Sri Lanka and a description of the data we collected to assess intergenerational relationships. This is followed by a discussion of several salient aspects of the aging process in Sri Lanka. Finally questions related to the structure of intergenerational exchange and support between the elderly and their children are addressed.

BACKGROUND: SOCIAL CONTEXT

This study of intergenerational relationships is located in a most interesting context. Sri Lanka, in 1990, had several characteristics generally associated with a modern society. Its birth rate was low (only slightly above replacement level fertility) and its death rate was low (expectation of life at birth was 70 years). The literacy rate was high (88% in 1985), and women enjoyed a relatively high social status. Universal free education and widely accessible health services have been available in the country since the 1940s.

Despite the demographic and social characteristics described above, Sri Lanka, surprisingly, is still a very poor country with a young age distribution. Per capita income in Sri Lanka in 1990 was $420 (U.S. dollars), which is only slightly higher than it is in India and Pakistan. Further, almost 80% of the population is still rural and engaged in agriculture. Reflecting the recency of the demographic transiton, the age structure of the population is still more characteristic of a developing country than a developed one. Only 4% of the population is over age 65, while 35% is under age 15. The respondents in this study, both the old and their adult children, have lived through a period of dramatic demographic and social change. Nevertheless, a large majority of both generations continue to live in rural areas with meager incomes.

Kalutara District, where our study was conducted, is located in southwest Sri Lanka—just south of the capital, Colombo. While there are several distinct regions in Sri Lanka, the Kalutara district is close to the national average on most social, economic, and health characteristics. Marriage and family patterns in the district mirror those of the country as a whole. About 80% of the population is rural, and a majority of workers are paddy cultivators or are employed on the organized plantations of rubber, coconut, spices, and tea. Almost all of those living in Kalutara are Sinhalese and Buddhist.

DATA

The data analyzed in this chapter come from two complementary sources. Qualitative data on aging in Sri Lanka was collected from focus group sessions conducted in December, 1990. Six distinct focus groups were formed according to the following criteria: females over 50; males over 50; females 25–49 with an older person in the household; females 25–49 without an older person in the household; males 25–49 with an older person in the household; and males 25–49 without an older person in the household. Each group had a moderator and six participants. Sessions lasted for about an hour and a half. The recording of each session was later translated into English and transcribed. Questions to the focus groups dealt with perceptions of the aging process and the nature of parent-child relationships in later life.

Quantitative data was collected from personal interviews with 432 respondents. A multistage, self-weighting probability sample survey of about 2700 households in Kalutara district was conducted in 1989 by the Family Planning Association of Sri Lanka (FPASL). Using the household rosters from this survey, we selected households of three types: Type 1, only adults age 55+ present; Type 2, only adults age 25–54 present; Type 3, adults in both age categories present. The sample design called for an interview with one older person in each of 40 Type 1 households. A quota of 150 was set for Type 2 households, with an interview from a randomly selected adult respondent. A similar quota (150) was set for Type 3 households, with one older person and one younger adult to be interviewed.

Locating households of Type 2 and Type 3 did not present any difficulty, and interviews were completed with approximately the number of respondents desired. Finding households that contained older persons living without a child present proved more difficult, despite the information available on household composition from the survey conducted a year earlier. In that survey, 10% of all households containing a person over age 55 did not contain any younger adults. In other words, it is uncommon for the elderly not to coreside with at least one child. Nevertheless, we identified enough households that appeared to be of this type to meet our quota. In the field, however, we were able to locate only 22 households containing older persons.

Extensive interviews were conducted with the survey respondents by trained interviewers working for the FPASL. The questions covered basic information regarding demographic, social, economic, and health characteristics of the respondent, as well as attitudes and views related to the aging experience. In addition, information was collected on other household members and on parents or children living outside of the household. Special attention was given to social and economic exchanges occurring between the respondent and these other persons. The rationale for collecting these data came from our desire to have rich data on intergenerational support between the elderly and their children (both those coresiding and those living in separate households). Collecting this data presented no special difficulties; however, analyzing them presents a greater challenge.

AGING OCCURS EARLY IN SRI LANKA

In Sri Lanka, as in all developing countries, the population is young. As mentioned above, only four percent of Sri Lanka's population is over age 65. But age 65 is not necessarily a meaningful marker of old age in this society. When asked to indicate the chronological age at which a person was considered old, no consensus emerged among our respondents. Only 12% reported an age in the range of 65 to 69, while 58% gave a younger age and 30% suggested 70 years or older as the beginning of old age. In addition to a majority of respondents, reporting that old age begins before 60, several other indicators suggest that changes associated with old age begin relatively early in the life course.

The participants in a focus group comprised of six women age 52 to 60 were asked about changes that occur when a man or woman reaches old age. Each woman in this group responded to this question with a personal observation about her own aging experience. Without exception, each woman indicated that she had already experienced a transition into old age. The salient changes associated with growing older noted by these women were declining ability to work and increasing dependence upon others. An excerpt from each woman's response in order to capture how pervasive their sense of personal aging follows:

Participant 1 (55 years old): "We used to work hard earlier. But now we do it with difficulty because of our old age."

Participant 2 (60 years old): "Still, I feel I can attend to the household work, although I am growing in years."

Participant 3 (56 years old):	"Earlier, I was employed as a coir worker, earning a lot of money. But now that I am old, I attend to the household work and partly do a little coir work to earn whatever money I can get."
Participant 4 (54 years old):	"Earlier, I used to work coir, but now that I am old and feeble I am unable to work. The employed children look after us."
Participant 5 (52 years old):	"It is three years after my husband's death.I live with my daughter. I have no income and have to depend on whatever my daughter brings home.
Participant 6 (60 years old):	"I live with much difficulty. Earlier, I used to do all the housework, but now I am unable to do any work. In passing my time, I look after my grandchildren in the way I can."

The sense of physical decline and increased dependency among these women (all 60 years old or less) suggests that social and cultural forces lead to early aging in this environment. Responses from participants in the older men's focus group reveal quite similar perceptions. One man stated: "A person will begin to feel these changes from the time he is 55 to 60 years. You get a little weaker and start noticing other changes, like teeth and eyes getting weaker." One man expressed his sense of loss in this way: "I had the strength single-handed to cut down huge trees, but now I do not have the strength to cut down even an arecanut tree." Another participant followed up, asserting, "then you become a real problem for young people." Others in the group then added supporting comments on how the physical changes associated with aging produced anger and irritability.

The survey responses showed a decline in physical functioning with age (Table 10.1). Several different measures of physical problems are included, in order to provide a general picture of when in the life course the negative effects of aging are experienced. As one might expect in a poor country, the overall prevalence of health-related problems is quite high. Only two-thirds of the adults reported their general health status as "good," "very good," or "excellent." Not surprisingly, the proportion who reported their health as "poor" or "fair" increased uniformly with age. This global measure of physical well-being suggests a fairly uniform increase in health problems after age 40 for both men and women. The more specific questions, however, indicate that the timing of perceived decrements in functional ability vary by type of problem.

Age-related decrements in vision are expected after age 40. The proportion reporting moderate or serious problems with vision in Sri Lanka jumps from about 10% among those under age 40 to over 50% of those age 40–49. Among the population over age 60, well over 80% report

Table 10.1. Percent of Population Reporting Physical Problems in Selected Areas, by Sex and Age

| Sex/Age: | (N) | | Percent Having Problems With | | |
		Health	General Vision	Walking	Heavy Work
Males					
<40	(50)	24	10	8	10
40–49	(55)	19	51	9	28
50–59	(47)	34	77	28	63
60–69	(43)	43	79	49	59
70+	(25)	52	88	79	96
Females					
<40	(50)	15	6	4	30
40–49	(37)	30	70	15	45
50–59	(46)	40	85	35	70
60–69	(34)	68	91	69	82
70+	(25)	81	92	75	100

vision problems. Information was not collected on how the deterioration of vision affected the lives of older persons. But, at a minimum, most of the population over age 50 was aware of a loss in this area.

A large increase in perceived problems with walking occurs after age 50. About one-fourth of the men and one-third of the women age 50–59 consider themselves to have some difficulty with walking, and the prevalence of this problem doubles among those in the next decade of life. Several other measures of physical problems (hearing problems, dental problems) similarly indicate that a large proportion of Sri Lankans is aware of experiencing substantial physical decline before reaching age 60.

Perhaps the best indicator we have of how early in the life course negative effects of aging are perceived comes from responses to a question about ability to engage in heavy work. The percentage of men reporting that they are unable to do heavy work or have a lot of difficulty doing it increases from 10% of those under age 40 to over 60% of those age 50–59. Among women, 70% of those in their fifties indicate problems in this area. Such widespread physical limitations among those under age 60 may have quite significant implications for a population in which physical labor is still the dominant type of work.

Additional evidence that significant life-course changes commonly occur for Sri Lankans as they move through their fifties and early sixties comes from data on work activities. Among men age 30–49, 16% report that they were not working in the past month. But the proportion out of the labor force doubles to 31% of those age 50–54, and further increases to 54% of those age 55–64. In other words, fewer than half of the men continue working past about age 60, and many are "retiring" before age 55. This pattern of reduced labor force participation suggested by cross-sectional data is confirmed by responses to a question asking men how their current level of work activity compared with that when they were age 50. Only 36% of those aged 55–64 reported that they continued to work as much as they did earlier, while 64% said they were doing "less" or "much less."

A similar question about changes in level of work given to household chores was asked of men and women. Among men age 55–64, 66% reported that they were doing less than they were at age 50, and among women 70% said they were doing less. Thus, changes both in self-reported physical condition and in activity patterns confirm what the focus-group participants were saying: People in Sri Lanka tend to make a transition into "old age" at relatively young ages. There is, to be sure, a great deal of heterogeneity within the population over age 55, and there does not appear to be any sharp demarcation between middle age and old age. Nevertheless, it is reasonable to consider the population over age 55 as old when studying patterns of intergenerational support in later life.

CONTRACTION OF SOCIAL LIFE IN OLD AGE

If entering old age tends to involve a reduction in amount of time spent working outside and inside the household, one might expect that some other activities would take on increased significance. The increased physical problems associated with growing old may force a reduction in other activities. Further, behavior in later life may be influenced by cultural norms that specify activities in which the old should or should not engage. Given these countervailing forces, it is difficult to anticipate how involvement in activities such as visiting friends, performing community service, and attending religious activities might change in later life.

Questions about how persons tend to change activity patterns in later life were asked in each focus group. There was most agreement about religious activities. Both younger and older men and women believed that religious activities increased after the demands of work and rearing children were past. Especially, it was felt that older women tended to increase their attendance at temple and observance of Sil. Results from the survey, however, indicate that this may be more of a stereotype than a reality (Table 10.2). While about one-fourth of the women past age 55 report an increase in their religious activities compared to the level exist-

Table 10.2. Changes since Age 50 Reported in Frequency of Visiting Friends and Attending Temple Services, by Age and Sex

Sex/Age	(N)	Percent Visiting Friends			
		More	*Same*	*Less*	*Lot Less*
Males					
55–64	(44)	2	39	45	14
65+	(50)	4	24	34	38
Females					
55–64	(27)	0	22	52	26
65+	(47)	0	11	53	34
		Percent Attending Temple Services			
Males					
55–64	—	20	52	25	2
65+	—	22	26	32	20
Females					
55–64	—	26	41	26	7
65+	—	23	32	23	21

ing when they were 50, an even larger percentage reported a decline in such activities. Quite similar patterns were observed among men, with more reducing rather than increasing their participation in religious activities in old age. Further probing is needed to understand these reported patterns. It is possible that personal religiosity does increase, but is not reflected in higher temple attendance because of physical limitations. But the survey data do not suggest any general movement toward increased social engagement in religious activities in later life.

A second area of interest involves time spent visiting and interacting with friends. Several younger women believed (perhaps wishfully) that in old age there would be more time for visiting with friends. More common, was the view that in old age "usually friends become less, but religious activities increase." When an older woman stated that "we have much less to do with friends and relatives," general agreement was expressed by others in the group. The survey results clearly support this view of a constriction in friendship networks with age. None of the women over age 55 reported more visiting with friends now than earlier in life, and only 15% reported stability in this area. Visiting with others occupies less time in old age for the great majority of men and women, and about a third of those past age 65 indicate that there has been a large drop-off in visiting.

A third sphere of activity involving community service did not receive much comment in the focus groups, except in the one comprised of older men. The conversation among these men was interesting. One participant noted that the old had more time to be involved, but the others objected to the notion that in old age they were doing more. "We may have more time, but we are not wanted now," one man countered. Another added that "most of the time they [the young people] do things as they want, and most of the people are forced to agree with them." A third man followed up, "I think we should let them [the younger adults] manage things and we should help." This sense that old age does not lead to more community participation is borne out by the survey results. Only 6% reported an increased level of community participation in later life, while 67% reported a decline.

The picture of aging in Sri Lanka developed thus far has focused upon losses. Physically, increasing age is associated with declining health, sensory loss, and decreased ability to engage in manual work. Further, the amount of time spent doing work and household chores tends to decline. There also is a contraction in such social activities as visiting with friends or engaging in community service. Significant decline in each of these areas occurs for many members of a cohort by age 55, and declines become increasingly prevalent as a cohort continues to age through later life. Given these multiple indicators of loss and decline, one might expect old age in Sri Lanka to be a very negative period of life.

SATISFACTION WITH LIFE IN OLD AGE

Do the elderly in Sri Lanka experience increasing economic problems and/or declining respect from others as a result of changes associated with aging? Data shown in Table 10.3 suggests that the decline associated with growing old does not lead to declining socioeconomic status. Complaints about inadequate income are less common among those age 55–64 than among the younger population. Dissatisfaction increases after age 65, but the proportion "very dissatisfied" is about the same as it is among the younger population. While the old in Sri Lanka tend to live on very low incomes (as do most people), there is no marked increase in severe economic problems in later life.

Responses to the question "How much respect do you receive in your family?" suggest that social devaluation is not common in old age. The highest proportion reporting that they receive "very little" or "not too much" respect occurs among younger women, while those receiving "very much respect" is highest among women age 55–64 and men over age 65. Overall, about two-thirds of the elderly feel that they are receiving a great deal of respect.

The mechanism for preserving the economic and social status of the

Table 10.3. Percent Distribution by Level of Satisfaction with Income and Amount of Respect Received from Family, by Sex and Age

Sex/Age	Income Satisfaction			Respect Received		
	Satisfied	Unsatisfied	Very Unsatisfied	Much	Some	Little
Males						
<55	47	35	28	66	16	18
55–64	54	30	16	64	22	14
65+	44	38	18	70	10	20
Females						
<55	51	36	17	56	22	22
55–64	68	21	11	71	18	11
65+	43	45	13	64	23	14

elderly in Sri Lanka was agreed upon by virtually all of the focus group participants. It is the family that buffers the elderly from experiencing economic hardship and humiliation as they experience the losses that accompany aging. In a variety of ways, the participants expressed a sentiment similar to that of an older woman, who said, "If the children are brought up well they will look after us, and we will be able to live a comfortable life." We turn now to explore more carefully the nature of intergenerational support between older persons and their adult children.

INTERGENERATIONAL SUPPORT: CORESIDENCE

Coresiding with a child in later life is an obvious form of intergenerational support. In a society where intergenerational coresidence is normative, the old who live with a child are expected to be advantaged compared to those who do not. Not only does coresidence facilitate support and interaction between the generations, but it also meets with social approval. In Sri Lanka, as in other Asian countries, most of the elderly do live with an adult child in the household.

In her review of data from a number of Asian countries, Linda Martin (1988) concludes that approximately three-fourths of the Asian elderly live in households containing an adult child. Highest levels of coresidence were found in rural India (90%) and Singapore (86%), while lowest levels were in Thailand (61%) and Malaysia (72%). Where information was available on which child the older persons were living with (Korea, China, and India), a strong preference for coresidence with a son was observed. Several studies (Caldwell et al., 1989; DeVos, 1989) suggest that Sri Lanka is similar to other Asian countries in having a high prevalence of coresidence, but different in not having a strong preference for sons over daughters. In the 1989 household survey in the Kalatara District which provided the sampling frame for this study, 90% of the households with a member over age 55 also contained a younger adult.

To examine effects of coresidence upon the elderly, we must have a sample of older persons living apart from any child for comparison. As previously noted, we attempted to obtain a sample of 40 older persons living apart from children by over-sampling households of this type. Our ability to locate only 22 such households in our sample confirms the other evidence that this is an uncommon arrangement in Sri Lanka. While the sample is too small for detailed analyses, a closer look at the old who were not coresiding with a child reveals circumstances that may produce this situation.

A majority of those not living with a child (13 of 22) did not have a child, either because of nonmarriage or childlessness within a marriage. In one case the old person was living with several of her grandchildren, so actually was in an intergenerational household. Three cases involved married couples who preferred to live independent from their children. In each of these cases, the older persons reported close relationships with their children and an intention to coreside with a child in case of widowhood. This leaves five cases of older persons living alone when they did not have a spouse and did have children. One of these was a 68-year-old man who was separated from his wife and, apparently, alienated from his family. The other four cases were widows, three of whom had only one child. Each of these widows reported a close relationship with a child, and it is not clear why they did not coreside. In any population, one expects to find some who do not conform to the general pattern. In Sri Lanka, surely, the emphasis should be placed upon how rare it is for older parents not to coreside with at least one child.

Coresidence with a child in later life is the preferred, as well as the actual, arrangement. Only about a fourth of the respondents felt that it was better for an older couple to live independent from their children, and even fewer (6%) felt that it was desirable for a widow or widower to live alone (see Table 10.4). In most cases the preference for intergenerational coresidence was as strong among the younger population as it was among the older population. Thus it does not appear that more recent cohorts are adopting attitudes that conflict with those of their parents. The only exception was a tendency for older women to be less inclined than younger adults or older men to favor older couples, living alone.

No strong preference for living with sons or daughters in later life is

Table 10.4. Percent Distribution by Preferred Living Arrangement in Later Life for Couples, Widows and Widowers, by Age and Sex of Respondents

Sex/Age	(N)	*Older Couples Should Live*				
		Alone	With Son	With Daughter	With Either	Depends/ Other
Male, <55	(129)	25	09	03	39	25
Male, 55+	(101)	31	10	10	30	20
Female, <55	(126)	27	06	06	36	25
Female, 55+	(76)	11	15	12	46	17
Total	(432)	24	09	07	37	22
Widow Should Live						
Male <55		05	00	34	38	24
Male, 55+		06	03	30	38	23
Female, <55		07	03	23	37	30
Male, 55+		08	10	33	33	16
Total		06	03	29	37	25
Widower Should Live						
Male, <55		05	06	18	44	27
Male, 55+		07	04	27	33	28
Female, <55		06	05	13	42	34
Female, 55+		10	14	22	29	25
Total		06	07	20	38	29

evident from this data. The largest response category for each hypothetical situation (older couple, widow, widower) was always "either a son or daughter," and another significant proportion indicated that the ideal arrangement would depend upon the particular situation. Among those who did state a gender preference for the child with whom an older couple would live, about an equal number chose a son as chose a daughter. However, when the question referred to the best arrangement for a widow, daughters were 10 times more likely to be preferred than sons. Daughters also were preferred over sons for widowers, although the contrast was not as extreme (about a three-to-one ratio). A reason for preferring daughters over sons for those who are widowed is suggested by comments offered by several focus group participants. They mentioned potential problems of daughters-in-law as caregivers to older, dependent persons. For example, a younger woman said, "I think . . . the best place is to be at your daughter's place, because the son's wife is an outsider." A younger man reported, "The daughter is usually at home, but in the case of a daughter-in-law, she will never like to attend to such work [caregiving]. If she does it at all, it will be with a lot of reluctance." In no case was concern expressed about problems of getting along with a son-in-law, who presumably is not expected to be involved in caring for an older person. However, the extent of concern over potential conflict with a son's wife should not be exaggerated—a majority of persons are open to living with either a son or daughter in later life. The most common approach is to evaluate the possible options, taking into account a variety of factors.

GIVING AND RECEIVING HELP

Exchanges between adult children and their older parents is a complex issue to study. How should "exchange" or "support" be conceptualized? It is clear that giving money is a form of exchange, as is giving other forms of material aid. But material support ranges from providing completely for the other person to occasional gifts of little value. Services (bathing, transportation, child care, and the like) also can be significant sources of support, but, again, there is a wide range in possible effort expended by the provider and in consequences for the receiver. Caring for grandchildren, for example, may be done by a grandmother for her own enjoyment, or it may be done sacrificially to help a child. Similarly, having an older parent watch one's children may have quite incidental consequences for a younger couple, or it may enable a young woman to work and thereby greatly increase the family's economic status. Beyond material support and services, socioemotional types of support may significantly affect quality of life. Those who provide social or emotional support may gain great satisfaction from the exchange, or they may experience it as a great burden. Receiving these types of support may enhance one's sense of significance and value, or they may lead to feelings of guilt (for being a burden). This study explores only a few of the many questions that can be raised about intergenerational exchanges.

The survey questionnaire asked about receiving and giving financial assistance, other goods, and services. Older persons were asked about these types of exchanges with adult children who were coresiding with them, as well as with children living in separate households. The number of interviews is too small to permit a very extensive multivariate analysis, but these exploratory data produce several interesting patterns. In addition, material from the focus groups provides useful insights into how exchanges between generations are perceived.

Overall levels of exchange with children reported by older persons are shown in Table 10.5. Responses regarding exchanges with children in the household are restricted to the old who coreside with children, while responses regarding exchanges with children living apart are re-

Table 10.5. Percent of Older Persons Reporting they Provide or Receive Support, by Coresidence Status of Children

Type of Support	Children In HH (N = 147)		Children Outside HH (N = 101)	
	Provide	*Receive*	*Provide*	*Receive*
Services	21	76	02	05
Money	27	57	03	52
Goods	26	37	02	34
Any support	43	88	03	52

stricted to the old who have children both inside and outside their households. The most striking result in this table is the much higher frequency of the old reporting that more support is received than is given. Twice as many older persons report receiving support from coresident children as report giving support to these children (88 vs. 43%). The contrast is greatest in the area of services, where 76% receive help but only 21% give help. Exchanges with children outside of the household are even more lopsided, as 52% receive support of money, goods, or services, but only three percent give their noncoresident children any of these forms of support.

Comparing differences by the coresidence status of the child leads to three additional observations. First, the exchange of services (help with chores, transportation, shopping, and the like) occurs almost exclusively within households. In terms of support received by the old, this is the area for which coresidence makes a huge difference. Older parents are 15 times more likely to receive caregiving services from children living in the household than from children living apart. Second, children who live separately are almost as likely as coresident children to provide material support (either money or goods) to their aging parents. This suggests that focusing solely upon the household when studying intergenerational exchanges gives a misleading picture of the actual situation. Adult children living separately frequently provide material assistance to their parents. Third, the giving of support to children almost always is limited to those children who coreside. As will be suggested later, this may be a somewhat misleading picture because it does not include one-time gifts of dowries and inheritances given to children at the time they leave home. But in terms of ongoing exchanges, support to children appears to end when the children leave home. It is also true, however, that a slight majority (57%) of older parents report giving no support to their coresident children.

Thus far, no attention has been given to the gender of the older person. But gender differences in the giving and receiving of support are

Table 10.6. Percent of Older Persons* Reporting Exchanges of Various Types with Coresident and other Children, by Sex of Respondent

| | Type of Support and Sex of Respondent | | | | | | | |
| | Services | | Money | | Goods | | Any Support | |
	Male	Female	Male	Female	Male	Female	Male	Female
Give to Children								
Coresiding only	16	26	37	04	35	08	42	28
Other only	02	00	02	02	00	04	02	00
Both	00	02	02	00	00	00	02	02
Neither	81	72	58	94	65	89	54	70
Receive from Children								
Coresiding only	72	83	26	32	16	28	47	47
Other only	00	02	21	21	09	15	00	06
Both	07	02	26	36	23	21	48	43
Neither	21	13	28	11	51	36	05	04

* Restricted to the 46 older men and 55 older women who had both coresiding and other children

marked, as shown by data in Table 10.6. Among the elderly, giving money or goods to adult children is primarily a male activity. Over 40% of the older men report giving money to a child, in contrast to only 6% of older women. Giving services to a child is more common among women than men. These differences reflect gender role differences in which men tend to control financial decisions while women are more engaged in household tasks and caregiving. On the receiving side, differences between older men and women tend not to be large. All but a trivial proportion of the older population report receiving some form of support from children. In general, however, women are slightly more likely to receive each of the various types of support. The greater support received by older women may result from more women than men being widowed (64 vs. 9%) and in greater need of support from children.

RECIPROCITY IN EXCHANGES

A number of focus group participants expressed grave concern about becoming a burden on their children in their old age. As one younger adult said, "we should not be a burden to our children. They will have their own problems." A young woman elaborated upon this theme: "I think it is better if we can save a least a small amount of money so that when we are old we don't have to depend on our own children. It's not that they will not look after us or anything like that, but . . . it will be very difficult for our children to manage with their salaries." This concern over the increasing cost of living for young families was noted by several persons, including an older man who said, "According to today's prices, the children can barely manage for their needs and it is unfair to expect money from them. But still they also do things for us. If they do not do so, society will look down on them." Note that the concern was not that children would fail to provide for their aging parents, but that the old would drain resources from children who were struggling to make ends meet. Ways in which the old are seen to minimize or avoid being a burden upon children are discussed below. But it is interesting to note first the negative consequences that were perceived to occur when the old really did become a burden.

A young man observed, "when a person grows old, his temperamental moods change, a certain amount of anger sets in, . . . most probably it is because he is unable to do certain things in the same way that it was done in his younger days." Similarly, a young woman, commenting on her old father, said he "doesn't like to admit that he is now old and unable to do work. Therefore he has developed a temper and is always finding fault with all of us." Still another young woman noted that sometimes "when a person gets into old age and is unable to get about, they suffer a lot mentally and finally fall sick. This is mainly because they hate to be a burden for their children." The view that old men became angry and/or sick when they became a burden on their children was expressed not only by younger adults—the older men observed these changes occurring in themselves. After one older man described the declining health and strength that accompany growing old, another man added, "then you become a real problem for your people." Another followed up, "and also then the person, if he had earlier been a nice person, begins to become troublesome and a real problem." Still a third added his experience: "Another thing is that as we get older, doctors ask you to take vitamins and more nutritious food and when you don't have the money to take these, you get angry and anger makes you get sick. These are our problems."

Everyone agreed that it was undesirable to become a burden upon others in old age. The negative situation of being a burden is avoided when the relationship can be viewed as involving reciprocity. When the old are giving as well as receiving support, the sense of being a complete burden is overcome. But what happens when one can no longer contribute anything to the relationship? One older man expressed a rather extreme view: "In old age you must have complete freedom and I would wish to die before I cannot manage by myself." But his view received a quick rebuttal from two other group participants: "One way our children can gain merit is by looking after and caring for parents, so I don't agree with you. If you become disabled, you must give that opportunity to the children." "I feel the same way. It is the duty of children to look after their parents." While no one likes the complete dependence of older persons upon their children, the duty of children to provide support remains largely unquestioned. As the daughter of parents who were still living independently in their seventies said, "When they are unable to manage on their own, one of us will have to bring them to our place."

As the focus groups discussed intergenerational relationships, the issue of reciprocity came up frequently. The ways by which the old are perceived to reciprocate for the support they receive can be grouped into three categories. First, the old earned the support of their children by providing good care for their children earlier in life; second, the old could do valued things to assist their children and improve the well-being of the household; and third, the one-time transmission of a dowry or inheritance to a child may balance the ongoing support that an old person receives in later life.

The extent to which respondents linked support received in later life to good child care provided earlier in life is impressive. This was a common theme expressed by men and women, young and old. Repeatedly, a connection was made between quality of childrearing and obligations to older parents:

(*Older woman*): "Because we have brought them up in the correct way, their feelings toward us will not change."

(*Older woman*): "We have to bring up our children well, to expect this return from them. It is very important."

(*Younger woman*): "We must always try to bring up our children properly. Then, only, they will be good to us when we are old. Otherwise they will neglect their elders and just go dump them into an elder's home."

(*Younger man*): "If the older people have done their obligations to the children, they in turn will look after them in their old age."

(*Older man*): "It is the duty of children to look after their parents. Of course, that depends on the way the children have been brought up."

What are the things a parent should do for a child to ensure faithful support in old age? The things mentioned most often were providing a good education, arranging a good marriage, and setting a good example. "Our first and main obligation should be towards our children. We should educate them and bring them up in the proper way. Only then will they see to our necessities in old age." This young woman then went on to explain how her care for an elderly parent was setting a good example for her children. In another group discussion, a participant stated that "it's our duty to find good partners for them [the children] and give them in marriage at the right age." Another participant agreed by saying, "If they don't get the correct partner, even at old age we won't have any peace of mind." Thus, one aspect of reciprocity is the balance seen between the earlier support that parents gave their children and the later support they receive from children.

The contributions of parents to children are not, of course, always restricted to the past. An older parent who coresides with a child may provide considerable support. Some older parents continue to work or receive pensions, in which case they can add to the household income. As one young male noted, "if an older person gets an income, any child will gladly keep the parent as it would not be a burden on him." Other older parents contribute by doing household chores. But, by far, the most salient role for the elderly involves child care. Repeatedly, respondents noted how valuable it could be to both themselves and their children to have an older parent living in the household. The sentiment expressed by this woman was echoed by others: "Especially now-a-days, it's a great asset to have grandparents at our own houses, as they look after our children while we are away from home." With a grandparent available to provide childcare, a woman in Sri Lanka can work outside the home to supplement the family income. Indeed, in some cases siblings compete over which one gets to have the parents live with them. One young mother who gave up her job when she had children, said, "It would be a great help for me if my mother could come and stay with my children so that I could start on a job again. But I don't like to ask her about this, as my brother, too, has this problem. My brother's wife also had to give up a job because of her two children." (The brother was in the process of arranging for his mother to live with him.)

A third form of reciprocity between the old and young is the provision of dowries and inheritances. Views in Sri Lanka of how parental property should be divided among children are varied. Some favor equal division, some favor the youngest child over the others, some favor sons over daughters, and so on. But there is widespread agreement that it is best for parents to settle questions about inheritance while they are still living. Frequently, the transfer of property to children occurs around the time of the children's marriages—as either a dowry or an inheritance. Group discussants indicated that the advantage of this approach was that it prevented misunderstandings and conflict among siblings. Another function of distributing property early is the obligation it gives children to care for their parents in late life. An adult child expressed this view in this way: "They must have a place [in our household], even if they have grown old. After all, they have left everything to

Table 10.7. Percent Distribution of Older Parents by Type of Intergenerational Exchange Reported, by Gender of Parent and Coresidence of Child

Type of Exchange	Coresiding Children		Noncoresiding Children	
	Male	Female	Male	Female
Give/receive	46	29	02	02
Give only	05	03	02	00
Receive only	40	62	47	47
Neither	09	06	49	51

us—their hard-earned money and even a little property. Therefore, we must always respect and regard them and look after them well." Older parents also are aware of the role that inheritance plays in reciprocity. As one older man, living with his 27-year-old unmarried son, put it, "this one, of course, will get married soon, but he will live with us and continue to look after us. Our house will one day belong to him."

A partial examination of the extent of reciprocity in intergenerational exchanges is possible using the survey data we collected. The several types of support (money, goods, services) are combined to form a measure of giving and/or receiving any support. Four possible patterns of exchange exist: giving and receiving, giving but not receiving, receiving but not giving, and neither giving nor receiving. The distribution of older men and women by the type of exchange relationship they report with children inside and outside the household is shown in Table 10.7.

Within the household, most exchanges involve either reciprocal exchanges or parents receiving but not giving support. Men more often than women report mutual exchanges with children, corresponding with the greater concern men expressed about being a burden upon adult children. As discussed earlier, very few older persons report giving any type of support to children who were not coresiding with them. About half of the respondents reported no exchanges with nonresident children, while half reported receiving support only. A major limitation of this approach to studying the extent of reciprocity in exchange relationships is the narrow conceptualization of support used. The focus group discussions made it obvious that much of the parental support occurred earlier in the life course. In particular, parents may be viewed as deserving support from children, based upon their earlier sacrifices to care for, educate, and arrange marriages for their children. Also, inheritance already bestowed upon children may balance the support currently received from children. Also missing, of course, are nonmaterial types of support that may enter into the subjective calculation of equity in exchanges between the generation.

Table 10.8. Percent Distribution of Older Parents by Type of Intergenerational Exchange within the Household, by Parents' Gender, Health Status and Economic Status

	Gender and Health Status			
	Males		Females	
Type of Exchange	*Good*	*Poor*	*Good*	*Poor*
Give/receive	52	38	52	18
Give only	04	06	05	02
Receive only	32	53	38	73
Neither	12	03	05	07
	Gender and Economic Status			
Give/receive	63	29	42	16
Give only	02	07	06	00
Receive only	29	51	45	78
Neither	05	12	06	06

It seems clear that persons prefer to maintain relationships with adult children in later life that involve continuing reciprocity. Thus, reciprocal relationships should be more prevalent among the elderly who have physical and economic resources that enable them to assist their children. We examined this hypothesis by comparing patterns of exchange by the self-reported health and economic status of older person. Health is labeled "good" if the respondent reported his or her general health as "good," "very good," or "excellent"; otherwise, it is labeled "poor." Economic status is labeled "adequate" if the respondent did not indicate dissatisfaction with it; otherwise, it is labeled "inadequate." The effects of health and economic status upon exchange patterns are shown with data in Table 10.8.

As expected, poor health and inadequate income in old age are negatively associated with current reciprocity in parent-child relationships. Reciprocity in relationships is reported by 52% of the older men and women who are in good health, but by only 38% of the men and 18% of the women with poor health. The bigger effect of health upon women is expected, since the primary support they give is service, rather than money or goods. Similarly, mutual support is two to three times more likely among older men and women when their economic status is considered adequate, rather than inadequate. The decline in reciprocity with failing health and economic status in old age is due to the declining ability of the old with these problems to assist their children. The children continue to support aging parents who cannot reciprocate.

CONCLUSION

The elderly in Sri Lanka are aware of experiencing losses that they attribute to the aging process. Decrements in physical functioning become increasingly prevalent after age 50, and these, in turn, lead to decreased involvement in work and increased dependence upon others for support. Losses also are reported in such social activities as visiting with others and engaging in community activities. As physical strength wanes and social life contracts, aging parents generally turn to their children for support. Most of the elderly coreside with at least one child, and most receive material support and/or services from their children. This arrangement, in which adult children support their parents in later life, appears to be accepted by all segments of the population.

While few question that adult children are obligated to care for their aging parents, many express concern about the strain that this support places upon the middle generation. Adults who have both dependent children and dependent, aged parents may encounter serious economic challenges in any society. Certainly this is the case in Sri Lanka, where incomes are low and aspirations to improved standards of living are high. In this context, no one wants the elderly to become a burden upon their children. This concern leads to the high saliency of the issue of reciprocity at this time. What can the elderly do for their children that will balance the support they receive from them?

The nurturing that older parents gave to their children in the past establishes a basis for deserving support in later life, and this is recognized as an important dimension of reciprocity. Past support, however, does not help meet the immediate needs of a family. The giving of dowries and inheritances when children marry also enters into the calculation of reciprocity, since these improve a child's standard of living. But on a daily basis, it is the older parent who continues to provide income to the household and help with child care or household chores who is perceived as an asset, instead of a burden. Over the next several decades, the ratio of elderly-to-young adults will increase rapidly. With this demographic change, it will be important to maintain and expand the productive roles played by the elderly in Sri Lanka.

ACKNOWLEDGMENTS

Amy Tsui was co-investigator on this project, and Victor de Silva organized and supervised the field work. Funding for this study was provided by the Carolina Population Center.

REFERENCES

Caldwell, J., et al. (1989). Sensitization to illness and the risk of death: An explanation for Sri Lanka's approach to good health for all. *Social Science Medicine, 28,* 365–379.

DeVos, S. (1989). The relationship between age and household type in Sri Lanka. Journal of Comparative *Family Studies, 20,* 291–307.

Martin, L. G. (1988). The aging of Asia. *Journal of Gerontology: Social Sciences, 43,* S93–113.

United Nations (1989). *Global estimates and projection of population by sex and age: The 1988 revision.* New York: United Nations.

11

Generational Relations and Their Changes as They Affect the Status of Older People in Japan

Kiyomi Morioka

INTRODUCTION

This chapter discusses the trend of postwar change in the pattern of living arrangements between parents and their married children in Japan. In those countries where the pattern of separate residence has been maintained for centuries, scholars have investigated such issues as frequency, chances for, or occasions of contact and mutual aid among close kin. In contrast, Japanese investigators have focused on the issue of changing living arrangements. Using previous research findings, I discuss the trends of change in both quantitative and qualitative terms and illuminate the Japanese side of generational relations in the later years of life.

Generational relations between aging parents and their children change through three successive phases: parents with child(ren) in the process of transition to adulthood, parents with married child(ren) in the early stage of family life cycle, and parents in the later years of life. In the first phase, parents assist their children. A survey conducted by the Economic Planning Agency of the Government of Japan in 1985, of married women in the Tokyo metropolitan area reveals that a great majority of the respondents regarded it as a parental responsibility to pay the major expenditures for their children's college education, and that more than half of them expected parents to pay some portion of expenditures (major or minor) related to the child's wedding ceremony, including a honeymoon tour and the purchase of furniture for a new household (Economic Planning Agency, 1986, p. 36).

In the second phase, too, parents assist the younger generation, particularly in the care of babies and young children of working mothers. Although statistical evidence on this issue is not available, child-care assistance is often reported by grandparents. Parents also provide sizeable financial assistance to the younger generation for the purchase of housing and other non-normative events. According to a survey by the Tokyo Metropolitan Institute of Gerontology in 1982, about one-third of old parents in the Tokyo area once gave funds for purchasing a housing lot or residence to their children who were residing separately (Okamura, 1984, p. 30).

In the third phase, the major direction of assistance usually is reversed. Presently, the elderly in Japan are greatly assisted by the social security system, including the public pension and the social welfare service (Morioka, 1986, p. 275). Still, many of them are supported in the households they maintain with coresident children (Honma, 1985, p. 62), and some of them are aided by a monthly allowance and/or occasional gifts from children living separately (Okamura, 1984, pp. 28–29). The affectional needs of aged parents in Tokyo may be satisfied to a greater or lesser extent by daily contact with coresident offspring or by the fairly frequent exchange of visits with children (Okamura, 1984, p. 28). Personal care to the sick widowed is provided mostly by coresident daughters-in-law (Takahashi, 1991, pp. 964–965).

Generational relations in the second and third phases thus vary significantly according to the living arrangements of parents and married children. Two patterns of living arrangements may be identified for elderly support in the third phase. One is the coresidence of aged parents and an adult child, married or unmarried. Even if the parents had two or more children, only one child remains in the parental household as the caretaker designated by the social norm governing living arrangements, or by choice and agreement among those concerned. The other is the separate residence of aged parents and married child(ren) living within a short distance of each other, as a result of choice and agreement or because of housing and occupational conveniences. A kin-family network formed among such parents and children functions as a support system for the elderly (Sussman & Burchinal, 1962). A parent may possibly be supported and taken care of by a child living far away, but residence of a child at such a great distance is a negligible model for elderly support. For this reason, coresidence or separate residence at a short distance as the dominant patterns of living arrangements between generations is proposed.

Historically, the Japanese have maintained the pattern of coresidence between parents and a married eldest son as the successor to household headship, and have kept, therefore, a stem family system known as *ie*.

This pattern has been characterized by parents' intensive contact with coresident offspring, on the one hand, and by estranged relations with married children living separately, on the other. After the end of World War II, however, the Japanese stem family system began to change drastically under the impact of postwar forces, including the conjugal family ideology as embodied in the Civil Code, revised in 1947, and the rapid economic growth in 1960s and 1970s. Accordingly, the pattern of living arrangements between the generations also has been altered.

THE JAPANESE STEM FAMILY SYSTEM

A stem family system prevailed in Japan up to the 1940s, with greater or minor variations by regions and social classes. Under this system, parents lived with one of their married children as heir, usually and preferably the eldest son, and formed one single household. To children other than the heir, two possible ways of completing the transition to adulthood were open: either establishing a new household as a branch (mainly for males), or entering an existing household by adoption (mainly for males) or by marriage (mainly for females). If both ways were closed, the child had to remain celibate in the parental household.

Around 1950, Toshimi Takeuchi, a well-noted Japanese rural sociologist, made a survey of household heads and their siblings (totaling 3,828) in 14 rural communities in terms of alternative patterns of completing the transition to adulthood (Takeuchi, 1969). His findings are summarized as follows (see Table 11.1).

For a decade following the end of World War II, the constituent unit of a rural community in Japan was still predominantly the household, founded by an earlier generation or newly founded by the present head. Every household, whether old or new, had a successor to the headship from among the head's children or else had to secure one by adoption.

Table 11.1. Distribution of Siblings of Household Head's Generation by Sex and by Patterns of Transition to Adulthood (%)

	Succession	New Branch	Adoption	Marriage	Unmarried*	Total (N)
Total	24.2	17.7	8.5	37.3	12.3	100 (3,828)
Male	41.4	30.6	15.1	0.0	12.9	100 (2,094)
Female	3.3	2.2	0.6	82.4	11.5	100 (1,734)

Source: Takeuchi, 1969, p. 14.
* Almost all of this category of population was expected to proceed to the categories of New Branch, Adoption or Marriage in due time. Only a few remained single in parental households for life.

The successor remained in the parental household with his wife and children, thus guaranteeing the persistence of the line of the household and family over generations. The alternative pattern of completing the transition to adulthood, as shown in Table 11.1, functioned within the framework of the stem family system and sustained it accordingly.

The stem family system in Japan differed from those in other Asian countries, such as Korea, and also from those in agricultural regions of western societies. It was unique in various features, such as succession and property transmission, adoption and marriage, retirement and elderly support. The most salient characteristics of the system in Japan appear in the emphasis placed on a linear continuation of family and household over generations, as manifested in the persistent preservation of the family name and ancestral rites. The above-mentioned differential intensity of intergenerational contact—that is, an intensive contact with coresident offspring combined with an estranged relation with the noncoresident children—is a behavioral manifestation of the cultural emphasis upon a lineal continuation of the family household from generation to generation.

The stem family system was maintained for centuries with material, legal, ideological, and situational backing. It was supported by the transmission of family property across generations, by a family enterprise based on the family property, by the Meiji Civil Code, by an ethical principle regulating generational relations (kō), and by an urgent demand for elderly support under the scarcely developed social security system.

The props of the stem family system have received a severe blow from the postwar reforms and developments in various sectors of Japanese society; consequently, the family system has been in decay. In contrast, the conjugal-family system has taken root firmly under the revised Civil Code, which was inspired by the conjugal-family ideology, and on the expanding chances of employment afforded by rapid economic growth. As a result of the interplay between the declining and rising family ideologies, a Japanese variant of the conjugal-family system has emerged with a characteristic of mother-centeredness rather than couple-centeredness.

The actual household form under the stem family system includes not only a stem family, but also, quite often, a nuclear family as was demonstrated by a study of the family life cycle (Morioka, 1973, p. 59). Demographic variables being equal, it is assumed that the ratio of stem family households or instances of generational coresidence would have been decreasing as a consequence of the decline of the stem family system and the concomitant appearance of the conjugal family system. In the following section, this quantitative aspect of the changing living arrangement between generations is reviewed, examining first ratios of people living with their married children and then those of married people living with their parent.

DECLINING RATIOS OF THE CORESIDENCE
OF PARENTS AND MARRIED CHILDREN

Ratios of Old People Living with
Their Married Children

According to the available data on the population of 65 years or older, the ratio of old people living with children, married as well as unmarried, was as high as about 80% in the 1960s, fell to the level of 70–79% in 1970s, to 69% in 1980, and to 60% in 1990 (Ministry of Health and Welfare, 1991b, p. 123). A decreasing trend is evident.

Table 11.2 shows the changes in living arrangements of the aged in the latest decade. Coresidence with married children has remained the dominant pattern for Japanese old people, but the ratio has decreased noticeably from 53 to 42%. However, a great increase of ratios has occurred for the aged forming old-couple-only households and one-person households, and a slight one for those coresiding with unmarried children. Old-couple-only households, which rank the second largest in ratio, will become one-person households through the death of a spouse, or coresidence with a married child by joining with his or her nuclear family. Coresidence with unmarried children (which ranks third) is likely to be transformed into coresidence with married children by the marriage of a coresident child, or into an old-couple-only household by the departure of all children.

A Japanese demographer, Kiyoshi Hiroshima, identified the factors

Table 11.2. Shifting Ratios of Those Age 65 or Older by Household Forms* (%)

Year	(1)	(2)	(3)	(4)	(5)	(6)	Total (N)**
1980	8.5	19.6	52.5	16.5	2.8	0.2	100 (10,729)
1985	9.3	23.0	47.9	16.7	2.8	0.2	100 (12,111)
1990	11.2	25.7	41.9	17.8	3.3	0.2	100 (14,453)

Source: Ministry of Health and Welfare, 1991b, p. 123.
* Household forms: (1) One-person household; (2) Household of old couple only; (3) Coresidence with married children; (4) Coresidence with unmarried children; (5) Coresidence with kin other than children; (6) Coresidence with nonkin.
** Thousands

responsible for the decreasing ratio of coresidence with married children. He found two factors: first, an increase in the proportion of married population among the aged (e.g., from 72% in 1975 to 80% in 1985 for men of 75–79 years old, and from 20 to 27% during the same period for women of the same age), and second a decrease of coresidence actualization rate (nearly 90% in 1970, 70% in 1980, and 65% in 1985). With regard to the first, he presented statistical evidence to show that the coresidence ratio of the married elderly is lower than those of the widowed and the divorced. Obviously, then, an increase in the married population ratio has contributed doubly to the recent shift of household forms—that is, to the increase in ratios of old-couple-only households, and to the concurrent decrease in ratios of coresidence with married children. Hiroshima found that the decrease in the coresidence actualization rate would reflect the changing attitude toward coresidence from a positive one to one less positive, and that it would have contributed to the recent decrease in ratio much more than the increase in proportion of the married population of the aged (1991).

Ratios of Married People Living with Their Parents

Under the stem family system, the ratio of coresidence seen from the perspective of a parent and that from a married child should coincide, if every parent had only one married child available for coresidence. On the average, however, each parent has more than one child. Consequently, the ratio seen from the child's perspective is assumed to be smaller than that from the parent's.

The following evidence partially supports the above statement. A survey conducted by the Prime Minister's Office in 1974 revealed that 55% of the respondents between 60 and 74 years old lived together with their married children, whereas only 38% of married men between 30 and 49 years old lived with their parents (Prime Minister's Office, 1975). There is a significant discrepancy in the ratios between the two samples.

Since such data on coresidence as comparable with that in Table 11.2 is not available, I refer as a substitute to the ratio of coresidence with parents directly after marriage, provided by the Fertility Rates Survey of the Institute of Population Problems, Ministry of Health and Welfare. The survey was conducted at five-year intervals in 1977, 1982, and 1987; a portion of this data is summarized by Hiroshima (1991). The ratio was as high as 60% for the around 1945 marriage cohort. In contrast, it has been about 30% for the 1965–1985 cohorts, a decrease from around 1945 to 1965, and also stagnation since 1965 up to the recent date are revealed here. The decreasing trend is as anticipated. How then can we explain the stagnation following the decrease? Hiroshima attempted to interpret it by referring to the countervailing effect of increasing coresidence feasibility rates and decreasing coresidence actualization rates (Hiroshima, 1991).

Under the Japanese stem family system, it was the rule for an eldest son, rather than a younger son or a daughter, to stay in the parental household. So what change has taken place in the normative, or at least preferred pattern in the context of a general decrease of coresidence ratio? Let us compare first the eldest son with other sons, and then sons with daughters in terms of coresidence with parents.

According to the Fertility Rates Survey, the coresidence ratio was 61% for the eldest son, nearly twice as large as the ratio for other sons (33%) in the 1955–59 marriage cohort. Both ratios for the two categories of sons decrease more in the later marriage cohorts, in the way the differences between the two become the smallest in the latest 1985–87 marriage cohort (35 vs. 23%). The preferential pattern for an eldest son has considerably been neutralized.

The gender preferential pattern concerns the rule of residence. The stem family system in Japan was predominantly viri-local in this regard. An uxori-local arrangement, except for families with women-centered businesses, was approved only when the parent had no sons, only daughters. By dividing coresident parents into husband's side and wife's side, we shall be able to discover to what extent the rule has been kept or neutralized.

Relying on the data derived from the Fertility Rates Survey again (see Hiroshima, 1991), and according to this data, the ratio of coresidence with husband's parents was 43% and that with wife's parents only 6% in the 1957–61 marriage cohort. The former decreases markedly in the younger cohorts, while the latter does so only slightly. As a result, the difference between the two has become smaller. A viri-local tendency is still manifest, but not so dominant as before.

Using a recent opinion survey administered to unmarried people of 18–34 years old, Hiroshima estimated that the ratio of married people living with their parents will decrease further, and that it will fall below 20% around the end of the present century (Hiroshima, 1991). We may conclude that the coresidence ratios for parents and for married children have decreased to a great extent in the past few decades. Concomitantly, the preferred coresidence pattern in terms of gender and birth order has faded away considerably.

WHY IS THE CORESIDENCE PATTERN MAINTAINED?

Japanese social scientists are impressed by the sharp decrease of generational coresidence ratios from 53 to 42% in the latest decade. By contrast, however, western scholars may regard 42% as a high coresidence ratio and ask why the pattern of coresidence with a married child is maintained. This question is addressed in the present section.

A generational coresidence rather than a separate residence was the arrangement convenient for children to perform their sacred obligations to keep family names respectable and to maintain continuity in ancestral rites. This was particularly true of upper-class families. For ordinary people who had neither famous family name nor a large property, generational coresidence was instrumentally functional or requisite in order to carry out a family enterprise and transmit it and the family fortunes to the succeeding generation. It was also the most efficient way of caring for the elderly with the limited resources available to them.

Regarding the aforementioned, two things should be apparent. One is a drastic decrease in the ratio of self-employed workers and family hands among all gainfully engaged workers, from 61% in 1950 to 25% in 1985. A large majority of contemporary family hands may be wives of the principal workers, not their adult children. If this is the case, only a very small portion of the population would have a family enterprise to transmit to the next generation.

The second is the postwar decay of the ethical principle regulating the relation with one's parents, known as filial piety or kō. In the prewar period, filial piety was internalized by young people fully through informal teaching at home and formal indoctrination in elementary schools. The ethics of filial piety told them to be dutiful to their parents and to be devoted to them, particularly in their very old age. It was a moral and ideological prop of the stem family system, and it also helped mitigate intergenerational conflict that may be caused or intensified by coresidence.

After the end of World War II, filial piety ceased to be taught or even discussed at home and in schools. The postwar school education of Japan stressed the ethics of modern citizenship, and left the traditional kinship ethics to the private sector. Nevertheless, parents of young children, having lost self-confidence due to changes in the value system after the defeat in 1945, rarely stressed to children the importance of filial piety. Thus the term kō, a cardinal virtue for the prewar Japanese, is now an obsolete word. Even college students are not necessarily familiar with the word, and only a few among them know its correct meaning.

In addition, postwar legal reform from the imposition of elderly support exclusively on an eldest son to a shared responsibility among children relieved the eldest son of the duty to live together with his parents. Nevertheless it failed to make other children realize their responsibility, and thus made the status of old people unstable in terms of the support to be extended by their children.

Why is the coresidence maintained, despite an extensive disruption of family enterprises to be transmitted over generations, the virtual decay of the *kō* morality, and the weakened sense of responsibility to support aged parents? Coresidence is the most effective way of coping with the task of elderly support with limited resources available, but people will not coreside with their aged parents if the sense of filial responsibility is faint.

Kikuko Kato (1988) tried to explain why a stem family comprised of two married couples comes into existence without the inheritance of family fortunes and/or the transmission of a family enterprise. Analyzing the data collected from 184 households in Sapporo in 1982–83, she reports that generational coresidence is an effective means to overcome successfully a set of real or anticipated crises that occur in family development, and that it is especially effective in the early and the later stages of life cycle. She points out the four conditions conducive to the formation of a generational coresidence as follows:

1. One couple or both are in a critical situation where it is difficult for them to perform developmental tasks or to proceed from one stage to the next, due to a shortage of manpower and/or material resources.
2. At least one couple possesses the resources necessary to assist its counterpart, the older one or the younger.
3. At least one couple has the flexibility necessary to modify the lifestyle established prior to coresidence. (Any couple tends to have a greater flexibility in the transition from one stage to the next.)
4. Both couples have a concept of "family" favorable for generational coresidence, and are connected with each other by an affectional tie.

According to Kato (1988), the coresidence of parents and a married child will dissolve if they fail to draw any positive benefit from coresidence. She summarizes the four conditions that tend to result in split and make the coresidence temporary, as follows:

1. When the task is performed or the critical transition accomplished. (In other words, no further benefit is expected from the coresidence.)

2. When the capacity for assistance has declined (e.g., due to a growing demand for space beyond the housing capacity.)
3. When an adjustment of life-style is difficult (e.g., due to a transference of the coresident child to a job at a distance.)
4. When a generational conflict or tension occurs.

Obviously, these four correspond precisely to the four conditions itemized previously. In addition, Kato significantly notes that the prerequisites for keeping a coresidence functioning satisfactorily include a positive stance for generational cooperation to secure financial, service, and affectional benefits, as well as some devices to avoid generational conflicts. As practical recommendations, she stresses an early beginning of coresidence, (e.g., marriage of the child concerned) and a partial separation of activity space between generations to avoid possible conflict (Kato, 1988).

Kato's research findings suggest that present-day long-term coresidence is made possible only when both parties, not just parents draw some vital benefits from the arrangement, including material assistance, instrumental services, personal care, and affectional gratification; and when emotional disharmony between generations, if any happens, can be dissolved, averted, or kept latent by a reasonable adjustment accomplished early in coresidence, or when an excessive daily contact that tends to produce tension between in-laws is avoided by separation of activity space.

Kato (1988) proposes to call the emerging variation of stem family "modified stem family." I should like to define it vis-à-vis the concept of a "classical stem family," adapted from Eugene Litwak's terminology (Litwak, 1960). In this chapter the stem family system as a cultural pattern or program for family building is discussed. In contrast, a stem family is an actual household form comprised of one couple in each succeeding generation connected by the father-son (or daughter) tie. (Under the stem family system, as already mentioned, other household forms may appear—a nuclear family very often, or even a joint family, though only rarely.) What was hitherto meant by stem family is a classical stem family.

Ideally, a classical stem family represents one single household with a lifelong coresidence of parents and a normatively designated married child, and without any meaningful separation between generations except a bedroom allocated to each couple. By contrast, a modified stem family is a voluntary alliance, temporary in nature, of two nuclear families in successive generations, making one composite household with a partial but vital separation between generations. The family that appeared under the stem family system is a classical stem family, while a modified stem family exists only under the conjugal-family system, which is the alternative pattern for contemporary Japanese. By definition, an impressive advent of modified stem families today signals the growing prevalence of the conjugal-family system rather than a persistence of the stem family system in Japan.

As to the benefits of the coresidence under the stem family system, only support for the elderly have been examined up to now. But Kato's findings reveal the benefits that a younger couple should have received in the form of child care, inheritance, and succession. These benefits may be small, however, compared with the tremendous sacrifices demanded of a daughter-in-law, the heir's wife.

Why was a lifelong coresidence possible without any separation of activity space between generations? Some reasons have already been suggested, and additional reasons will be addressed here. One is that the privacy was not cultivated, and remained in a primitive state. Privacy was virtually neglected, while great importance was attached to the communal life of a household. The other reason is that a young girl was socialized to perform the submissive role in the household she would join as a daughter-in-law.

Today, privacy is highly appreciated, and self-actualization is regarded as the goal, particularly by women who were in the past most inconvenienced by the neglect of privacy and who were forced to perform the "virtue" of self-sacrifice. The model of coresidence for the benefit of both parties and with a generational separation of activity space has been created through a prolonged process of adjustment and negotiation between the old demands and the new aspirations.

The present status of an activity-space separation within households, is summarized by Naoi (1984) based on a survey conducted by the Tokyo Metropolitan Institute of Gerontology in 1982, which studied three generations of women. The activity space may be divided into four areas: house equipment such as entrance, kitchen, bathroom, and toilet; a living room allocated at least to one couple for their exclusive use; budget, and instrumental services such as preparation of supper, washing of clothes, and shopping. The findings are as follows:

1. The ratio of the households with house equipment for separate use by each couple is 3% for an entrance, 6% for a kitchen, 2% for a bathroom, and 15% for a toilet. (A bathroom is separated from a toilet in an ordinary Japanese house.)
2. The ratio of the households that divide the payment of expenditures between two couples is 4% for food, 3% for dwelling, and 2% for light and heat.
3. The ratio of the households where instrumental services are car-

ried out separately by parents and the child's family is 11% for preparation of supper, 52% for washing of clothes, and 31% for shopping. (Naoi, 1984, pp. 35–38)

Michiko Naoi's (1984) report on sharing and separation did not adopt the second item as one of indexes to measure the degree of separation. But it is in this item that we can find the most widespread separation of activity space. The reservation of a living room for the exclusive use of old parents is not a modern invention, but was part of retirement in some regions, or among wealthy families in prewar Japan.

A survey conducted by the Prime Minister's office in 1974 reveals that almost all aged people living with married children have a room for their exclusive use (Prime Minister's Office, 1975, pp. 52,56). As the housing conditions of the Japanese have improved significantly in space as well as quality since the time of the survey, one room at least for the exclusive use of aged parents is an established pattern for coresidence today. Obviously, the relative size of living space for exclusive use varies according to the power relation with the younger generation, particularly the locus of house ownership. Nonetheless, a room used exclusively by one couple is the most visible evidence of activity-space separation and may be regarded as the almost universal basis of separation in other areas.

As discussed earlier, the coresidence ratio has declined drastically. The content or quality of coresidence has also changed considerably during the same period, as shown in the growing tendency for coresidence *not* to be limited to a male child and the eldest son, in the greater importance placed on choice and preference of those concerned, rather than on the traditional norms, and in the wider acceptance of activity-space separation between generations. It may not be an oversimplification to summarize the trend in coresidence as a movement from the norm-bound to the situation-bound.

SEPARATE RESIDENCE AND KIN FAMILY NETWORK

Needless to say, the decline of coresidence ratios is accompanied by the increase of separate residence ratios. In this section, the extent to which old people and their children live close to each other in both distance and frequency of contact is examined, and whether a kin-family network has emerged with aged parents as a focal point of contact.

Table 11.3, based on the 1986 and 1989 Basic Surveys of National Life

Table 11.3. Ratios of Elderly Age 65 Years or Older by Age Grades and by Distance to Nearest Children

Year	Age	Total (N)* %	(CR)	(S1)	(S2)	(S3)	(S4)	(NO)
1986	65–74	100 (7,851)	59.0	3.5	6.3	8.4	12.8	10.0
	75+	100 (4,775)	73.0	3.2	4.4	5.4	7.3	6.7
	Total	100 (12,626)	64.3	3.4	5.6	7.3	10.7	8.7
1989	65–74	100 (8,711)	54.5	3.8	7.6	9.5	15.0	9.6
	75+	100 (5,527)	68.5	3.9	5.7	6.7	8.8	6.4
	Total	100 (14,239)	60.0	3.8	6.8	8.4	12.6	8.4

Source: Ministry of Health and Welfare, 1987, pp. 132–133; 1991a, pp. 162–163.
* Thousands
Code: Distance to nearest children: (S1) On the same housing log; (S2) In the same neighborhood; (S3) In the same municipality; (S4) In other municipalities; (CR) Coresidence; (NO) No children and unknown.

by the Ministry of Health and Welfare (1987, 1991a) discloses a recent picture of old people in terms of the distance to children living closest to them. If all children are taken into account, the total picture of their spatial distribution will be more dispersed than that shown there.

According to Table 11.3, around 30% of old people live separately from children (S1+2+3+4), and the ratio tends to increase, as indicated earlier. The distance between parents and children is divided into four degrees from the nearest to the farthest: living on the same housing site (S1), in the same neighborhood (S2), in the same municipality (S3), and in other municipalities (S4). The distance of the first and the second degrees is close enough to allow daily contact. Assuming that frequent contact would be possible also in the third degree, I added up the three as the ratios of adjoining residence, and obtained 16% for 1986 and 19% for 1989. The ratio is definitely small if compared with that of coresidence, and we cannot argue that it is growing unproportionately to the total increase of separate residence, from 27 to 32%.

The old people are divided into two age grades, namely, young old (65–74 years) and very old (75 and over). Table 11.3 demonstrates a greater concentration existing in the coresidence ratio of the older age stratum for the two survey years. If this reflects an age effect rather than a cohort effect, it may signal the coresidence formed in the later years of life because of parents deteriorating health. This type of coresidence represents a compromise of the traditional pattern of the elderly support and the newly established pattern of a generational separation of residence.

Another age variation is significant. Among the old people living separately, the ratio of adjoining residence (S1+2+3) varies as age advances, from 58 to 65% for the 1989 sample. This is particularly true for those living on the same housing site (S1), as is shown in the variation from 11 to 16% for the same survey year. The tendency toward a closer residence may indicate an emergence of a separate residence at a short distance as an alternate, or as a minor pattern to complement the major one.

The National Survey of Old People conducted by the Ministry of Health and Welfare in 1984 (Ministry of Health and Welfare, 1985) provides us with two sorts of information about intergenerational contact. One concerns the time required for a person age 65 or older who lives separately to visit the child with whom the parent has the most frequent contact. It is less than 10 minutes for 30% of them, 10 minutes or more but less than half an hour for 20%, 30 minutes or more but less than one hour for 15%, and one hour or more for the remaining 35%. One out of two old persons living separately has at least one child within a 30-minute distance.

The other concerns the frequency of visits to and from the child with whom the parent has the most frequent contact. The ratios of old people by the degree of frequency are as follows: 26% for those with daily visits, 12% with two or three visits a week, 25% with several visits a month, 16% with one or two visits per three months, 11% with one visit or so per six months, 7% with one visit or so per year, and the remaining 3% without any visit during the preceding year. The ratio of the old people who have visits with the closest child several times or more a month is as high as just over 60%.

In conclusion, the findings of the two recent surveys by the Ministry of Health and Welfare (1989, 1991a) suggest that about half of the old people living separately from children keep fairly frequent contact with them, at least with the one living most closely. The major pattern of generational relations remains one of intensive contact between the elderly and one coresident child's family, though with some separation in space and time. Alongside of this, a new pattern has been emerging for the aged in frequent contact with children living closely, as is evident among old people without any coresident child.

Although the data available to us is not sufficient to confirm the emergence of a kin-family network as a new kinship pattern, it seems almost certain that some new pattern has been or is being formed. More data is required to disclose whether the new pattern is something like a kin-family network involving all children, with parents as the center of an alliance of aged parents with one married child living closely.

With regard to the gender of married children with whom parents tend to keep a frequent contact, one recent report on the Sapporo study in 1982 supposes the dominant status of daughters as a result of forces at work between generations (Mitani & Seiyama, 1985). Conversely, another recent report on the Osaka study in 1976–77 suggests that sons are dominant, and proposes the concept of "modified *ie*-like family" to denote a network of families connected by a patrilineal tie (Mitsuyoshi, 1986). Probably each of these contradictory research findings reflects the mixed reality in transition, focusing on either the more modernized aspect or the more traditional one. Further research is needed in order to establish the major trend in this regard.

CONCLUDING REMARKS: WHO TAKES ON THE TERMINAL CARE OF OLD PEOPLE?

In the previous sections, generational relations and their changes in terms of the living arrangements, which regulate the manner and the extent of contact and assistance between the generations were discussed. In the final section, terminal care of aged parents, assuming that some vital aspect of the generational relation would be manifested in the kinship status of the caretaker of dying parents, will be addressed.

The Survey of Old People Who Died Natural Death in August 1979 by the Ministry of Health and Welfare, (1981) supplies data concerning the principal caretakers prior to the death of those age 70 or older, as shown on Table 11.4. The materials were gathered from three prefectures representing different degrees of urbanization, but tabulated there as a whole. The relative distribution by household forms indicates an overwhelming concentration in the coresidence with a married child (74.7%), followed by the far smaller ratio (9.3%) of the old-couple-only household, the remaining three being almost negligible.

The form of household where terminal care is mostly provided by the adult members at home includes coresidence with a married child, old-couple-only, and coresidence with unmarried children. In more than 50% of the remaining two forms, the care is supplied by nonkin helpers—public, voluntary, or privately employed.

Among the first three forms, spouses are most commonly the principal caretaker in the old-couple-only households; spouses and coresident offspring are dominant in households with unmarried children; and daughters-in-law are dominant in those with married children. The ratio of the cases where offspring live separately or their spouses are recognized as a principal caretaker is quite small. This is especially true with the married-child coresident households (3.3%).

Among the remaining cases where the greatest assistance is provided by nonkin helpers, the "other" households are characterized by help from relatives other than offspring and their spouses (18.7%). One-

Table 11.4.   Ratios of Elderly Age 70 or over by Household Forms* and by Status of Principal Personal Caretaker, 1979

	(1)	(2)	(3)	(4)	(5)	Total
Spouse	—	78.1	19.8	31.2	3.6	24.1
Coresident offspring	—	—	18.7	43.7	6.5	16.9
Spouse of coresident children	—	—	45.9	—	3.6	34.7
Offspring living separately	24.7	7.3	2.8	4.7	6.5	4.4
Spouse of offspring living separately	7.1	4.4	0.5	3.9	3.6	1.5
Other relatives	7.1	2.4	1.9	0.8	18.7	3.1
Non-kin helpers employed or voluntary	51.7	6.3	4.3	10.2	54.6	9.8
No caretaker	9.4	1.5	6.1	5.5	2.9	5.5
Total (*N*)(i.e., elderly who died a natural death in Iwate, Osaka & Sage Prefectures in August, 1979)	3.9% (85)	9.3% (205)	74.7% (1,648)	5.8% (128)	6.3% (139)	100% (2,20 5)

Source: Ministry of Health and Welfare, 1981, p. 72.
* Household forms: (1) One-person household; (2) Household of old couple only; (3) Coresidence with married children; (4) Coresidence with unmarried children; (5) Others.

person households receive assistance from nonresident offspring or their spouses (31.8% in total), though a much smaller amount than anticipated.

On the whole, terminal care is provided mostly by coresident adult (female) family members. When domestic resources are scarce, care is provided from outside, particularly by nonkin helpers. The offspring living separately take the role of principal caretaker only in a critical situation where service is not available within the household. These providers are underrepresented in Table 11.4, possibly for two reasons: Because the data concerns the principal caretaker only, neglecting the role of assistant caretaker which noncoresident offspring may perform frequently; and because they tend to evade filial responsibility, perhaps as an aftereffect of the former asyametric relations—the estranged relation to noncoresident children in favor of intensive contact with the coresident child's family.

The model of living separately but closely, as an alternative pattern of the elderly support, is still in an extremely primitive stage of development and does not function well as a terminal care system. In contrast, generational coresidence, especially with a married child, is well suited for the task. But coresidence with a married child has tension built in, which may become manifest under the demanding task of prolonged care. The ratio of "no caretaker" is small but comparatively large for this household form, suggesting an abandonment of dying parents in spite of the relatively rich manpower resources. This may reflect domestic conflict deriving partly from in-law relations.

Finally, the social security policy and social welfare services are important not only as a substitute for the kin support system for the isolated old people. They also serve as an effective buffer to keep generational coresidence functioning positively by relieving it from the crushing task of prolonged care for aged parents who are ill.

REFERENCES

Economic Planning Agency. (1986). *Life plan for the Mass-Longevity Society.* Tokyo: Printing Bureau, Ministry of Finance.*

Hiroshima, K. (1991). A demographic analysis of the recent trend in the parent-children coresidence. *Journal of Population Problems, 200,* 50–66.*

Honma, S. (1985). Standard of living of the aged living with their children. *Social Gerontology, 22,* 42–62.*

Kato, K. (1988). A family developmental approach to the Japanese three-generation family. *Japanese Sociological Review, 155,* 56–70.*

Litwak, E. (1960). Occupational mobility and extended family cohesion. *American Sociological Review, 25,* 9–21.

Ministry of Health and Welfare. (1981). *The 1979 socio-economic study of demographic movement (death to old people).* Tokyo: Ministry of Health and Welfare.*

Ministry of Health and Welfare. (1985). *A summary report on the 1984 national survey of old people.* Tokyo: Ministry of Health and Welfare.*

Ministry of Health and Welfare. (1987). *The report on the 1986 basic survey of national life.* Tokyo: Ministry of Health and Welfare.*

Ministry of Health and Welfare. (1991a). *The report on the 1989 basic survey of national life.* Tokyo: Ministry of Health and Welfare.*

Ministry of Health and Welfare. (1991b). *The report on the 1990 basic survey of national life.* Tokyo: Ministry of Health and Welfare.*

Mitani, T., & Seiyama, K. (1985). "Asymmetry in the intergenerational relations of urban families." *Japanese Sociological Review, 143,* 51–65.*

Mitsuyoshi, T. (1986). "Changing structure of ie in the family of parents and children living independently." *Sociological Review of Kobe University, 3,* 36–55.*

Morioka, K. (1973). *A study of the family life cycle.* Tokyo: Baifukan.*

———. (1986). Changes in household forms and life style of the old people in Kakegawa City, 1973–84. *Quarterly of Social Security Research, 22,* 260–279.*

Naoi, M. (1984). Possible variables in a scale on nuclear unit independence. *Social Gerontology, 19,* 32–57.*

* denotes an English translation of the original Japanese title.

Okamura, K. (1984). Reciprocities between elderly mothers and their middle-aged daughters in separated household. *Social Gerontology, 19*, 18–31.*

Prime Minister's Office. (1975). *A Survey on elderly support*. Tokyo: Prime Minister's Office.*

Sussman, M. B., & Burchinal, L. (1962). Kin-family network: Unheralded structure in current conceptualizations of family functioning. *Marriage and Family Living, 24*, 231–240.

Takahashi, H. (1991). Aging and dying in the family. *Japanese Journal of Geriatric Psychiatry, 2*, 961–971.*

Takeuchi, T. (1969). *The family folkways and the Japanese family system*. Tokyo: Kouseisha-Kouseikaku.*

* denotes an English translation of the original Japanese title.

III

EPILOGUE

12

Generational Relations
A Future Perspective

Matilda White Riley and John W. Riley, Jr.

Just prior to the Delaware Conference on "Aging and Generational Relationships: A Historical and Cross-Cultural Perspective," we had returned from an international conference in Moscow (immediately following the coup against Gorbachev). In Moscow, we had been struck anew by the extraordinary challenge and the responsibility confronting scholars today. In this world fraught with revolution, crisis, and change, social scientists are literally living in a laboratory for studying social and cultural change. Clearly, it behooves us to integrate our studies of the past with worldwide contemporary studies, and to use this knowledge to anticipate the future and to help guide practical decisions as we look toward that future.

The Moscow conference was at the global level and focused on specific issues of medical demography. Beneath these specifics, however, lay cataclysmic questions about the generational impact of political and economic convulsions that are exposing the oncoming cohorts of young people to life styles undreamed of by their parents. The Delaware Conference was on the human, rather than the global, level. It focused directly on examination of personal relationships across generations. Throughout the world the numbers of older people are mounting.

That is yesterday's news. Yet, for tomorrow, there is deep current concern that changes in the very nature and meaning of the family portend loss of social support for the oldest generation.

HISTORICAL AND FUTURE PERSPECTIVES

Thus, for the present volume, the central questions are: How will adults relate to their elderly parents? Will there be harmony or cleavage between them? Will new norms of intergenerational commitment and responsibility emerge? Neither the present volume nor any other is likely to provide clear answers to such questions. However, these chapters offer many new insights into the cultural and historical forces that continue to shape intergenerational relations. Taken together, these chapters clearly aim toward two intellectual objectives we emphasized at the Delaware Conference:

- First, to identify principles for understanding how social change and cultural diversity influence generational relations in later life—either to strengthen or to weaken them.
- Second, to develop practical and policy-relevant conceptual and methodological implications for the future.

It is our hope that this brief epilogue will encourage readers of this volume to hold in mind this broad approach. More particularly, we want to extend the cultural and historical perspective to speak to the future perspective. Toward this end, we venture a radical proposition as to what the future of intergenerational relations might be. As a thought experiment for examining this proposition, we suggest three "ideal types" of kinship structure—no matter how radical their implications may be.

Our proposition for the future (for the sake of stimulating thought) is this: As traditional family forms break down, they will be replaced by new forms of kinship bonds—often transcending the household or the nuclear or extended family. There will be fewer ascribed and obligatory relationships, but more potential relationships for older people to choose from as needs arise.

IDEAL TYPES OF KINSHIP

In thinking about such an altered kinship structure in a possible future, we have elsewhere outlined one "ideal type" that we call a "latent matrix of kin relationships" (see Riley,1988; Riley & Riley, 1993). These relationships are no longer constrained by generation or age: That is, people of *any* age, within and across generations, may opt to support, love, or confide in one another. Then we contrast this latent matrix with two other idealized types of kinship structure: the "simple" and the "expanded."

We hold no brief for such a typology, save as a heuristic device. We have developed it while analyzing the accumulating body of family stud-

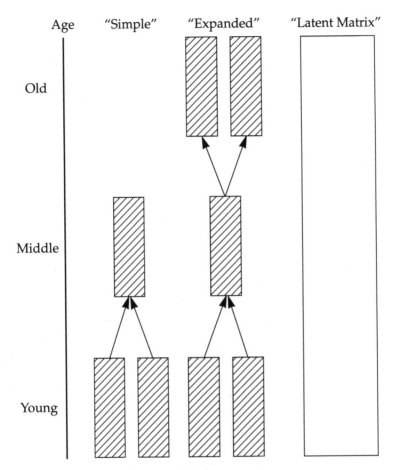

Figure 12.1. "Ideal types" of kin structures.

ies, many of them written by contributors to this volume. As "ideal types," they are, in Max Weber's sense, artificially simplistic; they may never exist (or have existed) in reality, but are an idealized selection from it. Yet (keeping in mind the truism that history is by no means unidirectional) we think of each type's key elements as either reflective of the reality of the past or prophetic of real directions for the future.

The primary distinguishing element among the three types lies in their generational structure. The "simple" type is composed of two generations of adults; the far more complex "expanded" type contains three generations of adults; and the "latent matrix" is so complex that the lines demarcating generations have become blurred—often completely indiscernible.

For each type of generational structure, we ask two questions: What are the predominant *bases* for personal relationships across generations (such as material resources, power, or influence)? And how do *social and cultural conditions* influence these structures and relationships?

"SIMPLE" TYPES OF KINSHIP

This volume contains several realistic approximations of the "simple," two-generational type. In this type, the offspring of the "oldest" generation are young adults (some with little children of their own). But, by contemporary standards, the "oldest" generation is not very old. There are exceptions, of course, but on average, the wife has died by the time the youngest child has left home.

As just one example, Stanley Brandes (in his earlier studies of Spain and Portugal before World War II, as described in Brandes, 1989) defines a simple structure of independent households: that of the parents and that of each adult offspring. He shows the elaborate procedures by which care of the aged parents was intertwined with the transmission of property. Ideally, these relationships involved the exchange of the parents' material goods for filial companionship and support in old age. Actually, however, the exchange all too often resulted in abuses of power by the older generation. And such relationships were unconstrained by the political or cultural forces of that time and place.

"EXPANDED" TYPES OF KINSHIP

Quite different studies (like some reported in this volume) reflect elements of the expanded, three-generational type of kinship structure. Consider what that added generation means for parent-offspring relationships! As one seminal example, Tamara Hareven's well-known earlier studies of the more recent cohort from the New Hampshire mill town dramatize these changes (Hareven & Adams, 1989; see also Hareven, 1982). Here the "oldest" generation are the parents of those late middle-aged people who were the "oldest" in the simple structure. As more members of each generation live to become old, increasing numbers of middle-aged couples have two or more elderly parents still alive (as demonstrated early by Uhlenberg, 1980). The adult offspring have had a long period of living independently of their children (in the so-called "empty nest" stage), while their elderly parents are growing old—a phenomenon that relates to some of the changes in coresidence discussed in this volume. And the very meaning of generational relationships has been altered, as parents and their offspring typically survive jointly for so many years that a mother and her daughter are only briefly in the traditional relationship of parent-and-*little*-child. During the several remaining decades of their lives, they become status equals. The power imbalance between them is redressed. Even when offspring are separated from one parent through divorce, their joint survival means that the two can still call upon one another if the need arises. Unlike the husband-wife link, the parent-offspring link cannot be destroyed by divorce.

Such expanded structures stem, of course, from the enormous increases in longevity during the twentieth century. Here there are *no* historical parallels: For the first time in all history, most people now live to be old. Moreover, coincident with increasing longevity, generational relations are also influenced by related transformations in fertility, the economy, education, standard of living, and the rise of the nation state. Much intergenerational dependency has been eliminated through public funds and private pensions, although families remain the major caregivers for that critical minority (but they are only a minority) of the very old who become disabled.

"LATENT MATRIX"

Turning now to the "latent matrix of kin relationships," which, for the purposes of our thought experiment, we postulate for the future, we foresee a new type of structure that has lost the sharp boundaries set by generation, age, or geography. Instead, the boundaries of the kin network have widened to encompass many diverse relationships, including several degrees of step-kin and in-laws, and also adopted and other surrogate "relatives" chosen from *outside* the family. We describe this type as a latent web of continually shifting linkages that provide the potential for activating and intensifying close kin relationships as they are needed.

TRACES OF THE LATENT MATRIX

Lest this ideal type seem purely fanciful, consider a few traces that (here we speak of the United States) are beginning to emerge in actuality:

Cohabitation

Among unmarried couples, cohabitation is becoming institutionalized in the cohorts of young people who will be old in the future. Nearly half of young people today have cohabited, a trend that may produce new forms of generational relationships (Bumpass & Sweet, 1989).

Surrogate Kin

In many guises, surrogates are taking the place of true kin relationships. For example:

- Children are increasingly being adopted (including adoption by homosexual couples), as in other times children often were adopted as heirs.
- Older people are sometimes adopted as foster parents.
- Close kin-like relations often develop with sympathetic aides in nursing homes or other formal care institutions.
- "Fictive" kin, including godparents and other nonrelatives, assume real obligations. Such fictive kin, traditional in racial and ethnic minorities, become increasingly significant with the rising numbers of minorities in the United States population.

(Of course, many of these elements also appear at other times and in other places, but their relative salience is renewed in the United States as traditional family bonds loosen.)

New Biosocial Relationships

Given the possible biosocial technologies of the future, the latent matrix may contain still unimagined relational structures. Even now it is possible for an offspring to have biological linkages to *two* mothers: one who donates the egg and a second who bears the child!

One personal example will illustrate this latent matrix. (The names here, but not the facts, are fictitious.) Our granddaughter, Susan (a Harvard alumna), cohabits with Ted (an astrophysicist at Harvard). They are not married, but they have a baby (our first great-grandson). Ted has been twice divorced, and has a daughter nearly as old as Susan. Susan has close bonds to this daughter and to both ex-wives, and often travels from Massachusetts to Texas to visit them. The question is: How is Susan related to all these "ex's"? There are no words in the English language for such relationships! Even more intriguing: Suppose one of us were suddenly stranded alone in Texas and needed a supportive relationship. It is not unimaginable that Susan's grandparent might seek out one of Ted's ex-wives for help—indeed, might eventually develop a close relationship to her. And what would that relationship be called? This may sound humorous, but it is nonetheless real. Again, there are no names, no concepts, for such linkages.

This example shows why we speak of the matrix as "latent" and volitional rather than obligatory. Many of the relationships remain latent, unless they are called upon. They form a safety net of significant connections to choose from in case of need. If a close relative is not available, a substitute often stands ready in the wings.

PORTENTS OF THE FUTURE

How nearly the generational relations of the future—in the United States and elsewhere—may, in reality, approximate this latent matrix will depend on many changes: changes in the economy and the polity of the diverse countries around the world, changes in the course of peace or war, and, above all, changes in culture and values. Will the oncoming cohorts of young people, as they grow old, sustain the recent focus on self and on material goods? Or will they instead develop norms of commitment to personal relationships and to a "good society"?

Such speculations bring us back to the central question with which we began: What will the future relationship be between older parents and their adult offspring? There are many dismal forebodings—about single-parent families, families separated by divorce, cohorts of people now old who (as in countries torn by World War II) are literally without *any* relatives. Yet we glimpse five potentially positive changes that, at least in the United States, have been transforming the nature of kin relationships:

1. The *power* balance has changed, now that for most of their long lives parents and offspring are status equals.
2. *Property* and material resources are no longer the predominant base of most generational relationships, now that support from the state and other institutions is expected to enhance the finan-

cial independence of the old. Instead, greater emphasis is being placed on social-emotional ties, companionship, intimacy, love.

3. Nowadays most (though not all) older people are reasonably *healthy*, and able to be largely self-sufficient.

4. Contemporary families are increasingly heterogenous in *age*, as divorce and re-marriage produce a range of step-kin and in-laws. This heterogeneity in age (hence also in cohort experiences) reduces the traditional age-graded "generation gap" as a source of potential strain and conflict.

5. The many *alternative* forms of relationship available today diffuse the traditional primary focus on the simple connection between parents and offspring, offering instead a wide choice of kinship bonds.

On the whole, we believe these five changes bode well for the future of generational relations. To be sure, the larger society (especially the organization of work and education, see, for example, Kohli, 1991) is still subject to numerous and strict age constraints, and hence to possible age-based tensions and cleavages. Yet the emergent kin connections bid fair to transcend any such divisiveness. They are more often optional rather than contractual or obligatory. And it is our view that they hold high promise of modulating, rather than exacerbating, whatever intergenerational strains, conflicts, or perceived inequalities the future may bring.

With all these changes swirling around us, we conclude with the obvious query as to the broader sociotemporal utility of such United States experience, and the equally obvious question as to the heuristic utility of our simplistic "ideal types." At least some answers to these questions are reflected in the excellent chapters in this volume, which significantly contribute to the two goals of enhancing *understanding* of changing generational relationships, and developing *practical and policy-relevant* implications for the future. We are indebted to the volume's editor, Tamara Hareven, for addressing it to these important objectives.

ACKNOWLEDGMENT

This paper, funded by the National Institute on Aging, is part of M. W. Riley's "Project Age and Structural Change (PASC)."

REFERENCES

Brandes, S. (1989). *Kinship and care of the aged in traditional rural Iberia.* Paper presented at the meeting of the Social Science History Association, Washington, D.C., November, 1989.

Bumpass, L., & Sweet, J. (1989). *National estimates of cohabitation: Cohort levels and union stability.* National Survey of Family and Households Working Paper No 2. Madison: University of Wisconsin.

Kohli, M. (1991). Labor market perspectives and activity patterns of the elderly in an aging society. In W. van den Heavel, A. Illsley, A. Jamieson, & K. Knipscheer (Eds.), *Opportunities and Challenges in an Aging Society.* Amsterdam: Elsevier.

Hareven, T. (1982). *Family time and industrial time.* Cambridge: Cambridge University Press.

Hareven, T., & Adams, K. (1989). *The second generation: A cohort comparison in assistance to aging parents in the United States.* Paper presented at the meeting of the Social Science History Association, Washington, D.C., November, 1989.

Riley, M. W. (1983). The family in an aging society: A matrix of latent relationships. *Journal of Family Issues, 4,* 439–454.

Riley, M. W., & Riley, J. W., Jr. (1993). Connections: Kin and cohort. In V. Bengtson & A. Achenbaum (Eds.) *The Changing Contract Across Generations.* New York: DeGruyter.

Uhlenberg, P. R. (1980). Death in the family. *Journal of Family History, 5,* 313–320.

Index